THE HOUSE OFFICER'S GUIDE TO ICU CARE

FUNDAMENTALS OF MANAGEMENT OF THE HEART AND LUNGS

Third Edition

THE HOUSE OFFICER'S GUIDE TO ICU CARE

FUNDAMENTALS OF MANAGEMENT OF THE HEART AND LUNGS

Third Edition

John A. Elefteriades, MD
William W. L. Glenn Professor of Cardiothoracic Surgery
Director, Aortic Institute at Yale-New Haven
Yale University School of Medicine
New Haven, Connecticut

Curtis Tribble, MD
Professor of Surgery
Chief, Division of Cardiothoracic Surgery
Medical Director of Transplantation
Vice Chair, Department of Surgery
University of Mississippi
Jackson, Mississippi

Alexander S. Geha, MD, MS
Professor and Chief Emeritus, Cardiothoracic Surgery
University of Illinois Medical Center at Chicago
Chicago, Illinois
Professor of Cardiothoracic Surgery
University of California San Diego Medical Center
San Diego, California

Mark D. Siegel, MD, FCCP, FACP
Associate Professor
Department of Internal Medicine
Pulmonary & Critical Care Section
Yale School of Medicine
Program Director, Traditional Internal Medicine Residency
Co-Chair, Adult Ethics Committee
Yale-New Haven Hospital
New Haven, Connecticut

Lawrence S. Cohen, MD, FACC
The Ebenezer K. Hunt Professor of Medicine (Emeritus)
Department of Internal Medicine (Division of Cardiovascular Medicine)
Yale University School of Medicine
New Haven, Connecticut

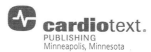

cardiotext.
PUBLISHING
Minneapolis, Minnesota

Third revised edition
© 2013 John A. Elefteriades, Curtis Tribble, Alexander S. Geha, Mark D. Siegel, and Lawrence S. Cohen

First edition published 1985. Second edition 1994

Cardiotext Publishing, LLC
3405 W. 44th Street
Minneapolis, Minnesota 55410
USA

www.cardiotextpublishing.com

Any updates to this book may be found at: www.cardiotextpublishing.com/titles/detail/9781935395683

Comments, inquiries, and requests for bulk sales can be directed to the publisher at:
info@cardiotextpublishing.com.

Library of Congress Control Number: 2012952060

ISBN: 978-1-935395-68-3

Printed in the United States of America.

To our families for their continued understanding.

Contents

Acknowledgments

We wish to express appreciation to Carol Syverson and Mike Crouchet at Cardiotext for their expertise and stewardship of this book.

Appreciation is expressed also to the hundreds of house officers and students who have provided feedback on this textbook and whose suggestions have strengthened the presentation. The innumerable positive comments from these users of this book have encouraged us in pursuing this Third Edition.

Appreciation is expressed to Ms. Marianne McCarthy and Ms. Carol Calini, our Academic Specialists in Cardiac Surgery at Yale, who have provided essential editorial assistance in the preparation of this Third Edition.

Foreword to the First Edition

It is said that the human brain, given free access to the world's libraries and now also to computer networks, has at its dendritic "fingertips" the capacity for retrieval of some 100,000 trillion bits (binary digits) of information. Surely, at least this much information has been processed across the cerebral cortex of most survivors of a medical education, if one takes into account all of their premedical acculturation and intensive postdoctoral training. Such a vast educational investment is not just pedantic overkill, for only through an understanding of the historical and theoretical bases of our knowledge of the complexities of health and disease can the most effective strategies for treatment and prevention, and especially their most effective advancement, become available.

Yet even when steeped in all this academic indoctrination, or perhaps because of it, when the neophyte first (and at long last) assumes some responsibility for a critically sick patient in an intensive care unit, he or she typically experiences a surge of insecurity and self-doubt. All of that massive background of theoretical knowledge, gleaned from texts, articles, lectures, and bits of prior exposure to patient care, suddenly becomes inadequate to deal with the often relatively simple but quintessentially critical moment-to-moment decisions that are unavoidable in the intensive care setting: whether to extubate or not, reoperate for bleeding or not, administer countershock or not, transfuse or not, call in the family or not, etc. There is simply no possibility of moving back to a given branch on the decision tree to test the other choices.

As with any other demanding activity, experience and practice bestow efficiency, accuracy, and self-confidence. Until that welcome milestone is reached, however, the novice to the stressful demands of decision making in the intensive care setting longs for a plain-talk, bare-bones listing of the variables comprising the algorithms whereby these decisions are reached.

This book succeeds to a surprising degree in achieving such a mission. It provides a condensation of these essential materials that is incapable of further reduction. Its facts and statements are (unlike the preceding comments) presented snappily and crisply in a down-to-business manner.

The challenging dilemma of any teaching program is the safe and efficient transition of the gulf between factual knowledge and its practical application. Acquisition of knowledge at the traditional, expensive school of trial-and-error must be minimized if the "error" component of that curriculum, with its legacy of tragedy and suffering, is to be avoided. A book such as this one would become a travesty if in any way it were used as a procedural manual intended to allow a technician without medical training to manage patients in intensive care. However, as a handbook for the student or house officer who already has broad knowledge of the basic tenets and theory of medicine, it is surely a most valuable resource.

Dwight C. McGoon, MD
Mayo Medical School
Rochester, Minnesota

Foreword to the Second Edition (abridged)

Although the word "doctor" is derived from the Latin, docere, to teach, few doctors of medicine are also gifted teachers. Fortunately, the 3 authors of this book are teachers in the finest tradition. For students, house officers, generalists, and specialists, all of whom are inundated with an exponentially increasing amount of information, this guide will be invaluable. Intensivists must make decisions expeditiously and implement therapy judiciously for fragile and severely compromised patients. With wisdom predicated on extensive personal experience, the authors of the *House Officer's Guide to ICU Care* succeed admirably in identifying the core aspects of problems encountered and provide practical guidelines for optimal diagnosis and treatment.

The word "care" in the title is pivotal. The guide is oriented toward the well-being of patients rather than technology for its own sake. Horrific circumstances, witnessed all too often, exemplified by a group of house officers gazing at machines displaying wave forms rather than at a patient who may be apneic, can be best avoided by lessons learned from the guide.

The term "guide" in the title reflects the authors' sensitivity to the importance of medical judgment. It avoids the pitfalls of "algorithmic medicine." The authors empower the reader to chart a course consistent with physiologic principles, astute observation, and practical therapeutics.

This edition follows the first after a 9-year interval. Despite its breadth, the information is assimilated readily. The authors' approach of first delineating underlying physiologic principles, then principles underlying therapy (including pharmacodynamics and operational aspects of devices), and only then describing how the agent or device is used (with specific dose regimens and guidelines for use of equipment), is indeed empowering. The diagrams of wave forms and operational features of complex equipment along with outlines for selection of appropriate therapeutic interventions are particularly helpful.

The book is eminently practical. For example, the authors discuss not only the use of ventilators and novel modes of ventilatory support but also practical aspects of weaning. They consider not only the impact of mechanical ventilation on hemodynamic recordings but also the consequent artifacts that may cloud interpretation. They consider not only electrophysiologic principles underlying arrhythmia but also often-overlooked phenomena, such as inducibility by Swan-Ganz catheters and other devices with a potential for serious mischief.

Even mundane topics, such as management of chest tube drainage systems and their visual monitoring to detect the physiologic hallmark of serious bleeding, are treated in a thoroughly scholarly fashion.

Perhaps of most importance, the *House Officer's Guide to ICU Care* is cohesive. Because the book is written by 3 knowledgeable clinicians steeped in clinical science and involved daily in the care of patients, it boasts remarkable clarity. The authors support their recommendations rigorously with references to the literature, but it is their collective wisdom that is particularly telling. These 3 teacher-physicians have made a monumental contribution to the improvement of patient care in an area in which the intelligent use of modern technology increasingly requires sophisticated judgment and expertise predicated on a broad base of knowledge of pathophysiology and therapeutics.

Burton E. Sobel, MD
University of Vermont College of Medicine
Burlington, Vermont

Foreword to the Third Edition

Operations make patients sick. Patients leave the operating room sicker than they were when they entered. Granted, there are long-term benefits, but surgery adds a wound to the disease being treated. Healing begins in the ICU. At last, John Elefteriades and his colleagues have updated and expanded the *House Officer's Guide to ICU Care*, which is just that. This small but comprehensive volume explains how to manage cardiothoracic surgical patients as they begin their journey to health. Patients are vulnerable and fragile immediately after modern major operations, and there are lots of ways to die during this period. Modern medicine has learned to foresee, identify, and prevent disaster and to treat it successfully when it occurs. To a medical student or junior house officer, the complexity of ICU care is daunting and the stakes are high. Yet chapter by chapter, this book explains in clear, direct language how to navigate this crucial period.

The beginning chapter describes basic physiology of respiration, mechanical ventilators, operation of ventilators, and potential pitfalls to avoid. The writing style is crisp, to the point, and clear. A careful read gives the reader an understanding of how mechanical ventilation works, what to monitor and watch for, and what to avoid. All of the information is practical and useful, and this characteristic continues throughout the entire volume. The next chapters address management of cardiac function in a well-organized sequence, beginning with arrhythmias. These chapters explain the pathophysiology of the multiple causes of inadequate cardiac output, various instruments used to monitor circulation, and the drugs and devices employed to gently nurse or support function of the newly repaired heart. Each chapter progresses in order: the subject of the chapter is defined; pathophysiology of abnormalities is described; diagnostic signs and clues are presented; and appropriate remedies are identified and explained. This simple outline is the unique quality that allows Dr. Elefteriades and his coauthors to successfully separate wheat from chaff without losing a kernel in the process. The preface reveals the new additions and needs no further introduction. The above paragraphs attempt to portray the practical and essential information packed into this small volume. There is no baloney, only steak. This book is a ready reference for managing patients during the critical period after major cardiac and thoracic operations. Contemporary ICU patients are sick; many are elderly and/or have serious comorbid diseases, but they can get well. Institutional ICUs caring for these patients would be wise to have a digital version of this book available on their computers.

L. Henry Edmunds, Jr., MD
Professor of Surgery
University of Pennsylvania School of Medicine

Preface to the First Edition

This guide is designed to fill the need for a practical manual for the care of critically ill patients. The emphasis is on the postoperative cardio-thoracic surgical patient, but nearly all of the information covered is relevant to medical and general surgical patients in intensive care as well.

The various chapters have grown out of lectures given to students and residents rotating through the Cardiothoracic Surgery Service at Yale University School of Medicine. Students and junior house officers have repeatedly emphasized their difficulty in finding written sources for the "hands-on" information contained in this manual. Included are sections that describe the practical use of mechanical intensive care equipment such as face masks, ventilators, pacemakers, the defibrillator, transducers, monitors, the Swan-Ganz catheter, the intra-aortic balloon pump, and chest tubes and drainage systems. Also included are practically oriented chapters on patient management. Treatment of arrhythmias, hemodynamic management, use of inotropes and afterload-reducing agents, management of postoperative bleeding, management of cardiac arrest and near arrest, and treatment of chest trauma are covered. Specific chapters provide a general approach and orientation to problems following noncardiac thoracic surgery, to acute aortic dissection, and to prosthetic heart valves and anticoagulation. Breadth of coverage is restricted largely to the cardiorespiratory systems.

The emphasis throughout this guide is to provide basic knowledge and to outline fundamentals in order to enable the physician starting out in caring for ICU patients to make reasonable management decisions—and to make them independently. At most medical centers, the ICUs are left in the care of junior physicians for significant periods of time when senior personnel are occupied in the operating room or elsewhere. Adherence to the principles outlined in this guide should prevent major errors from being made while junior staff exclusively are at the scene. It is hoped to convey, with this guide, most of what our junior house officers say is the considerable maturity in patient care they acquire while rotating through our Cardiothoracic Surgical Service.

Only our own proven methods of patient care are covered. Patient care patterns do vary from center to center. This guide is meant to provide the house officer with one sound method of handling each major ICU problem that may arise. This one viewpoint may be expanded or modified as the individual reader gains experience at his particular medical center.

While references to some experimental studies are included, no attempt is made to cover fully the primary experimental evidence behind all management fundamentals presented. At the end of each chapter, following the specific references, a list of selected readings with annotations is appended to guide the interested reader to further, more detailed information.

There exist already numerous comprehensive volumes for the intensive care specialist. The goal of the present guide is to provide an introductory manual that may be mastered in days or weeks in preparation for a particular ICU rotation.

It is hoped that the guide may be of use especially to medical students and junior house officers embarking on ICU responsibilities. The material covered is fundamental enough to be of value as well to intensive care nurses and nurses in training. Physicians' assistants and respiratory therapists, as well, may find the guide useful.

Throughout the text, key concepts are emphasized in bold print to allow easy identification and efficient review. Figures and diagrams are used liberally to amplify the text.

Preface to the Second Edition

The changes in the Second Edition fall into 2 general categories. The first is a thorough updating to reflect changes and advances in ICU care in the 9 years since the original publication. The second is an expansion in scope, beyond the specific care of the postoperative patient to that of the general care of the heart and lungs in medical as well as surgical patients.

Many new topics have been added to the text to reflect advances in care since the original publication. Arrhythmia surgery has emerged as a major field of endeavor, and a new chapter has been devoted to aspects of care after such operations. A new chapter covers cardiac assist devices that have become additional tools in the armamentarium for management of life-threatening pump failure. Material has been added to existing chapters to cover pressure support ventilation, the use of adenosine for supraventricular arrhythmias, the temporary external DDD pacemaker, changes in recommendations for conduct of cardiopulmonary resuscitation, use of noninvasive oxygen saturation monitors, synergistic use of amrinone and β-agonist inotropic medications, temporary pacing via the Swan-Ganz catheter, new intravenous and oral β-blocking and calcium channel blocking medications, aprotinin, heparin-induced thrombosis and thrombocytopenia, and the importance of the magnesium ion.

We discovered through direct feedback from house officers throughout the country that this text was being used not only by surgical housestaff but also by medical housestaff, including medical interns and residents and cardiology fellows, as well as by specialists in other fields who at times are called upon to care for ICU patients. It is this feedback that inspired the expansion of the scope of the text. Care of the postoperative cardiothoracic patient, the original focus, is still covered thoroughly. In addition, care of the medical ICU patient is emphasized as well. Much of the original material, such as ventilator management and care of arrhythmias, applies equally well to the medical patient. Additional chapters added specifically to expand the scope of the text include those on cardiac imaging in the acutely ill patient (including transthoracic echocardiography, transesophageal echocardiography, nuclear scanning, CAT scanning, and MRI imaging), management of acute coronary ischemia, acute management of valvular heart disease, and management of acute pulmonary disease.

The broadening of scope to include the medical ICU patient is reflected in the invaluable addition of Lawrence S. Cohen as an author of the book.

As in the First Edition, this is an introductory text covering what the house officer absolutely, positively needs to know to feel comfortable and to deliver safe, front-line care—especially during those many times when experienced leadership is not immediately on site.

Preface to the Third Edition

This Third Edition follows the last edition after more than 10 years. Thus, house officers and students have been using this small book for more than 3 decades. This version has been thoroughly revised to reflect the many changes in imaging, diagnosis, and treatment that have entered clinical practice in the intervening years. Extensive efforts have been made to preserve the conversational "mentor-to-trainee" tone that multiple generations of house officers have appreciated.

We have added talented new authors. Dr. Curt Tribble is a renowned cardiothoracic surgeon and editor whose experience and wisdom have enhanced the current revision of this textbook dramatically. Dr. Mark D. Siegel is a pulmonologist and intensivist who has contributed multiple important sections to this book and made certain that the important viewpoint of the pulmonary specialist is represented in the text.

The content of this book has been thoroughly revised and expanded. Specifically, the following additions and revisions have been implemented.

- New chapters have been added, covering sedation and analgesia, kidney injury and replacement therapy, and heart transplantation. These are all vitally important topics for the junior house officer.
- References and suggestions for further reading have been updated throughout the book.
- A new self-assessment tool has been added at the end of the book, with 3 tests that the reader can use to assess his assimilation of the information in this book.
- A concentrated "Emergency Response Sheet" of essential paradigms, drugs, and doses has been created and placed at the end of this book (pages 471–472). This can be copied so that it can be carried in the young doctor's pocket. This will keep him or her ready for immediate response to clinical emergencies.
- The chapter on ventilators and respiratory management has been brought up to date, with added sections on Bi-PAP, the ARDS protocol, the P:F ratio as a measure of adequacy of oxygenation, pressure support ventilation, the Rafferty maneuver for acute postoperative hypoxia, coordination of the patient with the ventilator, and the RSBI (rapid shallow breathing index) for assessment of readiness for extubation.
- The chapter on arrhythmias has been updated fully, with coverage of adenosine, amiodarone, and new therapeutic approaches.
- The chapters on temporary pacemakers and defibrillators have been updated to reflect the newest technological advances.
- The chapters on hemodynamic assessment and management have been updated, and the chapter on inotropic agents has been brought up to date, with an emphasis on the newly popular milrinone and vasopressin. We have also added a section on recognition and treatment of the newly appreciated vasoplegic syndrome.

- The chapter on the intra-aortic balloon pump (IABP) has been updated to reflect technological advancements in these devices.
- In the highly technological area of cardiac assist devices, the chapter has been updated to feature the modern miniaturized axial flow pumps.
- A quick reference table to guide the house officer has been added to the chapter on cardiac arrest and near arrest.
- The chapter on thoracic imaging has been extensively revised in recognition of the diminishing role of conventional angiography, which has been nearly completely superseded by CT, MRI, and echocardiography.
- The chapter on coronary ischemia has been developed anew, as so many changes have taken place over the last few years. The house officer will be able to differentiate ST elevation and non-ST elevation infarction and will become familiar with the proper roles for thrombolysis and acute angioplasty.
- A section on the importance of BNP in the evaluation of heart failure has been added to the chapter on valvular heart disease.
- The chapter on postoperative bleeding has been enhanced with user-friendly pathways and procedures outlines.
- The chapter on chest tubes and drainage systems has been updated and freshened, but it did not require major alteration. The fundamental principles have not changed since the early days of thoracic surgery.
- The chapter on chest trauma has been fully updated, including new information on lung contusion from flail chest and the FAST system for rapid sonographic evaluation.
- The chapter on acute pulmonary disease has been brought up to date with additional recent information on treatment of massive hemoptysis, acute bronchospasm, and pulmonary embolism.
- The chapter on management of aortic emergencies has been fully rewritten to reflect substantial advances in diagnosis and treatment since the Second Edition.

While we have expanded and enhanced the scope of this short textbook, we have maintained the original intent. Thus, this book is still a guide that can be read easily within a single 2- to 4-week ICU rotation. It is still a non-intimidating volume written in plain, simple language. This book is still aimed at providing you all the information you need to keep your patients safe, and not a word more. You can rest assured that—by applying the principles and guidelines presented in this book—you will treat your patients appropriately and that, though local patterns and preferences will vary, the general thrust of your care will be above criticism.

We hope that you will enjoy as you learn from this book—and that you will enter your ICU experience confident that you have a substantial base of knowledge and a basic approach that you can use initially and modify as you mature and are taught by your talented local faculty.

So, go ahead: Read, learn, enjoy, and build your confidence. Your patients will benefit.

VENTILATORS AND RESPIRATORY MANAGEMENT

The management of a patient on a ventilator is a topic that junior house staff often find confusing. Management decisions are quite simple if a few basic principles are clarified and categories of dysfunction are recognized.

The purpose of this chapter is to enable the house officer to manage any respirator problem on any patient. Initial consideration is given to basic physiologic principles regarding oxygenation and ventilation and the assessment of the adequacy and efficiency of these processes. Next, we discuss the practical respiratory parameters that must be set when a patient is first placed on a ventilator. Selection of the initial settings is clarified. Then the categories of dysfunction that may require changes in the initial settings are described, as is the method of changing the initial ventilator settings to correct these abnormalities. Next, we discuss weaning from the ventilator. Finally, we discuss some particular problems that are frequently asked about.

The House Officer's Guide to ICU Care: Fundamentals of Management of the Heart and Lungs, 3rd ed. © 2013 John A. Elefteriades, Curtis Tribble, Alexander S. Geha, Mark D. Siegel, and Lawrence S. Cohen, eds. Cardiotext Publishing, ISBN: 978-1-935395-68-3.

✚ PHYSIOLOGIC BACKGROUND

A respirator needs to ensure adequacy of 2 specific functions: oxygenation and ventilation. Oxygenation refers, of course, to maintenance of a satisfactory *arterial oxygen pressure* (pO_2). Ventilation refers to maintenance of a satisfactory *arterial carbon dioxide pressure* (pCO_2).

One basic principle in the management of ventilators is that these 2 essential functions, **oxygenation and ventilation, are separate and do not go hand in hand.** This independence is brought out by considering how oxygenation and ventilation vary with changing minute volume.[1] *Minute volume* is the product of *respiratory rate* and *tidal volume*. As can be seen from Figure 1.1, **oxygenation is, in fact, independent of minute volume until ventilation falls very low**—so low that severe atelectasis occurs. House officers frequently fail to appreciate this phenomenon and increase minute volume in an ill-conceived attempt to improve oxygenation. On the other hand, **CO_2 removal is directly dependent on minute volume.** It is this relationship that renders the terms "CO_2 removal" and "ventilation" synonymous with regard to ventilator management.

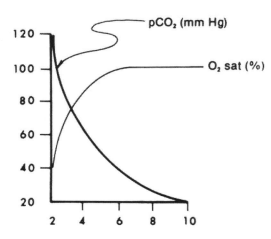

FIGURE 1.1

Relationship of arterial pCO_2 and arterial O_2 saturation to minute volume. Note that pCO_2 varies inversely with minute volume and that O_2 saturation is largely independent of minute volume until minute volume falls very low.

Source: Adapted from West JB. *Pulmonary Pathophysiology—The Essentials.* Philadelphia: Lippincott Williams & Wilkins; 2003.

Now, what constitutes adequate oxygenation? Beginners often feel that pO_2 should be maintained at the normal level of 100 mm Hg that they are taught in physiology. In fact, of course, oxygenation is adequate at much lower pO_2 levels. What must be preserved is oxygen-carrying capacity per unit of blood. The well-known O_2-hemoglobin dissociation curve (Figure 1.2) shows that at a pO_2 of 75 mm Hg, blood is 95% saturated, and at a pO_2 of 60 mm Hg, blood is 90% saturated.[2] Oxygen-carrying capacity is certainly well preserved at a pO_2 of 75 mm Hg and reasonably well preserved at a pO_2 of 60 mm Hg. So a pO_2 of 75 mm Hg is clearly adequate for all patients, and a pO_2 of 60 mm Hg is probably adequate for all patients except those with severely limited blood flow to key organs

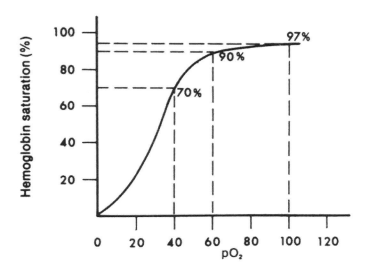

FIGURE 1.2

Oxyhemoglobin dissociation curve at 37°C and pH 7.4.

Source: Adapted from George RB. Alvcolar ventilation, gas exchange, oxygen delivery, and acid-base physiology. In: George RB, Light RW, Matthay RA, Matthay MA. eds. *Chest Medicine: Essentials of Pulmonary and Critical Care Medicine*. Philadelphia: Lippincott Williams & Wilkins; 2005:39-56.

(either from low cardiac output or from intrinsic vascular disease of the coronary arteries, extracranial cerebral vasculature, intestinal vasculature, or other specific vascular beds).

Next, what constitutes adequate ventilation? Here, no leeway can be tolerated from the normal parameters familiar from physiology. **In a patient on a ventilator, pCO_2 should be strictly maintained at normal levels—that is, at 40 mm Hg or less.** Often we maintain pCO_2 in the 30 to 40 mm Hg range. There is probably no need to alter settings to increase a pCO_2 in the 30 mm Hg range. Many forces in critically ill patients tend toward acidosis. The patient may develop metabolic acidosis from hypoperfusion, hypovolemia, or sepsis. Respiratory acidosis may occur for many reasons: the endotracheal tube may dislodge or leak, the ventilator may malfunction or become disconnected, or a pneumothorax or major atelectasis may develop. In all such cases, a baseline mild respiratory alkalosis, which is well tolerated indefinitely, will have a protective effect against the forces toward acidosis. Even in the face of total apnea, pCO_2 rises at about 3 mm Hg/min,[3] so that maintenance of a mild respiratory alkalosis in ventilator patients may allow the critical several minutes required to remedy a malfunction (to replace a dislodged endotracheal tube, for example).

Efficiency of ventilation is not commonly quantitated clinically, because ventilation is so efficient (by virtue of the greater ease of transport of CO_2 across the lung) that it suffers only in the preterminal stages of ventilatory dysfunction. Only very rarely is the house officer faced with critical impairment of CO_2 removal in patients on mechanical ventilation.

In severely ill patients, following both the efficiency of oxygenation and the adequacy of oxygenation may be required. The efficiency can be assessed by comparing the oxygen level provided in the alveolus to the oxygen level achieved in the blood. This parameter is quantitated as the $p(A - a)O_2$, the alveolar-arterial O_2 difference.

This can be calculated by putting the patient on 100% oxygen and measuring the arterial pO_2. At 100% oxygen, the alveolus will contain only 2 other gases: water vapor at a partial pressure of 47 mm Hg and CO_2 at a partial pressure of 40 mm Hg.[4] The sum of all partial pressures in the alveolus must equal atmospheric pressure. Thus,

$$p(A - a)O_2 = pAO_2 - paO_2$$
$$= (P_{am} - pH_2O - pCO_2) - paO_2$$
$$= (760 - 47 - 40) - paO_2$$
$$= 673 - paO_2$$

where pAO_2 and paO_2 are alveolar and arterial O_2 pressures, respectively. A normal $p(A - a)O_2$ is 60 to 80 mm Hg.[5] Thus in a normal patient on 100% O_2, arterial pO_2 levels of 600 to 620 mm Hg will be obtained. This is rarely realized in seriously ill ICU patients, in whom arterial pO_2 levels in the range of several hundred (on 100% O_2) are exceptionally good.

In patients with serious lung dysfunction, the $p(A - a)O_2$, if calculated on a daily basis, allows precise monitoring of the efficiency of oxygenation. Trends and consequences of treatment are noted sooner and are assessed more accurately if this parameter is followed.

Another parameter to assess the efficiency of oxygenation, which does not require the temporary administration of 100% oxygen during the test, is the P:F ratio. This parameter, like the A–a gradient, compares the inspired oxygen level to the achieved arterial pO_2. P represents the pO_2 (in mmHg) and F represents the fraction of inspired oxygen (as a decimal). So the P:F ratio is the pO_2 divided by the FiO_2. A P:F ratio of 285 or greater indicates "normal" oxygenation, while a P:F ratio less than 200 is diagnostic of severe pulmonary dysfunction. A well patient, for example, may show a pO_2 of 120 on an FiO_2 of 0.4, giving a P:F ratio of 120/0.4, or 300; this would represent normal efficiency of oxygenation.

Parameters to Set

When a patient is placed on a ventilator, as when returning to the ICU from the operating room, **the following parameters need to be specified for the respiratory therapist to set up the machine:**

- Mode
- Tidal volume
- Respiratory rate
- Fraction of inspired oxygen (FiO$_2$)
- Positive end-expiratory pressure (PEEP)

It is presumed that a volume respirator is being set. Pressure ventilators, because of greater uncertainty in delivery of a satisfactory tidal volume, are no longer frequently used in intensive care settings, especially in surgical or cardiac ICUs.

Mode refers to the modality by which the ventilator will cycle. Until earlier years, the available modes were mainly controlled ventilation and assisted ventilation. In controlled ventilation, the machine delivers a specified number of breaths per minute but does not allow the patient to breathe in between. In assisted ventilation, the machine senses the patient's inspiratory effort and delivers a breath at that time; in effect, it lets the patient decide when he needs a breath and then delivers that breath for the patient. Hybrids of these 2 modes are available as well.

In recent years, the *intermittent mandatory ventilation* (IMV) mode has been introduced. In this mode, the machine delivers a specified number of breaths per minute at regular intervals but allows the patient to take a breath freely between machine breaths. Despite common misconceptions, **there is not a patient in the hospital for whom IMV is not an appropriate mode of ventilation.** A very rare patient may be better served by one of the assist modalities,[6] but even these patients can be very safely managed by appropriately set and adjusted IMV. The inexperienced house officer will still encounter respiratory therapists or nurses who object to

IMV on certain patients—preferring, for example, controlled ventilation for paralyzed patients and reserving IMV for patients capable
of taking a breath. Those with this objection fail to realize that in
this mode, as in controlled ventilation, the specified breaths will be
delivered as reliably as in controlled ventilation. IMV need not be
reserved for patients who can breathe and can capitalize on the
feature of IMV that allows the patient to breathe freely between
machine breaths. In the vast majority of cases, feel free to set your
patient on IMV.

Tidal volume refers, of course, to the volume of air to be cycled
per machine breath. A normal tidal volume is approximately 5 mL/
kg body weight, for spontaneous breathing. **For setting a ventilator, tidal volumes of 10 to 15 mL/kg are used.** This holds for
newborns and infants as well as for adults. (For the very obese,
nonobese body weight for frame size should be taken into account.)
This 10 to 15 mL/kg represents an *initial* setting, to be modified
based on *arterial blood gas* (ABG) determinations, as discussed in
the next section.

Respiratory rate specifies the number of breaths per minute the
machine is asked to deliver. Rates of 8 to 12 are appropriate for
adults; 20 to 25 may be required for newborns; and 15 to 20 may
be necessary for small children. These represent *initial* setting
ranges at which these groups of patients are known to ventilate well;
modifications, again, are based on ABG results.

FiO$_2$ refers to the fraction of oxygen in the delivered air. This can
be expressed in percent (as in 28%, 50%, or 100% O$_2$) or in decimal
form (as in 0.28, 0.50, or 1.00 O$_2$). For initial settings after major
surgery, such as open heart surgery or major abdominal, thoracic,
or vascular procedures, an initial FiO$_2$ of 1.0 is appropriate. For
lesser procedures, an initial FiO$_2$ of 0.5 should provide an adequate
margin of safety for oxygenation. Again, initial settings will be modified based on ABG results.

PEEP refers to the amount of positive end-expiratory pressure
to be maintained in the airways. Most experts feel that some

physiologic PEEP is normally provided by an intact glottis. An endotracheal tube eliminates this normal physiologic mechanism responsible for keeping alveoli open. For this reason, most would agree that every patient should be maintained on at least 5 cm H_2O of PEEP.

ABG Contingencies and Parameter Resetting

The 2 functions the respirator must perform are oxygenation and ventilation. **Adequacy of oxygenation is assessed entirely based on the arterial pO_2. Adequacy of ventilation is assessed entirely based on the arterial pCO_2.** Thus, complex as ventilator management may seem to the beginner, all conceivable abnormalities of ventilator effectiveness can be grouped into 2 ABG contingencies (Figure 1.3).

These are the situations one must be prepared to handle:

- pCO_2 may be too high.
- pCO_2 may be too low.
- pO_2 may be too high.
- pO_2 may be too low.

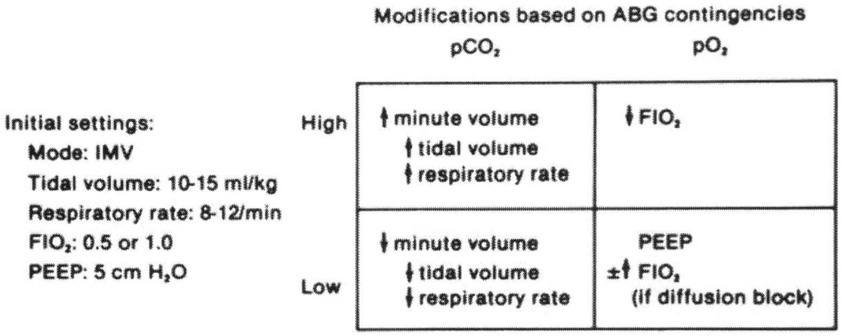

Modifications based on ABG contingencies

		pCO_2	pO_2
Initial settings: Mode: IMV Tidal volume: 10-15 ml/kg Respiratory rate: 8-12/min FIO_2: 0.5 or 1.0 PEEP: 5 cm H_2O	High	↑ minute volume ↑ tidal volume ↑ respiratory rate	↓ FIO_2
	Low	↓ minute volume ↓ tidal volume ↓ respiratory rate	PEEP ±↑ FIO_2 (if diffusion block)

FIGURE 1.3

ABG contingencies in ventilator management. Appropriate initial respirator settings indicated on left. Diagram on right indicates appropriate modifications for ABG contingencies.

If pCO_2 is too high, minute volume must be increased, either by increasing tidal volume or by increasing respiratory rate. As discussed earlier, pCO_2 varies inversely with minute volume, and increasing either tidal volume or respiratory rate will lower pCO_2. Now how does one choose which parameter to increase, tidal volume or respiratory rate? Here experience and judgment enter into the equation. If tidal volume is already at the upper limits of the suggested range, if peak inspiratory pressures are high, and if there is prominent chest expansion with each breath, one would be inclined to increase rate rather than volume. On the other hand, if the rate is already at the upper limits of the recommended range, if peak inspiratory pressures are low, and if chest expansion with each breath is not marked, tidal volume could safely and effectively be increased.

It should be noted that the adjustments described above presume that the pCO_2 is high despite proper functioning of the ventilator system. The pCO_2 may be high because the ventilator system is not delivering the prescribed minute volume. This may occur, for example, if there is a leak around the cuff of the endotracheal tube or in the ventilator tubing or connections, or if the endotracheal tube has been dislodged or was misplaced initially. When the pCO_2 is high, such problems must be checked for; it must be confirmed that the chest is moving and the breath sounds are good. The adjustments in tidal volume or respiratory rate are indicated once it is confirmed that the ventilator system is indeed delivering the minute volume initially set.

If the pCO_2 is too low, minute volume must be decreased, either by decreasing tidal volume or by decreasing respiratory rate. This is not a terribly serious condition, as it implies that one is ventilating the patient effectively—too effectively, in fact. As discussed earlier, mild respiratory alkalosis is desirable. We would not ordinarily decrease minute volume unless the pCO_2 fell below 30 mm Hg. The decision about which parameter to decrease—tidal volume or respiratory rate—centers on the same considerations as earlier: Is the rate already relatively high? Is the volume already relatively high? How are the peak inspiratory pressures? How prominent is chest expansion? Are good breath sounds heard bilaterally?

The issue of adjusting pCO_2 via dead space manipulation must be addressed. Some physicians will ask the therapist to add 6 or 12 inches of dead space to the ventilator tubing when the CO_2 is low. This seems to be done because of concern that lowering minute volume will adversely affect oxygenation. We have already established, however, that oxygenation is largely independent of ventilation. When this fact is appreciated, it becomes apparent that it is not necessary to use dead space to control pCO_2. Minute volume can be adjusted, and pO_2 will not suffer. In this way, certain dangers of dead space can be avoided. If a leak in the system should develop, the ventilation that is provided will not be wasted on increased dead space. When the patient is weaned from the ventilator, he or she will not inadvertently be left breathing through increased dead space. In our unit, dead space is *never* used to raise pCO_2.

What if pO_2 returns too high? This is not really a problem, as it signifies that the patient is oxygenating effectively—very effectively. If the pO_2 is high—that is, above the 75 mm Hg we established as adequate—this provides the opportunity to lower FiO_2. This is especially important if FiO_2 is above the potentially toxic levels of 0.5 or 0.6. If FiO_2 is below these levels and O_2 is still high, this is good, not bad; this implies efficient oxygenation. (We are not concerned here with the special matter of retrolental fibroplasia in newborns maintained at high blood pO_2.) No particular adjustment is required under these circumstances.

What if pO_2 returns too low? **If pO_2 is less than 75 mm Hg, especially if it is less than 60 mm Hg, serious hypoxia exists and remedial measures must be taken.** As will be made clear, **increasing FiO_2 is often not effective in postoperative patients; rather, the treatment for hypoxia is usually PEEP.**[7-10]

The overwhelming factor in postoperative hypoxia is atelectasis and its resultant ventilation-perfusion mismatch. Let us assume for illustrative purposes (Figure 1.4) that we group all the ventilated alveoli in one lung and all the nonventilated alveoli in the other. If the patient is on 50% O_2 by endotracheal tube (Figure 1.4A), conditions will be as follows. Blood entering either lung will be at mixed venous pO_2 and saturation levels—that is, at a pO_2 of 40 mm Hg and an O_2 saturation of 70%. Blood leaving the ventilated lung will be fully oxygenated in equilibrium with the alveolar pO_2, so that the effluent blood will have a pO_2 of about 300 mm Hg and an O_2 saturation in excess of 99%. Blood exiting the nonventilated lung will be unaltered, so that pO_2 will remain 40 mm Hg and saturation will be 70%.

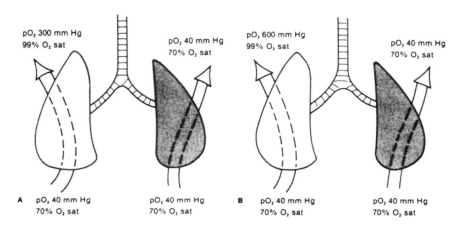

FIGURE 1.4

Model for conceptualizing ineffectiveness of increasing inspired oxygen concentration to treat ventilation-perfusion mismatch. All ventilated alveoli are assumed to be concentrated in nonshaded lung and all nonventilated alveoli in shaded lung. (**A**) Conditions on 50% inspired oxygen; (**B**) conditions on 100% inspired oxygen.

Now if the patient is placed on 100% oxygen (Figure 1.4B), conditions will be as follows. The blood flowing into either the ventilated or the nonventilated lung will have the same values as before—that is, the normal mixed venous values, pO_2 40 mm Hg and O_2 saturation of 70%. The blood leaving the ventilated lung will have a higher pO_2—say, 600 mm Hg—but the saturation will still be in excess of 99%. (This blood was already fully saturated on 50% inspired oxygen.) For the nonventilated lung, the effluent blood will still be fully desaturated; that is, pO_2 will be 40 mm Hg and O_2 saturation will be 70%. Thus, increasing the inspired oxygen in the face of postoperative ventilation-perfusion mismatch will *not* appreciably improve oxygenation. This is because blood exiting ventilated alveoli is fully saturated already, and blood exiting nonventilated alveoli does not come in contact with the increased ambient oxygen.

In this model, when blood from the 2 lungs mixes, half will be fully saturated and half will be fully unsaturated—just as before the FiO_2 was increased. (We have not considered here the amount of oxygen dissolved in plasma in addition to that bound to hemoglobin; this factor is negligible clinically.)

This very important principle regarding the ineffectiveness of increasing FiO_2 when there is ventilation-perfusion mismatch is confirmed graphically in Figure 1.5, which plots resultant arterial pO_2 against shunt fraction. Shunt fraction represents that blood passing through unventilated alveoli. The severity of the shunt increases along the *x*-axis of the graph. The isobars represent different levels of alveolar O_2 (in mm Hg). As can be seen, even very high levels of inspired O_2 are ineffective in raising pO_2 when major shunting prevails.

To improve oxygenation, the nonventilated lung must be expanded; the ventilation-perfusion mismatch must be corrected. The key to accomplishing this is positive end-expiratory pressure, or PEEP, which alters the balance of forces toward

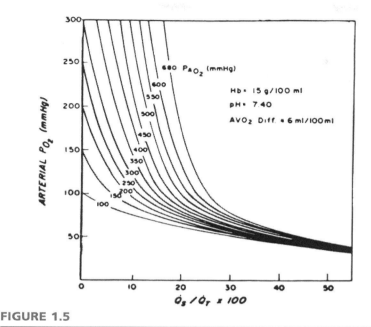

FIGURE 1.5

Arterial pO_2 as a function of shunt fraction (Q_s/Q_t) at different levels of FiO_2.
Source: Adapted from Shoemaker WC, ed. *Textbook of Critical Care*. Philadelphia: Elsevier/Saunders; 2011.

preserving alveolar expansion. PEEP is usually begun at 5 cm H_2O. This is more or less a safe, physiologic level for all patients. PEEP can be added in increments of 2.5 or at most 5 cm H_2O.[8,9] At times, as much as 20, 25, or even 30 cm H_2O of PEEP may be required for a given patient. Most patients, however, are adequately handled by PEEP levels from 5 to 12.5 cm H_2O. Details concerning the dangers of PEEP will be covered later in this chapter.

In fairness, despite this emphasis on use of PEEP rather than increasing FiO_2 levels, there are certain settings in which it may be necessary to increase FiO_2 as well. This is the case, for example, where there is a block to diffusion of oxygen across the respiratory membrane, as in congestive heart failure and interstitial edema from adult respiratory distress syndrome. PEEP is effective in restoring ventilation-perfusion matching and may even alter the balance of forces away from interstitial edema, but it cannot overcome a severe diffusion block. In such a setting, it may be necessary to increase FiO_2 significantly.

The "Rafferty maneuver." When patients come out of OR after cardiac surgery, their lungs have been deflated (while on cardiopulmonary bypass) for 1, 2, 3, or even more hours. These lungs are likely to be profoundly atelectatic. The anesthesiologist, when resuming ventilation at the completion of cardiopulmonary bypass, usually watches the surgical field to confirm that the lungs are reexpanding properly. He usually gives several large breaths for this purpose. But there is no way to be sure that the atelectasis has been expanded. Major atelectasis may persist on arrival in the ICU. In fact, **hypoxia after an uncomplicated cardiac surgical procedure is almost always due to persistent atelectasis.** For this, we use the Rafferty maneuver. We obtain an anesthesia ventilator bag (Jackson-Reese or equivalent) and inflate the lungs to a pressure of 40 or 50 cm H_2O. This is a very high airway pressure. The BP will fall from decreased cardiac return at those airway pressures. When we see the BP fall, we know that we have maximized the airway pressure and the lung expansion. It is not uncommon to see the pO_2 go from very low to fully normal in the minute or so that it takes to perform the Rafferty maneuver. This maneuver will work wonders for your patient and will make you seem like a hero to the ICU staff. You should inflate the lungs several times as described, watching the O_2 saturation on the monitor. You will see the saturation improve right in front of your eyes. Be careful not to maintain the high airway pressure too long, for fear of persistent hypotension. Be on alert for pneumothorax in patients with severe COPD.

Coordination with the ventilator. An oft-overlooked factor is whether the patient is coordinating with the ventilator. A patient who is tachypneic and out-of-sync with the ventilator will not achieve good blood gases. It is important to inspect the patient, his spontaneous respiratory effort, and his chest wall motion with each machine breath. If the chest does not move rhythmically and in sync with the ventilator, ventilation will be inefficient, and CO_2 may rise or O_2 may fall. This situation needs to be corrected. In a critically ill patient just out of the operating room, it may be best to sedate and/or paralyze the patient so that the machine does the breathing for him. You may achieve an immediate improvement in arterial blood gases. For patients not so critically ill—as those on long-term ventilation—the respiratory therapist may be able to help you select a modality that will achieve synchronization of spontaneous and machine breaths without sedation or paralysis; the assist-control mode or a mode of high-pressure support (see below) may achieve this purpose.

ARDS protocol.[11] **This protocol is intended for patients with severe hypoxia, a pulmonary edema pattern on CXR, and no direct evidence for cardiogenic pulmonary edema.** These patients can be said to have noncardiogenic pulmonary edema and may progress to what is termed "acute respiratory distress syndrome," indicative of severe pulmonary injury (often from cardiopulmonary bypass, infection, inflammation, transfusion, or lung trauma). For such critically ill patients with adult respiratory distress syndrome, a pattern of low tidal volume, high-frequency ventilation—avoiding pulmonary barotrauma—has become popular at most institutions. Tidal volume is usually as low as 6 mL/kg and respiratory rate is often 30 or greater. This method of ventilation has become nearly a fanatical religion, and the house officer will often be asked—or urged—to implement the so-called ARDS protocol. It is important to recognize that this protocol is based largely on one study that showed a mild survival benefit. Do not feel the need to implement this protocol without consultation with senior staff. The ARDS protocol does not achieve any immediate benefits; rather, it strives to attain a mild survival benefit in the long term over conventional ventilation. The ARDS protocol, by its very nature, involves accepting high pCO_2 and respiratory acidosis, with some inherent dangers from hypoventilation. For this reason, we advise not instituting the ARDS protocol urgently, but rather, enlisting experienced advice as to its applicability in a specific patient.

✚ WEANING FROM THE VENTILATOR

As is well appreciated, a patient must be surgically and hemodynamically stable in order to be safely weaned from the ventilator. Weaning and extubation are guided by (1) ABGs and (2) respiratory mechanics. Most patients can be taken from IMV 8 to IMV 4 to "blow-by" (oxygen delivery only, without positive pressure ventilation) with ABGs being checked along the way. **If pO_2 exceeds 75 mm Hg and pCO_2 is less than 45 mm Hg at each setting, weaning can proceed.** It is important to maintain some positive end-expiratory pressure even when the patient is on blow-by. A usual PEEP level is 5 cm H_2O for this purpose. **It is important not to leave a patient on blow-by for prolonged periods;** usually blow-by should be in effect no longer than 45 minutes, as the work of breathing is increased by the resistance to movement of air through the endotracheal tube. **Breathing spontaneously through a long tube is an intrinsically unphysiologic situation.** (Skeptics should try to breathe through a straw for a prolonged period.) If ABGs are acceptable at 45 minutes on blow-by with 5 cm H_2O positive airway pressure, this constitutes a satisfactory trial. For uncomplicated postoperative cardiac patients, as brief a blow-by trial as 20 or 30 minutes will suffice.

It is customary for the respiratory therapist to assess the respiratory mechanics during weaning or while the patient is on blow-by. The therapist will usually measure

- Tidal volume
- Vital capacity
- Negative inspiratory force

during spontaneous ventilation. Tidal volume is often quite low and is not used as a criterion in our unit. If vital capacity is of the order of the tidal volume used during ventilation—that is, 10 to 15 mL/kg—mechanics are considered satisfactory for weaning or extubation. (This is much less than a normal vital capacity, of course.) A negative inspiratory force of –25 to –30 cm H_2O is considered satisfactory. It must be kept in mind that the mechanics recorded are highly dependent on patient understanding and cooperation for the exercise.

A more recent criterion for extubation is the *rapid shallow breathing index* (RSBI).[12,13] This index values low respiratory rate and good tidal volume as indicators of readiness for extubation. Specifically, the rapid shallow breathing index is determined by dividing the respiratory rate (or frequency) by the tidal volume (in liters). The lower the respiratory rate and the larger the tidal volume, the lower will be the RSBI. An RSBI below 105 is generally considered satisfactory for extubation. You are probably breathing right now (despite the exciting nature of reading this book) at a rate of about 8 breaths per minute. You are probably moving a tidal volume of 500 cc per breath. This gives you an RSBI of 8/0.5 = 16. This is an excellent RSBI. Your patient on a weaning trial, however, may be breathing at 40 breaths per minute and moving only 200 cc per breath. This would give him an RSBI of 40/0.2 = 200. This represents a very bad RSBI—one not permissive of extubation. This RSBI will be a valuable resource for the house officer. It represents a quantitative measurement of the comfort of respiration; this parameter will supplement your clinical judgment while you build experience in evaluating respiratory status. The RSBI can be followed serially as a patient improves his breathing status.

If ABGs and respiratory mechanics are satisfactory, extubation may safely be carried out. It must be recognized as well that although the beginner should not wean or extubate patients with unsatisfactory ABGs or mechanics, the experienced ICU physician often chooses to do so. Without this decision, certain patients might never satisfy weaning and extubation criteria. With careful judgment by experienced physicians, the vast majority of extubations under such circumstances are successful.

For more chronic patients, who have had difficulty weaning from the ventilator with traditional methods, the so-called "pressure support" modality may be of benefit. In this modality, the patient breathes spontaneously, but the ventilator provides a preset positive pressure during inspiration to decrease the patient's work of breathing. The house officer can specify the level of pressure support—usually 10 to 25 cm H_2O. This pressure support also overcomes the increased work of breathing due to the endotracheal tube. Patients can stay on pressure support ventilation for hours. Over a period of hours or days, the degree of pressure support can be decreased, aiming toward extubation when substantial pressure support is no longer required. Pressure support ventilation is discussed in more detail below.

This chapter has covered how to set the ventilator initially, how to adjust respiratory parameters for the 4 categories of blood gas abnormalities, and how to withdraw mechanical ventilation, for essentially any patient in the hospital. What remains is to address special problems in respiratory management that are important for the neophyte.

✚ SPECIAL PROBLEMS
Oxygen Toxicity

It is important to remember that **oxygen toxicity does not occur unless FiO_2 is maintained above 0.5 or 0.6 for more than 24 hours.** Thus, placing the patient on 100% O_2 initially after returning from the operating room until a set of ABGs is obtained is not dangerous. Likewise, placing the patient on 100% O_2 for 20 minutes to calculate $p(A - a)O_2$ is not dangerous, and increasing FiO_2 briefly to treat an emergency is mandatory and *not* harmful.

However, a patient left on 70% O_2 overnight unnecessarily after a coronary bypass will begin to accumulate significant periods of high O_2 ventilation. We make every attempt to get the FiO_2 to 0.5 or lower by using PEEP and by accepting a pO_2 of 75 mm Hg (or occasionally 60 mm Hg) as soon as possible after surgery. With this management outlook, if a particular patient should develop problems subsequently, he will not have accumulated time at dangerous FiO_2 levels.

PEEP Complications

PEEP is not without toxicity. A well-known toxic effect of PEEP is barotrauma—that is, the tendency for PEEP to increase peak inspiratory pressures and cause pneumothorax or pneumomediastinum. In a patient on positive pressure ventilation, of course, a pneumothorax from a parenchymal lung leak may expand rapidly and produce tension and hemodynamic compromise. Handling of this emergency is discussed in Chapter 16, Chest Trauma. The point to be emphasized here is that PEEP results in an increased end-expiratory lung volume and, consequently, decreased lung compliance. Thus the higher the PEEP level, the greater the increment in pressure associated with a given tidal volume.

Normal patients, when ventilated with tidal volumes in the range described, will have peak inspiratory pressures of 25 to 30 cm H_2O. The house officer should follow peak inspiratory pressure, which is displayed with each cycle by a gauge or display on the ventilator. Barotrauma does not occur when peak inspiratory pressure is less than 50 cm H_2O; barotrauma is seen in 8% of patients when peak pressure is 50 to 70 cm H_2O and in 43% of patients when peak pressure is greater than 70 cm H_2O. Most ventilators have a pop-off valve to prevent development of high pressures. The level for pop-off is set by the therapist, usually in the range of 60 to 70 cm H_2O.[14] Above this pressure, an alarm sounds and the remaining tidal volume is vented and not delivered to the patient. Rarely, in critically ill patients with severe impairment of compliance, it may be necessary to disable or readjust the pop-off in order to ventilate the patient adequately. In such a setting, the risk of pneumothorax must be accepted. The patient may even develop bilateral pneumothorax and have bilateral chest tubes placed in order to be ventilated adequately.

PEEP may have significant hemodynamic consequences as well.[7-9] Not only is the pressure of PEEP delivered into the bronchial tree, but some of the PEEP pressure is transmitted to the thorax and mediastinum. Positive pressure in the thorax and mediastinum discourages filling of the right heart, and consequently of the left heart. By the Starling mechanism, stroke volume and cardiac output suffer. This is the basis for the **well-known depression of cardiac output by PEEP.** Blood pressure may fall and urine output may decrease. A patient with a normal heart may well tolerate 10 or 15 cm H_2O of PEEP without difficulty. Patients with sick hearts, especially postoperative cardiac patients, may tolerate PEEP very poorly. In a sick, postoperative mitral valve patient, 5 cm H_2O of PEEP may make the difference between a stable low-output state and frank cardiogenic shock.

The house officer should note as well that PEEP can artificially alter observed filling pressures. (See Chapter 5, Hemodynamic Monitoring and the Swan-Ganz Catheter.)

Thus PEEP is useful and important, but dangerous. Its respiratory and hemodynamic consequences must constantly be kept in mind. Bear in mind also that positive pressure ventilation in and of itself, even without PEEP, has the same respiratory and hemodynamic consequences described earlier for PEEP, especially when peak inspiratory pressure is high. From this point of view, spontaneous ventilation, with the normally negative intrathoracic pressures, allows better cardiac filling and cardiac output than does positive pressure ventilation.

Mask O$_2$

The beginner often fails to realize that the designations of various face masks (40%, 60%, 100% mask) are nominal only. Many studies have demonstrated the limitations of such O_2 delivery systems.[15-18] In fact, **it is impossible reliably to deliver greater than 50% O_2 except by endotracheal tube.** This has been determined by sampling tracheal O_2 in patients on various types of O_2 delivery apparatus. Nasal prongs have been shown to increase FiO_2 only insignificantly above room air levels. Even "100%" face masks do not deliver much more than 40% or 50% actual oxygen concentration. (Even the so-called "non-rebreather" masks, despite misconceptions, cannot deliver high FiO_2 without extraordinarily high low rates of 90 L/min or more, which are not practically feasible.) Face masks do not seal perfectly and in fact are designed so that the patient draws in air with each breath. If a normal inspiration lasts one second and involves movement of 500 mL of oxygen-enriched air, this represents an instantaneous flow of 30 L/min. It would be impractical to supply flows of this magnitude for face masks. A corollary of these observations is that one need not worry about O_2 toxicity in patients on a face mask. (This regards actual O_2 toxicity to the lung. The well-known, though uncommon, suppression of hypoxic drive for ventilation in patients with chronic lung disease may occur with a face mask.)

Absorption Atelectasis: Loss of the Nitrogen Stent

That increasing the FiO_2 may not improve oxygenation has already been explained. There is a way in which increasing the FiO_2 may actually impair oxygenation. When a patient is on 100% oxygen, there is no nitrogen in the alveolus. Nitrogen normally present in the alveolus, by virtue of its poor absorbability, provides some intra-alveolar positive partial pressure that acts as a so-called "nitrogen stent" for the alveolus.[19] On 100% oxygen, or to a lesser extent on other high-oxygen concentrations, this nitrogen stent is lost or diminished. Atelectasis, called *absorption atelectasis* in this setting, may occur. Oxygenation may actually deteriorate. This is another factor in favor of using PEEP instead of raising FiO_2 to combat hypoxia.

Pressure Support Ventilation

A recent change in patterns of weaning patients from mechanical ventilation has been the advent of *pressure support ventilation* (PSV),[20] a new modality that has become popular with house officers and respiratory therapists and one that has been incorporated into the setting menus of nearly all commercial ventilators. Traditional long-term weaning patterns have been T-piece weaning (in which the patient is allowed to breathe completely without ventilator support for progressively longer periods of time) and IMV weaning (in which the number of breaths provided by the ventilator is progressively decreased). Both T-piece weaning and IMV weaning are often supplemented by conventional low-level positive end-expiratory pressure.

Pressure support ventilation is a new and different modality in which, although the ventilator delivers no set mechanical breaths whatsoever, it senses the initiation of the patient's spontaneous breath and delivers a specified amount of pressure support during that breath. This support is like a "boost" or "tail wind" for the spontaneous breath, which makes the breath easier for the patient. The amount of pressure support can be varied over a continuous spectrum. High support corresponds to 15 to 30 cm H_2O, and low support corresponds to 5 to 8 cm H_2O. The pressure support increases the flow rate and the tidal volume significantly beyond what the native breath itself would achieve (Figure 1.6). At high levels of pressure support, the work of breathing is nil and ventilation is fully supported mechanically. The house officer must remember, however, that unlike IMV, PSV does not deliver a single preprogrammed breath, so an apneic patient, or one with inadequate respiratory drive, will not receive adequate ventilation. As the amount of PSV is decreased, the patient takes on more of the workload of breathing. At low levels of PSV, the positive pressure serves mainly to counteract the excess resistance of the endotracheal tube and ventilator as compared to the normal resistance without a tube.

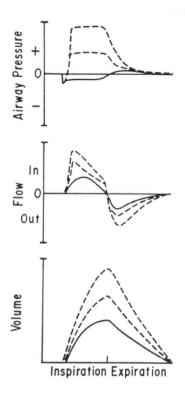

FIGURE 1.6

Schematic representation of airway pressure (top panel), airflow (middle panel), and lung volume (lower panel). Solid lines depict a spontaneous breath without pressure support. Dotted lines depict two levels of pressure-support ventilation. Note higher airflow and larger volume of breath with pressure. Note also the patient's continued negative-pressure effort when unassisted, compared to the brief period of such patient effort when PSV is used.

Source: MacIntyre NR. Respiratory function during pressure support ventilation. *Chest.* 1986;89(5):677-683. Reproduced with permission from the American College of Chest Physicians.

Several paradigms for selection of initial setting of pressure level for high-level support in PSV have been proposed. One method is to apply one-third of the maximum inspiratory pressure observed during mechanical ventilation. (For example, the maximum inspiratory pressure for a given patient during conventional IMV ventilation is 45 cm H_2O; the initial pressure level selected for PSV is one-third of 45, or 15 cm H_2O.) Another method is to experiment with different levels of pressure support at the time of institution of PSV to determine and select that level of pressure support that yields a normal tidal volume for mechanical ventilation (ie, 10 to 12 mL/kg).

Although most centers use PSV for specific weaning trials of finite duration, some physicians maintain patients on PSV around the clock, gradually and progressively decreasing the amount of pressure support as the patient improves and strengthens.

Pressure support ventilation is intended for application not to the standard patient (eg, the uncomplicated postcardiac surgical patient who is weaned quickly from the ventilator the morning after surgery), but to the more complicated or precarious patient who can be expected to require at least several days to wean from the ventilator. PSV is intended not for use while the patient is acutely ill, but for use later in recovery, when hemodynamics have stabilized and acute lung problems (atelectasis, edema, infiltrates) have cleared or improved. PSV clearly decreases the work of breathing. Patients respond very favorably, probably reflecting an improved coordination with the ventilator compared to IMV. In IMV, the prescribed breaths are interposed according to the machine's timing cycle. In PSV, the patient determines timing, depth, and frequency of breaths, with "boosting" of each breath by the pressure support. Dyspnea is minimized and patient comfort is dramatically improved. Nurses and allied personnel sense this feeling of improvement and respond favorably to PSV.

Although proponents argue for widespread application of PSV because of increased patient comfort and theoretical advantages, detractors point out that there is absolutely no clinical evidence that weaning is better or more effective with PSV[21] than with conventional modalities. Debate continues actively. Personal and institutional preferences abound. Progressively wider application of PSV has indeed become commonplace, and the house officer must be familiar with the characteristics of this promising new modality of ventilation.

Bi-PAP

Bi-PAP, or *bi-level positive airway pressure*, aims to support ventilation—without an endotracheal tube—in patients whose respiratory status is marginal.[22] This modality provides 2 levels of support, a high level during inspiration (to augment the native breath), and a low level during expiration (to keep the airway open and permit easy exhalation). Bi-PAP machines are usually set in an assist mode, in which they sense the patient's own breathing efforts and facilitate those. The modality, of course, relies on proper fit of the mask and patient tolerance.

The most common settings for use of Bi-PAP are (1) in patients admitted with respiratory failure but not yet requiring intubation and mechanical ventilation and (2) in patients previously extubated who are struggling and heading toward reintubation.

The authors are skeptical that a course of Bi-PAP can prevent reintubation in a struggling patient headed in that direction. CO_2 removal may be enhanced by improved chest excursion, and O_2 can be improved by diminished atelectasis. However, these beneficial effects are usually transient, disappearing when the Bi-PAP is stopped. There is little or no evidence to support the position that Bi-PAP is any more than a temporizing measure in postoperative patients; this modality does not seem to prevent reintubation.

Bi-PAP is simply not appropriate for prolonged use. If a patient requires prolonged support of ventilation, this is best accomplished with an endotracheal tube and a ventilator.

Bi-PAP is fraught with dangers. Patients needing Bi-PAP support are struggling by definition. They may drift in and out of consciousness. Patients may vomit into the mask and aspirate, often terminally. The Bi-PAP may produce dangerous gastric distention, from passage of tidal volume into the esophagus instead of the trachea. We have even seen gastric distention so severe as to produce gastric perforation. Bi-PAP interferes with communication by the patient. It produces a sense of claustrophobia in many patients.

It is important for the house officer to have Bi-PAP in his or her armamentarium, but he must be aware of its limitations and vigilant regarding its potential complications.

REFERENCES

1. West JB. *Pulmonary Pathophysiology—The Essentials*. Philadelphia: Lippincott Williams & Wilkins; 2003.

2. George RB. Alveolar ventilation, gas exchange, oxygen delivery, and acid-base physiology. In: George RB, Light RW, Matthay RA, Matthay MA, eds. *Chest Medicine: Essentials of Pulmonary and Critical Care Medicine*. Philadelphia: Lippincott Williams & Wilkins; 2005: 39-56.

3. Alfery DD, Benumof JL. Anesthesia for thoracic surgery. In: Miller RD, ed. *Anesthesia*. New York: Churchill Livingstone; 1981:925-980.

4. Guyton AC. Physical principles of gaseous exchange: diffusion of oxygen and carbon dioxide through the respiratory membrane. In: Guyton AC. *Textbook of Medical Physiology*. Philadelphia: WB Saunders; 1971:470-480.

5. Dunnill RPH, Crawley BB. *Clinical and Resuscitative Data*. Oxford: Blackwell; 1977.

6. Hudson LD. Intermittent mandatory ventilation (IMV). *Pulmonary Perspect*. 1984;1:5-7.

7. Snyder JV, Carrol GC, Schuster DP, Culpepper J, Klain M. Mechanical ventilation: physiology and application. *Curr Probl Surg*. 1984;21(3):1-87.

8. Shelhammer JH, Natason C, Parrillo JE. Positive end expiratory pressure in adults. *JAMA*. 1984;251(20):2692-2695.

9. Luce JM. The cardiovascular effects of mechanical ventilation and positive end-expiratory pressure. *JAMA*. 1984;252(6):807-811.

10. Winter PM, Miller NJ. Oxygen toxicity. In: Shoemaker W, Thompson W, Holbrook P, eds. *Textbook of Critical Care*. Philadelphia: WB Saunders; 1984:218-224.

11. Acute Respiratory Distress Syndrome Network. Ventilation with lower tidal volumes as compared with traditional tidal volumes for acute lung injury and the acute respiratory distress syndrome. *N Engl J Med*. 2000;342(18):1301-1308.

12. Crawford J, Otero R, Donnino M, Garcia J, Khazal R, Lenoir T. Rapid shallow breathing index—a key predictor for noninvasive ventilation. *Critical Care*. 2007;11(Suppl 2):169.

13. Segal LN, Oei E, Oppenheimer BW, et al. Evolution of pattern of breathing during a spontaneous breathing trial predicts successful extubation. *Intensive Care Med.* 2010;36(3):487-495.

14. Peterson GW, Baier H. Incidence of pulmonary barotrauma in a medical ICU. *Crit Care Med.* 1983;11(2):67-69.

15. Shapiro BA, Harrison RA, Wolfson JR. *Clinical Application of Blood Gases.* Chicago: Yearbook; 1977.

16. Gibson RL, Corner PB, Beckham RW, McGraw CP. Actual tracheal oxygen concentrations with commonly used oxygen equipment. *Anesthesiology.* 1976;44(1):71-73.

17. Poulton TJ, Corner PB, Gibson RL. Tracheal oxygen concentration with a nasal cannula during oral and nasal breathing. *Respir Care.* 1980;25(7):739-741.

18. Schacter EN, Littner MR, Luddy P, Beck GJ. Monitoring of oxygen delivery systems in clinical practice. *Crit Care Med.* 1980;8(7): 405-409.

19. Vinocur B, Artz JS, Sampliner JE. Monitoring of respiratory status. In: Berk JL, Sampliner JR, Artx JS, Vinocur B, eds. *Handbook of Critical Care.* Boston: Little, Brown; 1976:57-86.

20. MacIntyre NR. Pressure support ventilation: effects on ventilatory reflexes and ventilatory muscle workloads. *Respir Care.* 1987; 32:447-457.

21. Hughes CW, Popovich J Jr. Uses and abuses of pressure support ventilation. *J Crit Illness.* 1989;4:25-32.

22. Esteban A, Frutos-Vivar F, Ferguson ND, et al. Noninvasive positive-pressure ventilation for respiratory failure after extubation. *N Engl J Med.* 2004;350(24):2452-2460.

2

ARRHYTHMIAS

This chapter presents a simplified, fundamental approach to the management of acute alterations in cardiac rhythm. The perspective is primarily that of the care of the postoperative cardiothoracic patient, where many of the arrhythmias are most frequently seen. The principles are applicable as well in the coronary care unit and in the general surgical or medical intensive care unit.

After an initial listing of data to be gathered in assessing a rhythm disturbance, discussion is divided into 3 sections: bradycardias, supraventricular arrhythmias, and ventricular arrhythmias.

The House Officer's Guide to ICU Care: Fundamentals of Management of the Heart and Lungs, 3rd ed. © 2013 John A. Elefteriades, Curtis Tribble, Alexander S. Geha, Mark D. Siegel, and Lawrence S. Cohen, eds. Cardiotext Publishing, ISBN: 978-1-935395-68-3.

✚ GENERAL APPROACH TO ARRHYTHMIAS

There are several questions that house officers must ask themselves in evaluating any arrhythmia:

- **What is the rhythm?** This question is of obvious importance.
- **Is it hurting the patient?** Different arrhythmias cause different degrees of physiologic disturbance. Some need urgent treatment (as in rapid atrial fibrillation with alteration in vital signs, or in ventricular fibrillation). Others may require no additional treatment at all (as in recurrence of atrial fibrillation with a controlled rate in an already digitalized patient).
- **What is causing the arrhythmia?** House officers are usually quite thorough in investigating factors that may be responsible for arrhythmias. These include the following:
  - ○ **Electrolytes.** Potassium is especially critical. In settings of ventricular irritability or digitalis administration, serum potassium should be maintained at 4.5 mEq/L or greater. Magnesium levels are also important to replete aggressively. In general, magnesium tends to be lost in parallel to potassium. Postoperative cardiac surgical patients, due to their polyuria, are often severely magnesium-depleted. Most ICUs will have standing orders for magnesium supplementation. Many surgeons give magnesium empirically and routinely into the pump just before weaning cardiopulmonary bypass, figuring that the magnesium is almost certain to be low. The house officer should be aggressive in repleting potassium and magnesium, both to prevent and to treat ventricular ectopy. Remember that both electrolytes can be toxic. **Potassium can cause asystole**—that is, after all, how we stop the heart during cardiac surgery (the

"cardioplegia" is potassium-rich). **Magnesium can cause cessation of breathing.** In the early postoperative phase, the patients are usually intubated and ventilated, so this is not a great issue. Cardiac ICUs will have strict policies regarding administration of potassium and magnesium. **We recommend no more than 20 mEq of KCl over 1 hour and no more than 2 g MgSO$_4$ over 1 hour.**

- ○ **ABGs.** Hypoxia certainly can cause arrhythmias, as can acidosis.
- ○ **EKG.** A 12-lead EKG must be evaluated for evidence of ischemia as the factor causing the arrhythmia.
- ○ **The Swan-Ganz catheter.** One factor that is often overlooked is the Swan-Ganz catheter. The tip of this catheter can drop back through the pulmonary valve, into the right ventricle, and irritate the myocardium, causing ventricular ectopy. A loop of catheter also may cause ectopy if it rubs on the ventricular wall. This must constantly be kept in mind, especially when ectopy is unexpected from the patient's general physiologic condition and when ectopy occurs in runs of PVCs with entirely normal intervening periods. In this setting, the ectopy may be accompanied by a change in the Swan-Ganz trace, from that typical of pulmonary artery placement to a right ventricular configuration. The catheter must be withdrawn from the heart into a central venous position if it is thought to be the cause of life-threatening ectopy. (See Chapter 5, Hemodynamic Monitoring and the Swan-Ganz Catheter, for further discussion of Swan-Ganz catheter positioning.) Even a CVP line, a TPN line, a PICC line, or a dialysis catheter may on occasion cross into the right ventricle from the ideal venous location, irritate the ventricle, and cause significant ventricular ectopy. The house officer should keep this possibility in mind as well.

- **Is digitalis involved?** Digitalis excess can cause essentially any arrhythmia. In our ICU, we review in detail the complete "digitalis history" whenever an arrhythmia occurs. This involves ascertaining exactly how much digitalis was given when—including preoperatively, intraoperatively, and postoperatively. Digitalis levels may help as well.
- **How do I treat it?** Only after the preceding questions are asked and answered can a treatment plan be formulated appropriately. The following discussion covers particular treatment of specific arrhythmias.

✚ BRADYCARDIAS

The house officer should have a clearly organized armamentarium for the management of bradycardias, for these arrhythmias can be acutely life-threatening. The approach outlined here is valid for essentially all bradycardias, including sinus bradycardia, nodal bradycardia, and slow ventricular rhythm.

When does a bradycardia require treatment? Many patients exhibit slow rhythms but tolerate them well and do not require urgent intervention. Any cardiac ward, for example, frequently carries elderly patients whose pacemaker generators have failed. Most do not require any treatment other than semielective pacemaker generator replacement. Heart rate, of course, is a major determinant of cardiac output (output equals the product of heart rate and stroke volume). If cardiac output is maintained despite bradycardia, urgent treatment is not required. In the acute setting, adequacy of cardiac output is assessed by blood pressure and level of consciousness. If blood pressure is satisfactory, without dizziness, lightheadedness, or disordered mentation, cardiac output is likely to be satisfactory. If these criteria are not met, cardiac output is unsatisfactory, and urgent treatment must be begun.

Even if blood pressure and consciousness are maintained, in most cases bradycardia should be treated if the rate is below a certain absolute level. **If the pulse is less than 45/min, and certainly if it is less than 40/min, treatment should be administered.** Very few hearts, especially in the elderly or those with ischemic or valvular heart disease, can increase stroke volume enough to maintain cardiac output for sustained periods at pulse rates in this range. Furthermore, with pulses this slow, dangerous ventricular foci may supervene.

There are 3 cardinal stages to the acute treatment of serious bradycardias (Figure 2.1).[1]

1. **The initial treatment of choice is atropine.** This drug acts as a parasympatholytic agent to speed and encourage supraventricular, junctional, and ventricular foci and to promote *atrioventricular* (A-V) conduction.[2] Atropine is available as atropine sulfate in single-dose syringes containing 0.5 or 1.0 mg. The initial dose is 0.5 mg IV. An effect should be realized in 2 to 3 minutes. The dose should be repeated if no response is seen within this time. This drug is safe and should be used liberally. If no response is seen after the second dose, additional doses are unlikely to be effective, and one should move on to the second stage of treatment.

2. **If atropine is ineffective, the second drug of choice is isoproterenol (Isuprel).** If the parasympatholytic agent atropine is not effective, a β-agonist is required for its β-chronotropism. As is discussed in Chapter 7, Isuprel has a strong, almost pure β-activity. This makes it the next agent of choice in severe bradycardias. A convenient method of administration is by drip (2 mg/500 mL; again, see Chapter 7, Continuous Infusion Agents). The drip is initially run quite fast (30, 60, or 120 mL/h or greater, if required) until a pulse response is seen. The drug should be

effective within minutes. It is important to slow the drip as soon as a pulse increment is observed, as untoward effects may be seen. Any patient can be thrown into ventricular fibrillation if Isuprel is infused fast enough. The infusion should be adjusted to achieve a safe rate, usually 60 mL/h or less.

3. **If Isuprel is ineffective, further pharmacologic efforts are futile and emergency cardiac pacing is indicated.** Pacing can be done with an external pacemaker, or a temporary transvenous pacing lead can be placed. All physicians should know how to place temporary pacemakers. This is covered fully in Chapter 3, Temporary Pacemakers.

It should be kept in mind that most postoperative cardiac patients have temporary pacemaker wires placed directly into the right ventricular myocardium and brought through the skin. These should be used, if available, when a postoperative cardiac patient requires temporary pacing.

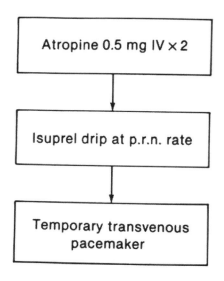

FIGURE 2.1

Stepwise management of urgent bradyarrhythmias.

✚ SUPRAVENTRICULAR ARRHYTHMIAS

Supraventricular arrhythmias include sinus tachycardia, premature atrial contractions (PACs), atrial fibrillation, and atrial flutter (Figure 2.2). Paroxysmal atrial tachycardia (PAT), seen commonly in healthy, young patients, is rarely encountered following cardiac surgery. PAT and its variant MAT (multifocal atrial tachycardia) will not be specifically covered. When seen postoperatively, these rhythms can generally be approached as discussed later for atrial flutter.

Sinus tachycardia, PACs, atrial fibrillation, and atrial flutter in the postoperative cardiothoracic patient are all points on a spectrum of postoperative supraventricular irritability. Sinus tachycardia and frequent PACs often presage atrial fibrillation or flutter. A given patient may be in atrial fibrillation at one time and atrial flutter at another; over a period of days, the patient may convert back and

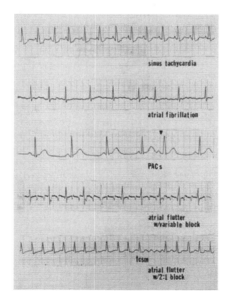

FIGURE 2.2

Supraventricular arrhythmias: illustrative EKGs (csm: carotid sinus massage).

forth from fibrillation or flutter to sinus rhythm, often with sinus tachycardia or PACs intervening.

Similar irritability can be seen in the coronary care unit with myocardial infarction or pericarditis; of course, these supraventricular arrhythmias can also be seen in the coronary care unit in the setting of valvular heart disease, or *de novo*, without other primary structural heart disease.

In the case of noncardiac thoracic surgery, the more extensive the procedure, the greater the incidence of these supraventricular arrhythmias; that is, the incidence of arrhythmia is higher for pneumonectomy than for lobectomy, and higher for lobectomy than for simple exploration. Even in exploration without resection, however, there is a definite incidence of these arrhythmias. Although many causes have been postulated (direct irritation of the atrium, irritation of the pleura, disruption of parasympathetic atrial innervation), no clear explanation has been substantiated. It appears, however, that roughly one-half of patients undergoing pneumonectomy and one-third of patients undergoing lobectomy develop these arrhythmias.

Much research has been directed into determining why supraventricular arrhythmias are seen so commonly after cardiac or thoracic surgery. Some have postulated that the venous cannula irritates the atrial pacemaking tissue. Withdrawal from rate-controlling antianginal medicines may be a factor in allowing tachycardias to develop. More recently, evidence suggests that conventional cardioplegia does not effectively quiet atrial activity, so that atrial pacemaking tissues may be rendered ischemic and irritable on that basis.[3] In any case, at least a third of coronary bypass patients will develop these arrhythmias postoperatively. For patients with mitral valve dysfunction, supraventricular arrhythmias are part and parcel of the long-standing valvular heart disease with atrial enlargement. If the mitral patient has not already developed atrial fibrillation preoperatively, chances are that it will develop postoperatively.

Much effort has been directed toward developing methods to prevent these postoperative arrhythmias, but no clear-cut solution has emerged. Prophylactic digitalization has yielded mixed results.[4-6] Various protocols for resumption of β-blockers postoperatively appear promising.[5-7] A meta-analysis, combining data from many studies on therapeutic strategies to prevent postoperative atrial fibrillation, concluded that

- Digitalis alone does not prevent postoperative atrial fibrillation.
- β-blockers do discourage postoperative atrial fibrillation.
- The combination of digitalis and β-blockers discourages postoperative atrial fibrillation more effectively than either drug administered alone.

Until more reliable prevention is available, these supraventricular arrhythmias will continue to be one of the cardiothoracic surgeon's most common problems.

Sinus Tachycardia

Sinus tachycardia usually has a physiologic cause; that is, the cardiovascular system attempts to compensate, to increase cardiac output, by increasing heart rate. The cause may be fever, pain, hypoxia, hypovolemia, low cardiac output, congestive heart failure, pulmonary embolus, or another primary disorder. The treatment for sinus tachycardia is that of the underlying physiologic disorder.

Fever and pain are especially common postoperative causes. Occasionally, however, a postoperative cardiac surgical patient will demonstrate sinus tachycardia, although he or she is well in all other respects: the patient is not febrile and has no severe pain; vital signs, physical examination, and urine volume suggest good cardiac output; hematocrit is stable; and chest x-ray and electrocardiogram are satisfactory. The cause for tachycardia in this setting is not at all clear. Some believe that withdrawal of β-blockers and calcium antagonists (given preoperatively for angina) may be responsible. In any case, in this setting, when the patient has sinus tachycardia and all investigations fail to disclose any physiologic abnormality, it is permissible to treat the tachycardia with β-blockers. Usually, 25 mg of metoprolol (Lopressor) orally, 4 times daily will suffice. Often this medication can be discontinued after several weeks without recurrence of tachycardia.

Premature Atrial Contractions

PACs in themselves are not dangerous. They are supraventricular beats conducted along standard pathways from the A-V node downward, so they produce a coordinated ventricular contraction. Usually, unless they occur very early in the cardiac cycle, PACs produce an effective pressure pulse and thus do not adversely affect cardiac output. Unlike PVCs, they do not presage life-threatening ventricular arrhythmias. However, as indicated, frequent PACs, especially after cardiac or thoracic surgery, portend impending atrial fibrillation; this requires prophylactic treatment to discourage atrial fibrillation and encourage rate control if and when atrial fibrillation supervenes.

Atrial Fibrillation

When a young, healthy patient develops atrial fibrillation, the rate of ventricular response can be quite rapid, at times as high as 180/min to 200/min.[8] In the elderly, sick patient, ventricular response is usually on the order of 140/min to 160/min. Although a young, healthy heart may be able to maintain cardiac output at rates in this range, most hospitalized and postoperative patients cannot compensate. Tachycardia occurs at the expense of diastole. Stroke volume is decreased because filling time is short. In addition, increased heart rate leads to increased myocardial oxygen demand, and the shortened diastolic time results in decreased coronary flow and hence decreased oxygen supply. This alteration in myocardial oxygen supply and demand results in myocardial ischemia, with its negative

TABLE 2.1   Treatment of Atrial Fibrillation by Level of Urgency

Urgency Level	Signs	Treatment
Level I	• Pulse: 120-140/min • BP: >100 mm Hg • Satisfactory level of consciousness • No angina	Digitalis or β-blocker (or calcium channel blocker)
Level II	• Pulse: 140-160/min • BP: 80-100 mm Hg • Possible dizziness • Possible mild angina	Digitalis or IV β-blocker or calcium channel blocker
Level III	• Pulse: 140-160+/min • BP: <80 mm Hg • Impaired level of consciousness • Angina	DC cardioversion

inotropic effect also contributing to decrease the stroke volume. **Atrial fibrillation with a rapid response represents a serious insult to the patient's physiology. The goal in acute management is not to restore sinus rhythm** (which, even if achieved, cannot usually be maintained) **but to effect control of rate.**

We have found it useful to separate patients with new-onset atrial fibrillation into 3 categories of urgency (Table 2.1).

Level I (relatively nonurgent).

A postoperative coronary bypass patient goes into atrial fibrillation on postoperative day 1. His rate is 135/min; blood pressure is 120/80 mm Hg. He is awake, alert, and responds appropriately to questions. He has no chest pain.

This patient falls into the first, lowest category of urgency. Treatment may be via digitalis, via β-blockers or calcium channel blockers, or via both digitalis and β- or calcium channel blockers.

Digitalis treatment. Traditionally, the treatment for such a patient has been rapid digitalization. Although there are alternatives in the present era, treatment with digitalis is fully acceptable even today. **Digitalis is the only available drug that slows ventricular response without adversely affecting myocardial contractility.** Several schemes of administration can be used. One rule of thumb is that digoxin, 0.9 mg/m² of body surface area, given intravenously in divided doses over 24 hours, will effect satisfactory digitalization. For practical purposes, for the average-sized adult, 0.5 mg IV initially and 0.25 mg IV every 6 hours for 2 or 3 additional doses (a total digitalizing dose of 1.0 to 1.25 mg) will usually digitalize adequately without overdosing. Subsequently, a daily maintenance dose, usually 0.25 mg IV or orally, can be started.

A particular patient may not slow with the initial 0.5-mg IV dose. Here the pharmacokinetics of intravenous digitalis come to bear. **Onset of action for intravenous digoxin takes as long as 30 minutes; peak effect may not occur for 90 to 120 minutes.**[9] Thus one should not expect an immediate or rapid effect. Likewise, **digoxin doses should not in general be given at intervals of less than 2 hours; otherwise the full effect of previous doses may not be realized and toxicity from additive effect may be induced.**

A very important point is that digoxin levels have little bearing on the acute management of new-onset atrial fibrillation. **The best indicator of adequacy of digitalization is the rate of ventricular response in atrial fibrillation.** Digitalis can be administered with impunity (with the preceding caveats as to dosage intervals) until the rate is controlled to 120/min or less.[1] Digoxin levels are not routinely available on an emergency basis. The levels are always tremendously high when drawn shortly after intravenous doses.

Thus if a particular patient does not slow after the initial digoxin dose, additional drug may be given, usually 0.25 mg IV, every 2 hours until the heart rate slows. The rate should be slowed at least to 120/min. Often we will slow the response to 90/min to 100/min to optimize ventricular filling between beats and lower myocardial oxygen demands.

This paradigm presumes that the rhythm is indeed atrial fibrillation. The impunity in dosage does not hold for other rhythms. Also, some reasonable maximum limit must be placed on the amount of digitalis administered. In our unit, no more than 2.5 mg of digoxin is administered in one 24-hour period.

Blocking medication treatment.[10,11] In the current era, it is often chosen to use blocking medications—either β-blockers or calcium channel blockers—instead of digitalis for the treatment of postoperative atrial fibrillation. For this Level I mild category of atrial fibrillation, the oral route may suffice. Metoprolol (Lopressor), 25 mg every 6 hours, may be started. Within 1 or 2 hours, the heart rate in atrial fibrillation will start to come down, as the β-blocker induces a higher degree of block through the A-V node. If response is too slow, supplementation with IV Lopressor (usually 2.5 to 5 mg at a time, up to about 10 mg per session) may help to achieve more rapid control. It is also acceptable to use a calcium channel blocker instead of a β-blocker. We usually employ diltiazem (Cardizem), starting at 30 mg every 6 hours orally and titrating up as needed (but not to exceed 60 to 90 mg q 6 h). Again, rate control can be expected to improve within an hour or two. Either the β-blocker or the calcium channel blocker is acceptable. The calcium channel blocker may be preferable in patients with a history of asthma or severe COPD, so as to avoid triggering bronchospasm with the β-blocker. Please note that the goal in the early treatment of postoperative atrial fibrillation is rate control, not conversion to normal sinus rhythm. In fact, it is questionable whether either β-blockers or calcium channel blockers contribute to conversion of postoperative atrial fibrillation. The atrial fibrillation tends to convert back and forth to normal sinus rhythm on its own; we have not really been impressed with any increased rate of conversion with either β-blockers or calcium channel blockers.

Amiodarone treatment. Amiodarone is another alternative for rate control in this setting. **Amiodarone does contribute to conversion to normal sinus rhythm,** in addition to effecting rate control. **Amiodarone is a powerful and potentially toxic medication,** covered in its own section below.

Level II (somewhat urgent).

A postoperative coronary bypass patient goes into atrial fibrillation on postoperative day 1. Heart rate is 160/min; blood pressure is 90/50 mm Hg. The patient is awake but somewhat confused. He feels some mild chest discomfort coming on.

This patient is clearly in greater jeopardy than the one described earlier. He qualifies for our second level of urgency.

As with the first patient, digitalis is one good option for control of ventricular response for this patient. Digitalis should be given immediately, as previously. However, this patient cannot wait the 30 minutes it may take for digitalis to act. His rate needs to be slowed quickly. Two categories of drugs are available for intravenous use that can slow the ventricular response within minutes: β-blockers and calcium antagonists. The β-blocker of choice is usually metoprolol (Lopressor), and the calcium antagonist of choice has been diltiazem (Cardizem). Both categories of agents can be used effectively.

Lopressor can be counted on to slow the rate reliably and in gradual fashion. **It is important to realize that the intravenous dose of Lopressor is much smaller than the oral dose, with a rough equivalency of 1 mg IV to 10 mg orally.** Errors have been made, with junior house officers giving an oral dose intravenously. **Lopressor is administered as a 2.5-mg to 5-mg IV push every 3 to 5 minutes until the desired slowing of rate is achieved.** (In the very early hours after surgery, it may be best to start with 1 mg). Up to 10 mg can be given at intervals in one session. Administration should be stopped when the rate reaches 120/min or less. Again, the goal is not to restore sinus rhythm but to control the ventricular response.

Diltiazem can also be used effectively. The effect from diltiazem may be more dramatic—a sudden slowing of rate or, at times, a conversion to sinus rhythm—but less controlled than that of Lopressor. Diltiazem may be given as 15 to 25 mg IV over several minutes, with the dose repeated in 15 minutes, if necessary. Diltiazem can also be given intravenously at a rate of 5 to 15 mg/h; this provides secure, titratable rate control. **Note the "Rule of 15s" for diltiazem[11]: Give 15 mg initially. Repeat in 15 minutes. Start a drip at 15 mg per hour.**

Important points to remember are the following:

- Both categories of agent (β-blocker or calcium channel antagonist) can cause bradycardia and heart block. If the patient is a postoperative open heart patient, the pacing wires should be connected to an external pacemaker set on the stand-by mode. If no pacing wires are available, measures should be taken to ensure that the drugs and equipment necessary for treating bradycardias (see earlier) are available.

- Intravenous β-blockers and calcium antagonists are not ordinarily used together, for their combined negative chronotropic and inotropic effects can be overwhelming in certain patients.[12] Asystole may occur.[12,13] In our unit, if intravenous β-blockers are chosen initially, intravenous calcium antagonists are not used for 4 hours, and vice versa. The experienced physician may make exceptions to this rule in selected cases.

- The use of β-blockers and calcium antagonists described earlier is crisis intervention. Once the rate is slowed or conversion to sinus rhythm is attained, the life-threatening condition is averted. However, when the β-blocker or calcium antagonist effect wears off, the arrhythmia is likely to recur, because the propensity for rapid rate is still present. This is why concurrent digitalization may be helpful. Beginning an oral dose of β-blocker (often Lopressor, 25 mg po q 6 h) or calcium antagonist (usually diltiazem, 30 mg po q 6 h) can help to maintain sinus rhythm and to ensure a controlled rate if atrial fibrillation recurs. Various new long-acting β-blockers and calcium antagonists are now available that allow the convenience of once-daily or twice-a-day dosing.

The guidelines we have given in this section for the treatment of postoperative atrial fibrillation can be applied as well to the treatment of new onset atrial fibrillation in medical patients being seen in the emergency department or in the medical intensive care unit or the coronary care unit.

See Table 2.2 for a listing of drug and dose options for the urgent treatment of atrial fibrillation.

Level III (urgent).

A postoperative coronary bypass patient goes into atrial fibrillation on postoperative day 1. His heart rate is 180/min. He loses consciousness, and his blood pressure falls to 60 mm Hg systolic. Just before losing consciousness, he complained of chest pain and clutched his chest.

This patient is acutely threatened. He is in a higher category of urgency than either of the 2 patients described thus far. The treatment for rapid atrial fibrillation with severe compromise of vital signs is direct current (DC) cardioversion.

Details regarding use of the defibrillator are reviewed in Chapter 4, The Defibrillator. Atrial fibrillation usually responds quite well, with return of normal sinus rhythm at a controlled rate. Following cardioversion, intravenous digitalization is in order, because the arrhythmia is likely to reappear. Oral maintenance Lopressor (or other β-blocker) or diltiazem (or other calcium antagonist) may also be instituted for further suppression and rate control.

In recent years, multiple new intravenous drugs have become available for the control of the ventricular response in atrial fibrillation, including both β-blockers and calcium antagonists. (See Table 2.2.)

TABLE 2.2   Drugs for Administration for the Control of Ventricular Response in Atrial Fibrillation

2.2A Oral Administration		
Digitalis	Digitalize with 1.25 mg total (0.5 mg initially followed by 0.25 mg q 6 h for 3 more doses). Note: After initial 0.5-mg dose, other doses can be given at 2-hour intervals, if necessary, for rate control, but at no less than 2 hours between doses.	
Amiodarone	(See Table 2.3.)	
	Starting dose	**Maximal dose**
β-blockers		
Metoprolol (Lopressor)	12.5-25 mg q 6 h	50 mg q 6 h
Calcium antagonists		
Diltiazem (Cardizem)	30 mg q 6 h	60-90 mg q 6 h
2.2B IV Administration		
Digitalis	Digitalize with 1.25 mg total (0.5 mg initially followed by 0.25 mg q 6 h for 3 more doses). Note: After initial 0.5-mg dose, other doses can be given at 2-hour intervals, if necessary, for rate control, but at no less than 2 hours between doses.	
Amiodarone	(See Table 2.3.)	
	IV bolus (over 3 min)	**IV infusion**
β-blockers		
Metoprolol (Lopressor)	2.5 mg (up to 10 mg)	NA
Esmolol (Brevibloc)	0.5 mg/kg	0.05-0.2 mg/kg/min
Calcium antagonists		
Diltiazem (Cardizem)	15-25 mg (0.25 mg/kg)	5-15 mg/h

Esmolol[14] is a very useful, short-acting cardioselective β-blocker for IV administration. It has a quick onset of action and a similarly short duration of action after discontinuation (half-life 9 min). The calcium antagonist diltiazem, as discussed above, is available in intravenous form for both bolus and continuous infusion. Diltiazem has a long duration of action (half-life 3.4 h). Titration of infusion rate to therapeutic effect is key with both esmolol and diltiazem. Care should be exercised in administration to patients with underlying hemodynamic compromise not directly related to rapid ventricular response. Choice among the agents listed in Table 2.2 is largely based on individual or institutional preference. The use of IV bolus or continuous infusion agents is limited to the period of time required for oral treatment with β-blockers or calcium antagonists to take effect.

Atrial Flutter

Atrial flutter represents another point on the spectrum of supraventricular arrhythmias. A given patient may have PACs at one moment, fibrillation at another, and flutter at still another. The atrial rate in flutter is about 300/min. Fortunately, conduction is usually 2:1 or less; that is, only one-half or fewer of the impulses reaching the A-V node are conducted to the ventricle.

The treatment of atrial flutter closely parallels that of atrial fibrillation. The objective, as with fibrillation, is control of rate rather than restoration of sinus rhythm. The same categories of treatment for the same general levels of urgency apply. The following points regarding atrial flutter should be kept in mind:

- Flutter is underdiagnosed by the house officer. Especially in a postoperative open heart patient, a perfectly regular rhythm with a ventricular response of 150/min is flutter with 2:1 block much more often than not. Flutter waves may not be seen at 2:1 conduction; carotid sinus massage to increase block even transiently to 3:1 conduction will clearly show flutter waves (see Figure 2.2). With 2:1 conduction, this rhythm is often mistaken for sinus or PAT. Of note as a distinguishing feature is the paroxysmal nature of flutter as opposed to sinus tachycardia. If the rate jumps suddenly to 150/min, that argues for flutter and against sinus tachycardia.

- In atrial flutter, unlike in atrial fibrillation, digitalization cannot be guided with impunity by the ventricular rate. Although the ventricular response gradually decreases with digitalization in atrial fibrillation, atrial flutter may be resistant to digitalis, and a sudden increase in block may occur, or another manifestation of digitalis toxicity may be seen.[1] If block changes from 2:1 to 3:1 initially, and then suddenly with more digitalis to, say, 10:1, the ventricular response will only be 30 min. It is best with flutter to give just a calculated appropriate total dose of digitalis in divided doses and then to use other agents. Here digoxin levels may be helpful on subsequent days.
- Atrial flutter is exquisitely sensitive to cardioversion. Usually 10 joules suffice to convert to normal sinus rhythm.
- Atrial flutter may at times be treated very effectively with overdrive pacing.[15] At centers where house staff are familiar with this technique, conversion to normal sinus rhythm may be accomplished quickly and easily. (Again, see Chapter 3 for details.) Even if overdrive pacing is used, digoxin with or without β-blockers or calcium antagonists should be begun for easier rate control when the flutter recurs.

On subsequent days, after the acute problems of new-onset fibrillation or flutter have been controlled, some physicians may choose to add an anti-fibrillation drug aimed at maintaining sinus rhythm. Amiodarone is the usual choice for this purpose. This decision will usually be made by a senior physician caring for the patient. On occasion, senior physicians may recommend some other potent anti-arrhythmic medication intended to discourage atrial fibrillation, such as sotalol (Betapace). Sotalol and other anti-arrhythmic medications may prolong the QT interval and in this way encourage serious ventricular arrhythmias. Specifically, the particular arrhythmia known as *torsades de pointe*, deriving its French name from the undulation of the electrogram away from and then close to the

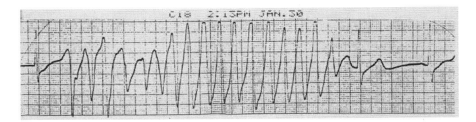

FIGURE 2.3

Torsades de pointe.

baseline, is a serious variant of ventricular tachycardia that can be seen from sotalol or other potent anti-arrhythmics (Figure 2.3).

The QT interval must be followed carefully, often daily. A prolongation in the QT interval often precedes proarrhythmic toxicity. The QT interval is measured from the beginning of the QRS complex to the end of the T wave. The QT interval must be adjusted for heart rate, as the interval normally decreases with increasing heart rate. The QTC, or corrected QT interval, is calculated by dividing the QT by the square root of the R-R interval. (Contemporary automated EKG machines print out the QT and QTC directly.) A QTC of greater than 400 msec should raise concern over the potential for proarrhythmic toxicity.

There has been a high level of interest among house officers recently in the antiarrhythmic agent adenosine. Adenosine (the naturally occurring nucleotide in intravenous form) is unique in that it is metabolized in seconds (half-life less than 10 sec). **Adenosine causes very transient interruption of conduction through the A-V node. This interruption lasts only seconds, so it is virtually impossible to cause any lasting harm by administration of this drug.** Contrary to a burgeoning reputation that this drug is a panacea for all manner of supraventricular arrhythmias, in fact, adenosine is useful therapeutically only for *paroxysmal supraventricular tachycardia* (PSVT). This abruptly occurring rhythm is often seen in young patients without structural heart disease. This is a reentrant tachycardia that depends on a circular conduction of impulses through 2 pathways between the atrium and ventricle. Wolff-Parkinson-White syndrome patients, and others, can develop such reentrant supraventricular tachycardias. By virtue of interruption of the A-V node limb of the reentrant circuit, adenosine is extremely effective at terminating PSVT and restoring sinus rhythm. **The dose of adenosine is 6 or 12 mg given by IV bolus.** Despite misconceptions to the contrary, **aside from a transient slowing of ventricular response, atrial fibrillation and atrial flutter are not impacted in any lasting fashion by administration of adenosine.** Although this transient increase in degree of block, may, like carotid sinus massage, make the fibrillation or flutter easier to recognize on EKG, there is no direct therapeutic benefit.

It should be kept in mind that, by 1 or 2 months after open heart surgery, except in patients with long-standing arrhythmias or valvular heart disease, the postoperative supraventricular irritability disappears. β-blockers, calcium antagonists, antiarrhythmics, and even digitalis can usually be discontinued at this point.

✚ VENTRICULAR ARRHYTHMIAS

The discussion of ventricular arrhythmias will be divided into 3 sections: premature ventricular contractions (PVCs); ventricular tachycardia; and ventricular fibrillation (Figure 2.4).

Premature Ventricular Contractions

Ventricular ectopic beats are threatening in 2 ways: They impair cardiac output, and they presage more serious ventricular arrhythmias. Unlike PACs, PVCs do not originate supraventricularly and do not propagate along specialized conducting tissues. For this reason, the cardiac contraction with a PVC is less "coordinated" than with a supraventricular beat. This can usually be seen in the arterial trace as a drop in arterial pressure, or a total lack of pressure spike, for the ectopic beat. As is well known, PVCs may be the forerunner of ventricular tachycardia or ventricular fibrillation.

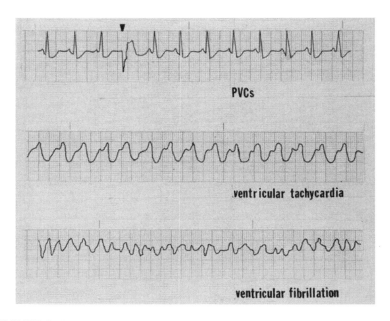

FIGURE 2.4

Ventricular arrhythmias: illustrative EKGs.

In the postoperative coronary patient, as in the patient with acute myocardial infarction, the general irritability of the heart argues for aggressive treatment of PVCs. **If the PVCs are frequent (more than 6/min), multifocal (manifested by multiple EKG configurations), or occurring in couplets or runs, treatment should be undertaken.**

The first-line drug for ventricular ectopy is lidocaine. The initial dose is 1 mg/kg (given by IV push). This is usually followed by a continuous infusion at 1 to 4 mg/min. An additional bolus of 0.5 mg/kg can be administered, along with an increase in the drip rate, if the initial bolus and drip do not control the arrhythmia.[16] Lidocaine does cause CNS effects (especially seizures) in high doses; administration at 4 mg/min should not be maintained any longer than absolutely necessary. **Lidocaine is a very effective drug.** Control of the PVCs is usually seen within

1 or 2 minutes. If lidocaine does not control the arrhythmia, chances are that other agents will not. However, amiodarone may be considered (see below).

If neither lidocaine nor amiodarone is effective, chances are the ectopy will not respond to drugs.

Ventricular Tachycardia

Ventricular tachycardia refers to a rapid, usually regular, wide-complex rhythm of ventricular origin. House officers often fail to appreciate that ventricular rhythms may at times sustain good hemodynamics. Although each contraction is not as coordinated as a normally conducted beat, it may produce a satisfactory stroke volume. After all, ventricular pacing, which is so commonly instituted for maintenance of cardiac output in patients with bradycardia or heart block, produces essentially a ventricular rhythm.

If hemodynamics are maintained by the ventricular rhythm, the treatment of choice is lidocaine. Particulars of administration are the same as for PVCs.

If hemodynamics are not sustained in ventricular tachycardia, the treatment of choice is electrical conversion. Details regarding the use of the defibrillator are covered in Chapter 4, The Defibrillator.

Ventricular Fibrillation

Ventricular fibrillation, with its chaotic, constant myocardial contractions, can never sustain hemodynamics. The treatment for ventricular fibrillation is immediate defibrillation. Immediate cardioversion without hesitation is likely to restore the rhythm and save the patient's life. The house officer must not hesitate. With every passing second, the chances of rhythm conversion and recovery diminish. If there is a delay in obtaining and implementing the defibrillator, chest compressions should be begun (see Chapter 11, Cardiac Arrest and Near Arrest).

The early postoperative period after cardiac surgery and the period following an acute myocardial infarction represent times of severe ventricular irritability. The operated heart has been handled,
incised, cannulated, cooled, warmed, and sutured. It is far from
surprising that it is irritable. In addition, the postoperative period is
one of electrolyte flux. Polyuria after bypass can exceed 1 L/h.
Forty or 60 mEq of potassium may be lost with each liter, sometimes within 1 hour. The patient may be very cold, especially after
procedures that involve deep hypothermic circulatory arrest (as in
aortic arch surgery); **cold is markedly proarrhythmic.** For all these
reasons, ventricular fibrillation may develop after cardiac surgery,
even in patients who are otherwise perfectly well. The arrhythmia
must be detected immediately, recognized immediately, and treated
immediately by defibrillation. On any cardiac service, in the course
of 1 year, at least several patients will have fibrillated, been defibril-
lated immediately, and recovered without problem, being discharged at the usual time. The key here is immediate recognition by
the house officer, followed by defibrillation; hesitation may result in
mortality.

✚ AMIODARONE

Amiodarone is a powerful, useful, but potentially very toxic drug.[17-19]
We have mentioned above its role in both atrial fibrillation and
ventricular arrhythmias. This drug has become the standard of
choice for ventricular tachycardia and ventricular fibrillation, as well
as being very popular for atrial fibrillation. The house officer should
be very familiar with this drug, yet respectful and mindful of its
great toxic potential.

   **Amiodarone has multiple favorable electrophysiologic prop-
erties: It decreases membrane excitability, decreases the rate of
the sinus node, and slows conduction through the A-V node.
Amiodarone also acts as a β-blocking drug.**

In long-term administration, amiodarone is poisonous. It causes pulmonary toxicity, hepatic toxicity, and turns the patient's nose a specific blue color. Pulmonary and hepatic toxicity can be lethal with long-term administration. The long-term toxicity is not so much an issue for the house officer, who deals more with the use of amiodarone in the acute setting.

Amiodarone is a peculiar drug in the sense that it has an extraordinarily long half-life. After achieving a steady state, it takes months for the drug to leave fatty tissues and wear off.

In terms of acute toxicity, amiodarone is a potent vasodilator and a negative inotrope; with both these effects, amiodarone can cause serious or life-threatening hypotension. Amiodarone can also cause profound bradycardia, which can be life-threatening. Amiodarone also has an uncommonly strong predisposition for adverse interactions with other important medications. Amiodarone interferes with the clearance of Coumadin and digoxin. Coumadin should be adjusted down when amiodarone is started, and digoxin should be reduced or discontinued.

Because of its peculiar pharmacodynamics, amiodarone requires a loading dose and then a maintenance dose (Table 2.3). Without a loading dose, amiodarone would require weeks to months to become effective. For oral loading, as in the case of low-acuity postoperative atrial fibrillation, we give 300 to 400 mg bid for 2 weeks. The usual maintenance dose is 100 to 300 mg bid. **For intravenous loading, as in the case of high-acuity atrial fibrillation or serious ventricular arrhythmia, we give a 150-mg bolus over 10 minutes,** followed by an infusion of 1 mg/min for 6 hours, followed by a maintenance infusion of 0.5 mg/min. The infusion can be continued at this maintenance rate, with levels followed in case of prolonged administration. The house officer should be aware that he can give a repeat 150-mg loading dose in case of recurrence of severe arrhythmia.

TABLE 2.3   Amiodarone Rx

Oral	Load	300-400 mg bid x 2 wk
	Maintenance	100-300 mg bid
IV	Load	150-mg bolus (10 min) 1 mg/min x 6 h
	Maintenance	0.5 mg/min

Because amiodarone has now become part of the standard resuscitative protocols, and because amiodarone is now used frequently for the treatment or prevention of atrial fibrillation,[17-19] it is vital that the house officer be intimately familiar with this drug—both in terms of its powerful beneficial actions, and also in terms of its virulent toxicity.

The prevention of atrial fibrillation has been an elusive holy grail of cardiac surgery for decades. Many approaches have been tried (β-blockers, antiarrhythmics, anti-inflammatory agents, statins, novel pericardial drainage techniques, etc), but many have been abandoned or not widely adopted. There is general enthusiasm for β-blockers and pockets of enthusiasm for sotalol. We use β-blockers aggressively at our institution but still suffer from frequent postoperative atrial fibrillation. Results in the literature are mixed. β-blocker administration is helpful, but far from a panacea.

Finding a cure to prevent postoperative atrial fibrillation is a noble cause, as the arrhythmia is frightening to patients and families, its treatment has dangers, it causes consternation to the attending surgeons, and it prolongs hospital stay and increases costs of hospitalization. One interesting study found that many cases of postoperative ventricular fibrillation arose out of atrial fibrillation; the atrial fibrillation was seen as providing an extremely rapid provocative stimulus (delivered through the A-V node) constantly irritating the ventricle, much like the deliberate electrical stimulation in an electrophysiolic study (EPS). Of all the agents tried for the prevention of atrial fibrillation after open heart surgery, amiodarone has seen the greatest success and widest implementation. One common regimen involves the administration of 10 mg/kg/day amiodarone for 1 week preoperatively, with 200 mg/day for 10 days postoperatively. This approach halved the incidence of atrial fibrillation (and also favorably reduced the rate of atrial fibrillation in those patients who did develop the arrhythmia).

By rigorously asking the key questions enumerated at the start of this chapter in all cases, the house officer can be assured of not overlooking significant data points in terms of causation of arrhythmias. By gathering data in this way and applying the principles outlined for specific arrhythmias, one can be assured of providing appropriate care for acute disturbances of cardiac rhythm.

REFERENCES

1. Kirklin J, Daggett WM, Lappas DG. Postoperative care following cardiac surgery. In: Johnson RA, Haber E, Austen WG, eds. *The Practice of Cardiology*. Boston: Little, Brown; 1980:1110-1132.

2. Innes IR, Nickerson M. Drugs inhibiting the action of acetylcholine on structures innervated by postganglionic parasympathetic nerves (antimuscarinic or atropinic drugs). In: Goodman LS, Gilman A, eds. *The Pharmacologic Basis of Therapeutics*. New York: Macmillan; 1970:524-548.

3. Smith PK, Buhrman WC, Levett JM, Ferguson TB Jr, Holman WL, Cox JL. Supraventricular conduction abnormalities following cardiac operations. A complication of inadequate atrial preservation. *J Thorac Cardiovasc Surg*. 1983;85(1):105-115.

4. Tyras DH, Stothert JC Jr, Kaiser GC, Barner HB, Codd JE, Willman VL. Supraventricular tachyarrhythmias after myocardial revascularization: a randomized trial of prophylactic digitalization. *J Thorac Cardiovasc Surg*. 1979;77(2):310-314.

5. Roffman JA, Fieldman A. Digoxin and propranolol in the prophylaxis of supraventricular tachydysrhythmias after coronary artery bypass surgery. *Ann Thorac Surg*. 1981;31(6):496-501.

6. Csicsko JF, Schatzlein MH, King PD. Immediate postoperative digitalization in the prophylaxis of supraventricular arrhythmias following

coronary artery bypass. *J Thorac Cardiovasc Surg.* 1981;81(3): 419-422.

7. Mohr R, Smolinsky A, Goor DA. Prevention of supraventricular tachyarrhythmia with low-dose propranolol after coronary bypass. *J Thorac Cardiovasc Surg.* 1981;81(6):840-845.

8. Kowey PR, Taylor JE, Rials SJ, Merinchak RA. Meta-analysis of the effectiveness of prophylactic drug therapy in preventing supraventricular arrhythmia early after coronary bypass grafting. *Am J Cardiol.* 1982;69(9):963-965.

9. Moe GK, Farah AE. Digitalis and allied cardiac glycosides. In: Goodman LS, Gilman A, eds. *The Pharmacological Basis of Therapeutics.* New York: Macmillan Co; 1970:677-708.

10. Prystowsky EN, Benson DW Jr, Fuster V, et al. Management of patients with atrial fibrillation. A statement for healthcare professionals. From the Subcommittee on Electrocardiography and Electrophysiology, American Heart Association. *Circulation.* 1996;93(6): 1262-1277.

11. King DA, Dickerson LM, Sack JL. Acute management of atrial fibrillation: Part I. Rate and rhythm control. *Am Fam Physician.* 2002;66(2):249-256.

12. Urthaler F, James TN. Experimental studies on the pathogenesis of asystole after verapamil in the dog. *Am J Cardiol.* 1979;44(4): 651-656.

13. Benaim ME. Asystole after verapamil. *Br Med J.* 1972;2(5806): 169-170.

14. Shettigar UR, Toole AG, Appunn DO. Combined use of esmolol and digoxin in the acute treatment of atrial fibrillation or flutter. *Am Heart J.* 1993;126(2):368-374.

15. Waldo AL, MacLean WAH, Karp RB, Kouchoukos NT, James TN. Entrainment and interruption of atrial flutter with atrial pacing: studies in man following open heart surgery. *Circulation.* 1977;56(5): 737-745.

16. McIntyre KM, Lewis AJ, eds. *Textbook of Advanced Cardiac Life Support.* Dallas: American Heart Association; 1981:VIII-l-VIII.

17. Ho KM, Lewis JP. Prevention of atrial fibrillation in cardiac surgery: time to consider a multimodality pharmacological approach. *Cardiovasc Ther.* 2010;28(1):59-65.

18. Creswell LL, Schuessler RB, Rosenbloom M, Cos JL. Hazards of postoperative atrial arrhythmias. *Ann Thorac Surg.* 1993;56(3): 539-549.
19. Gu S, Su PX, Liu Y, Yan J, Zhang XT, Wang TY. Low-dose amiodarone for the prevention of atrial fibrillation after coronary artery bypass grafting in patients older than 70 years. *Chin Med J.* 2009;122(24):2928-2932.

SUGGESTED FURTHER READING

Davis EM, Packard KA, Hilleman DE. Pharmacologic prophylaxis of postoperative atrial fibrillation in patients undergoing cardiac surgery: beyond beta-blockers. *Pharmacotherapy.* 2010;30(7):749, 274e-318e.
Looking toward the future.

Ho KM, Lewis JP. Prevention of atrial fibrillation in cardiac surgery: time to consider a multimodality pharmacological approach. *Cardiovasc Ther.* 2010;28(1):59-65.
An up-to-date review of the data.

Gu S, Su PZ, Liu Y, Yan J, Zhang XT, Wang TY. Low-dose amiodarone for the prevention of atrial fibrillation after coronary artery bypass grafting in patients older than 70 years. *Chin Med J.* 2009;122(24): 2928-2932.
Illustrative of the success attainable with amiodarone.

Benaim ME. Asystole after verapamil. *Br Med J.* 1972;2(5806):169-170.
Urthaler F, James JN. Experimental studies in the pathogenesis of asystole after verapamil in the dog. *Am J Cardiol.* 1979;44(4):651-656.
These two articles will serve to give the house officer a healthy respect for the dangers of combining β-blockers and verapamil.

3

TEMPORARY PACEMAKERS

The postoperative cardiac patient, the patient with coronary ischemia, and the post myocardial infarction patient are all at risk for bradycardia. Regarding the postoperative cardiac patient, the cooling associated with cardiopulmonary bypass, the cardioplegia, and the ischemia during the cross-clamp period all may affect the pacemaking tissues and conducting system of the heart. Patients who have had valve surgery may have operative injury to, or edema of, the His bundle, which can lead to sudden heart block. Furthermore, hypotension of any cause in the postoperative period may lead to hypoperfusion of the heart and cause bradycardia.

Thus the house officer who cares for acutely ill patients must be prepared to treat a sudden bradycardia at any time. The general management of bradycardia has been covered in Chapter 2, Arrhythmias. The postoperative cardiac patient almost always has temporary epicardial pacing wires placed specifically to allow reliable pacing in case of postoperative bradycardia. This chapter will concentrate on the basics of pacing with these wires and with other temporary systems and on the use of the temporary external pacemakers themselves.

The House Officer's Guide to ICU Care: Fundamentals of Management of the Heart and Lungs, 3rd ed. © 2013 John A. Elefteriades, Curtis Tribble, Alexander S. Geha, Mark D. Siegel, and Lawrence S. Cohen, eds. Cardiotext Publishing, ISBN: 978-1-935395-68-3.

✚ OPERATIVE PLACEMENT OF PACING WIRES

The epicardial wires placed at the time of cardiac surgery are insulated, except at the tip, near the curved needle (Figure 3.1). The curved needle is used to pass the wire through the myocardium. The ventricular wire is usually placed in the anterior wall of the right ventricle at a spot free of fat where the myocardium shows clearly (Figure 3.2). The curved needle is then cut off, the wire is positioned so that the uninsulated portion is in touch with the heart muscle, and it is secured. The end with the straight needle is passed through the body wall, and the wire is secured to the skin to prevent dislodgement. The sharp tip is cut off, and the remaining portion of the straight needle serves as a contact. At the time of discharge, the wire can be easily pulled out by gentle traction. A separate ground wire is placed in the skin only (with the curved needle end). Again, care is taken that the uninsulated portion is actually in touch with the skin.

Atrial pacing wires are placed somewhat differently. Because of the thin atrial wall, the wire is not passed through but is affixed to the atrial surface by suture.

When not in use, the external contacts of the pacing wires should be insulated from external electrical forces. This can be done by securing the needles between two pieces of tape or by putting them

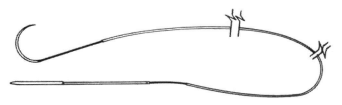

FIGURE 3.1

Epicardial pacing wire.

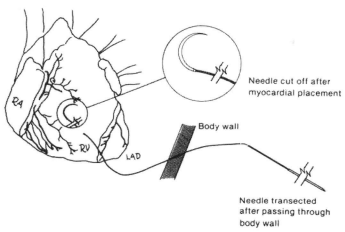

Needle cut off after
myocardial placement

Body wall

Needle transected
after passing through
body wall

FIGURE 3.2

Operative placement of ventricular pacing wire.

into a test tube or plastic needle sheath or underneath a plastic skin adhesive. Without this precaution, an electrical short circuit from bedside electrical equipment could conceivably be conducted to the heart.

A given patient may have no pacing wires at all (straightforward cases only) or may have any of a number of combinations of grounds, atrial wires, and ventricular wires. At the time of operation, the surgeon decides which wires might be needed postoperatively. It should be noted that a ground wire can be placed at any time, even in the ICU. If need be, an ordinary EKG skin electrode can be used as a ground.

Most hospitals have conventions that allow the house officer to recognize which wire is which. For example, at some centers, a ventricular wire will be brought to the left side of the chest and an atrial wire will be brought to the right. The ground wire can be recognized because it ends at the skin. Because the overall length of the wires is the same, the ground can also be identified as the wire with more length outside the body.

✚ EMERGENCY PLACEMENT OF PACING WIRES

Emergency placement of pacing wires may be required if bradycardia occurs in an ICU patient who does not have epicardial pacing wires already in place. For this reason, the house officer must become familiar with the emergency placement of temporary wires. Two general approaches are available: transvenous and transthoracic.

Transvenous Approach

For placement of a transvenous pacing wire, central venous cannulation is carried out as for intravenous access or central venous pressure (CVP) monitoring.[1] The flow-directed temporary transvenous pacing catheter has an inflatable balloon near the tip, just like a Swan-Ganz catheter (Figure 3.3). The pacing catheter is advanced to CVP position in the right atrium. At this point, the balloon is inflated and the catheter is advanced further. Just as for the Swan-Ganz catheter, the bloodstream carries the balloon and catheter tip through the tricuspid valve into the right ventricle. A sharp further advancement until resistance is felt will engage the tip in the right ventricular trabeculae. At times, the bloodstream will carry the tip through the ventricle to the pulmonary artery; in such a case, withdrawal into the ventricle will be necessary before advancement into the trabeculae. As this is a blind procedure, it is not possible to be absolutely certain of position. (Fluoroscopy is rarely immediately available in the ICU setting.) With some experience, the house officer can get the feel of the procedure. When some (low) spontaneous heart rate is present, the flow-directed catheter can be passed with a reasonable chance of success. If no spontaneous heartbeat at all exists to carry the flow-directed balloon, successful placement is unlikely, as the catheter tends to pass straight through the right atrium into the interior vena cava.

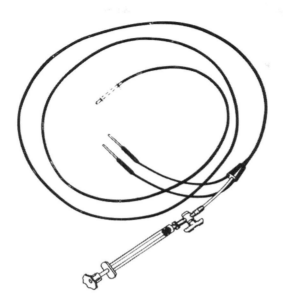

FIGURE 3.3

Temporary transvenous pacing catheter.

Systems have been described for monitoring the intracardiac EKG by attaching the end of the temporary pacing wire to a 12-lead EKG machine; this can allow identification of position in the ventricle on the basis of EKG characteristics.[2] Such monitoring can be cumbersome in emergencies, especially for a beginner. It may be more efficient just to pass the catheter as well as possible and then to connect it to the pacemaker to see if effective pacing is achieved; if not, the catheter is repositioned.

One common misconception is that a pacing spike on the monitor means that the tip of the catheter is in the heart. This is not true in the slightest. A pacing spike can be seen with the catheter tip anywhere in contact with body fluids. It is observation of a wide-complex QRS depolarization following the pacing spike that confirms proper contact with the ventricular myocardium.

Transthoracic Approach

In desperate circumstances, as when no effective heartbeat exists to carry a flow-directed catheter, a transthoracic pacing wire may need to be placed (Figure 3.4). The right ventricle is punctured by needle via a subxyphoid approach similar to that for pericardiocentesis. A specially designed wire is passed through the needle into the ventricle. Pacing is then instituted as for other catheters. This approach obviously is dangerous and should be used only when no alternative exists.

A

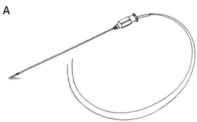

B

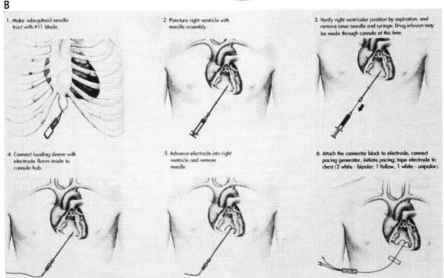

FIGURE 3.4

(**A**) Temporary transthoracic pacing wire. (**B**) Technique for placement.

✚ THE PACEPORT SWAN-GANZ CATHETER

A useful piece of equipment is the Paceport Swan-Ganz catheter (Baxter Healthcare Corporation; Irvine, CA). This device is a Swan-Ganz catheter that can provide cardiac pacing as well. The concept takes advantage of the fact that, with the Swan-Ganz catheter properly positioned in the pulmonary artery, for most patients a port 19 cm back from the tip of the catheter lies in the right ventricle. A pacing wire specifically designed for passage through this port is used to pace the heart (Figure 3.5). This device can provide extremely quick access to the right ventricle for pacing. Until pacing is required, the Paceport Swan-Ganz is used just as any other Swan-Ganz catheter for hemodynamic monitoring and cardiac output determination. Use of this model of Swan-Ganz catheter is recommended for circumstances in which the need for pacing appears likely or possible.

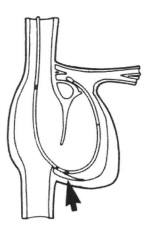

FIGURE 3.5

The Paceport Swan-Ganz catheter. Schematic representation shows the pacing wire protruding through the proximal (RV) port and making contact with the right ventricular endocardial surface.

Source: Reproduced with the permission of Edwards Lifesciences, Irvine, CA.

✚ THE EXTERNAL TRANSCUTANEOUS (ZOLL) PACEMAKER

It has been known for many years that it is feasible to pace the heart by applying a current between contacts placed on the skin external to the body—by selecting electrode locations that provide a current trajectory that intersects with the heart. In fact, many of the earliest attempts at cardiac pacing involved such systems. These systems fell out of favor—because of their unreliability and, especially, pain associated with pacing—with the advent of fluoroscopy and transvenous pacing systems.

Recent technical advances have made possible reliable and comfortable transcutaneous pacing[3] and have led to a resurgence of this modality. The current system (Zoll) involves two large electrodes placed anteroposteriorly over the left chest (Figure 3.6). An external console develops the current applied to the electrodes. The desired heart rate is set on the console, as well as the current output. (Current output of 40 to 100 mA is usually required, compared to the 1 to 2 mA required for pacing through a transvenous catheter.) Current level is set so as to provide reliable pacing but minimize

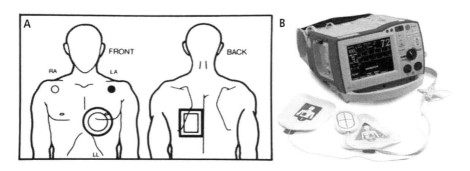

FIGURE 3.6

The external transcutaneous (Zoll) pacemeaker. (**A**) Electrodes in place in anteroposterior position. (**B**) The external console.

Source: Reproduced by permission of ZMI Corporation, 500 West Cummings Park, Woburn, MA.

pain. The device can be set in a "demand" mode, so that it fires only when bradycardia is occurring.

The house officer should be aware that the mere delivery of the stimulus by the external pacemaker can give the appearance of eliciting a QRS complex while not actually capturing the heart. This is true even of transvenous pacemakers but poses more of a problem by virtue of the high-current, long-duration stimulus required for external pacing. It is crucial to confirm the capture of the heart muscle by feeling a pulse synchronous with the pacemaker spikes or confirming a pressure pulse on the arterial line tracing.

The external transcutaneous pacemaker (Zoll) can provide very quick access to electrical pacing of the heart in emergencies. Transcutaneous pacemakers are now found in most emergency rooms, coronary care units, recovery rooms, and post cardiac surgery units. They are usually incorporated into a single unit that provides both defibrillation and pacing. **The transcutaneous system should be used, when available, in preference to transvenous placement and transthoracic puncture.** In fact, transcutaneous pacing has largely supplanted transvenous and transthoracic pacing in the ICU environment. A brief period of discomfort from pacing is a small price to pay for restoration of a life-supporting heart rate, especially in emergencies where the patient has a reduced level of consciousness. Once hemodynamic stability is restored, a transvenous temporary pacemaker can be placed in a precise manner under fluoroscopic control in the catheterization laboratory or in the operating room, to provide more reliable and more comfortable pacing.

✚ OPERATING THE PACEMAKER

A commonly used external temporary pacemaker generator is shown in Figure 3.7. The two knurled knobs on the pacemaker are for securing the ends of the pacing cables, which in turn are connected to the pacing wires themselves. The sense and pace lights indicate what the unit is doing for each beat—sensing or pacing.

1. Pace/Sense LEDs
2. Lock/Unlock Key
3. Lock Indicators
4. Rate Dial
5. Atrial Output Dial
6. Ventricular Output Dial
7. Menu Parameter Dial
8. Parameter Selection Key
9. Menu Selection Key
10. Pause Key
11. Power On Key
12. Power Off Key
13. Emergency/Asynchronous
    Pacing Key
14. Lower Screen
15. Ventricular Output
    Graphics
16. Atrial Output Graphics
17. Upper Screen
18. Rate Graphics
19. Setup Indicators
20. DDI Indicator
21. Low Battery Indicator
22. Setup Labels

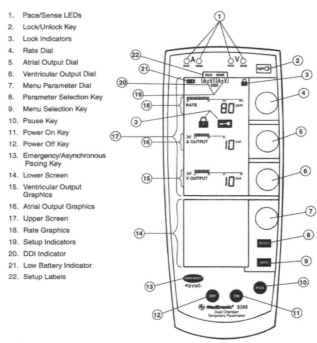

FIGURE 3.7

Temporary external pacemaker generator (schematic). Numerical legend shows controls and displays.

Source: Reproduced by permission of Medtronic, Inc, Minneapolis, MN.

✚ OPERATING PARAMETERS

There are several parameters (set by scrolling an on-screen menu) for the physician to adjust:

- The *rate* control is self-explanatory. Most units will allow 30 to 180/min. A reasonable initial setting for a bradycardic patient might be 70 or 80/min. In a patient who is not currently bradycardic but who had shown heart block in the early postoperative period or who is at risk for heart block after myocardial infarction, the rate might be set at 45 or 50/min. In this way, the patient's heart would be allowed to beat spontaneously but would be protected from a life-threatening low rate if heart block should recur.

- The *output* control allows the current of the pacing stimulus to be adjusted, usually in a range from 0 to 20 mA. In an emergency, the output should be set to maximum. Output can, in fact, usually be left at maximum. Another safe approach is to turn down the output until capture is lost and then double that for a safe output setting. If the skin is being used as ground, the patient may feel an electric shock at the skin site; this may require turning down the output somewhat. One must, of course, be sure to ascertain that the ventricle is still captured at the lower output setting. Output can be set for both the ventricle (the critical chamber to pace) and the atrium (the augmenting chamber).

- The *sensitivity* adjustment allows the sensitivity of the pacemaker to be modulated. At the lowest sensitivity, called "asynchronous," the pacemaker does not listen for a spontaneous heartbeat at all; the pacemaker will fire regularly at the set rate regardless of intrinsic cardiac activity. At full sensitivity, or "demand" setting, the pacemaker will not fire if a spontaneous beat occurs before the scheduled time for the next paced beat. The gradations between these two extremes control the height (in millivolts) that a spontaneous QRS complex must achieve to be recognized by the unit. **Usually, a demand setting will be used.**

- The *mode* setting determines the modality in which the pacemaker functions. Modality is designated by a code system that can be intimidating to the house officer. A three-letter code is utilized (Table 3.1). The first letter represents the chamber paced. V stands for ventricle, and A for atrium. The second letter represents the chamber sensed. Again, V stands for ventricle, and A for atrium. The third letter represents the mode of function. D stands for dual (pacing and sensing), and I stands for inhibited only. There are two common mode settings with which the house officer needs to be familiar: **DDD stands for full dual chamber sensing and pacing mode, and VVI stands for only single**

(ventricular) mode. In DDD, the pacemaker listens to both chambers and paces either atrium or ventricle if either is lagging. In VVI, the pacemaker listens to and paces only the ventricle. (Occasionally, we may use AAI pacing, in which the pacemaker only senses and paces the atrium; such a setting should only be selected if it is confidently known that the native conducting system will conduct the atrial pacing to the ventricle.) This is all a bit intimidating to the beginning house officer. **Fortunately, the pacemaker comes on in DDD mode with appropriate initial settings for all parameters when it is turned on; this DDD default mode is appropriate in nearly all acute settings.** Further refinements can be made in conjunction with an attending physician, depending on his particular preferences.

TABLE 3.1 Pacemaker Code Nomenclature

I	II	III
Chamber(s) Paced	Chamber(s) Sensed	Mode of Response
V = Ventricle	V = Ventricle	T = Triggered
A = Atrium	A = Atrium	I = Inhibited
D = Dual (A and V)	D = Dual (A and V)	D = Dual (Triggered or Inhibited)

DDD—Paces and senses both chambers (atrium and ventricle), triggering or inhibiting as necessary.

VVI—Paces and senses ventricle only, inhibiting when there is a spontaneous ventricular impulse.

AAI—Paces and senses atrium only, inhibiting when there is a spontaneous atrial impulse. *Appropriate only when there is reliable native conduction through the A-V node.*

- The *A-V delay* determines how long the pacemaker will wait to sense normal conduction of a beat to the ventricle; if the pacemaker does not "hear" a conducted ventricular beat during this time, it will pace the ventricle, to ensure safety. The default A-V delay is usually around 240 msec. It is rare for the house officer to need to adjust this. The attending physician may shorten or lengthen the A-V delay in certain instances (eg, to permit spontaneous conduction, even if delayed, through the patient's own conducting system).

In a way, it was easier for all involved when the pacemaker had just a few knobs, for adjusting rate, output, sensitivity, and A-V delay. Modern external pacemakers are built on a computer-like platform, and menus need to be scrolled for adjustment. This can be time-consuming and dangerous in an emergency setting. We recommend that the house officer become intimately familiar with the particular pacemaker used in his unit upon beginning his ICU rotation, so that he does not fumble or scramble when an emergency arises—and pacing emergencies will definitely arise. *Fortunately, the default settings that come into play automatically when the pacemaker is turned are fully appropriate for nearly any emergency setting.*

Polarity

The negative pole of the pacemaker should go to the heart and the positive pole should be the ground. This is contrary to what one would expect for an electrical ground. The best way for the house officer to remember this arrangement is to recall that electrons exit from the negative pole of a battery. Better capture occurs when this electron flow hits the heart directly.

Multiple Ventricular Wires

If more than one ventricular wire is present, either can be used as positive or negative. A patient who has discomfort at the skin site with paced beats can be converted to two ventricular leads (if two are available); this will eliminate any discomfort.

Atrial Wires

If the patient has intact atrioventricular (A-V) conduction and has atrial wires in place, it is usually preferable to pace atrially. This preserves A-V synchrony and atrial kick. Also, **the native His-Purkinje system creates a more coordinated ventricular squeezing and wringing action from the left ventricle than a paced beat.** A coordinated native beat actually wrings the blood (like wringing a wet towel) from the apex toward the aortic valve, twisting counter-clockwise as well as contracting toward the center. One can picture how the complex, multifascicled native conducting system illustrated in Figure 3.8 would produce a much more efficient contraction than the single epicardial impulse also illustrated in the diagram. If heart block exists, of course, ventricular pacing must be used, as the atrial impulse will not be conducted. Connections for the atrial wires are made similarly to those for the ventricular. Negative goes to the atrium; positive goes to skin ground. If two atrial wires are present, either can be used as positive or negative.

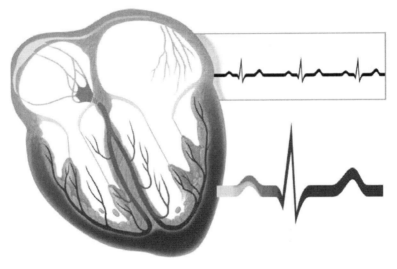

FIGURE 3.8

An electrocardiogram showing the conducting system of the heart. The fine biological "wires" conduct the heartbeat in sequence from the upper to the lower chambers of the heart.

Asynchronous Pacing

If it is ever necessary to use the asynchronous mode, the danger of precipitating ventricular tachycardia is remote. The house officer usually has heard of the R-on-T phenomenon precipitating ventricular tachycardia or ventricular fibrillation. This is a rare phenomenon. If need be, the house officer can pace a patient asynchronously if the demand mode should not work reliably. Asynchronous would correspond to DOO in the pacing terminology (pacing atrium and ventricle, not listening to anything) or VOO (pacing ventricle, not listening to anything). We recommend that **any periods of asynchronous pacing be limited to the shortest time possible, so as to minimize the risk of an R-on-T phenomenon.** Senior help should be enlisted to restore pacemaking function to demand (full sensitivity) mode.

Deterioration of Temporary Epicardial Wires over Time

The epicardial wires usually function very well in the early postoperative period. Over 7 to 10 days, however, exit block may occur. Scar tissue and edema at the sites of the wires on the myocardium may insulate the wires electrically from intact muscle. It may become difficult or impossible to capture the myocardium. The R wave heard by the sensing system may diminish in amplitude, leading to improper sensing, with the possibility of the R-on-T phenomenon. In such cases, different combinations of wires may be tried, following the preceding guidelines. One wire may function perfectly when another has exit block or poor R wave.

In case of dysfunction in the pacing system, the house officer must check all components carefully. The wires must be identified correctly and must be connected appropriately, the connections must be tight, and all programmable parameters must be set properly. A careful examination and some common sense will usually produce proper pacing.

Advantages of DDD Pacing

Fully physiologic pacing, which senses and paces both the atrium and the ventricle, has been available in permanent implantable pacemakers for years. This type of pacing is called "DDD" in the international nomenclature.

Despite this sophistication in implantable units, technology has only more recently been incorporated into temporary external units. Currently, the technology of full, physiologic DDD pacing is available in external temporary units.[4] These units can sense and pace not only the ventricle, but also the atrium. This can be a tremendous advantage if the atrial rate is irregular and if the A-V conduction varies. A heart rate is set for the DDD pacemaker. If a spontaneous atrial beat occurs within the time of the heart rate allotment, the pacemaker does not deliver an atrial stimulus. The unit then listens for a ventricular QRS. If one is sensed, no ventricular pacing stimulus is delivered; if none is sensed, a ventricular pacing stimulus is delivered with the specific A-V delay. If no atrial beat occurs within the time of the heart rate allotment, an atrial pacing stimulus is delivered; the unit then listens again for a ventricular QRS. In essence, the unit listens to and/or paces both chambers as required.

The additional settings required for the DDD external unit (as discussed above) are atrial sensitivity and atrial output. Also, the mode is specified by the house officer—that is, either ventricular (called VVI in the nomenclature), atrial (called AAI), or dual chamber (DDD).

Especially in patients who have heart rates that compete with the paced rate, the DDD pacemakers are optimal, providing A-V synchrony despite the beat-to-beat variability of the intrinsic heart rhythm. Atrial R-on-T is prevented, as is ventricular R-on-T.

Overdrive Pacing

In addition to their usefulness in bradycardias, external pacemakers can be useful in selected tachyarrhythmias, for so-called overdrive pacing.[5,6] The principle involved is to overtake a tachyarrhythmia by pacing the affected chamber faster than the intrinsic tachycardia; upon discontinuation of pacing, the tachyarrhythmia is often found to have been interrupted, with normal sinus rhythm supervening

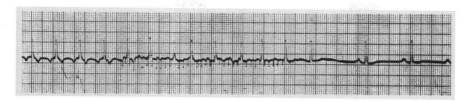

FIGURE 3.9

EKG demonstrating successful overdrive pacing to terminate supraventricular tachycardia. Note atrial flutter at beginning of strip. The downward spikes in the middle of the strip represent rapid atrial overdrive pacing. Normal sinus rhythm supervenes when rapid pacing is terminated.

Source: Reproduced with permission from Harthorne JW. The physiology of cardiac pacing. *Intelligence Reports in Cardiac Pacing and Electrophysiology.* 1984;3:1.

(Figure 3.9). It may be necessary to overdrive at very rapid rates (eg, 300/min or more for atrial flutter). The DDD external units in current use have a special mode for this purpose.

Overdrive pacing is most effective for supraventricular tachycardias, especially atrial flutter. At some centers, this is the preferred treatment of postoperative atrial flutter.[7] Even ventricular tachycardia can be treated at times in this way. **Only organized rhythms can respond; atrial or ventricular fibrillation is never ameliorated by overdrive pacing.**

The overdrive pacing technique has serious inherent dangers and should not be undertaken independently by the junior officer; experienced supervision is required.

Complexity

The house officer should not expect to understand pacing fully at first blush. This would be an unrealistic expectation. Using the guiding information in this chapter in clinical practice, supplemented with teaching from senior house staff and faculty, should produce familiarity within one or two cardiac ICU rotations.

REFERENCES

1. Vander Salm TJ. *Atlas of Bedside Procedures.* Boston: Little, Brown; 1979.
2. Schnitzler RN, Caracta AR, Damato AN. "Floating" catheter for temporary transvenous ventricular pacing. *Am J Cardiol.* 1973;31(3): 351-354.
3. Zoll PM, Zoll RH, Falk RH, Clinton JE, Eitel DR, Antman EM. External noninvasive temporary cardiac pacing: clinical trials. *Circulation.* 1985;71(5):937-944.
4. Ferguson TB Jr, Cox JL. Temporary external DDD pacing after cardiac operations. *Ann Thorac Surg.* 1991;51(5):723-732.
5. Fisher J. Pacing for tachycardias. *Resident Staff Physician.* July 1980.
6. Waldo AL, MacLean WA, Karp RB, Kouchoukos NT, James TN. Entrainment and interruption of atrial flutter with atrial pacing: studies in man following open heart surgery. *Circulation.* 1977;56(5): 737-745.
7. Harthorne JW. The physiology of cardiac pacing. *Intelligence Reports in Cardiac Pacing and Electrophysiology.* 1984;3:1.

SUGGESTED FURTHER READING

Craig, K. How to provide transcutaneous pacing. *Cardiac Insider.* 2006;36:22-23.
A practical guide, written by a nurse, and very well illustrated, describing the specifics of utilizing external transcutaneous pacemakers.

Brady, WJ Jr, Harrigan RA. Evaluation and management of bradyarrhythmias in the emergency department. *Emerg Med Clin North Am.* 1968;16(2):361-388.
A comprehensive, thoughtful review.

Overbay, D, Criddle, L. Mastering temporary invasive cardiac pacing. *Crit Care Nurse.* 2004;24(3):25-32.
A well-illustrated, comprehensive, practical review.

4

THE DEFIBRILLATOR

As discussed in Chapter 2 (Arrhythmias), cardioversion and defibrillation are important techniques for the management of acute disturbances of cardiac rhythm. Cardioversion refers to the delivery of a
depolarizing electrical impulse synchronized with the patient's EKG; defibrillation refers to the delivery of a depolarizing impulse randomly, without synchronization with the EKG.

The techniques of cardioversion and defibrillation should be within the
armamentarium of the house officer, especially if he or she is to treat coronary care or postoperative cardiac patients. All too frequently, unfortunately, the house officer's first responsible application of cardioversion or
defibrillation comes during an emergency for which he or she is not prepared. This chapter aims to clarify important basic concepts regarding
these techniques. In addition to assimilating the following material, the
house officer should spend time with the particular defibrillator used in his
own intensive care unit; a review of the instruction manual and a run-
through with the controls are important.

*The House Officer's Guide to ICU Care: Fundamentals of Management of
the Heart and Lungs,* 3rd ed. © 2013 John A. Elefteriades, Curtis Tribble,
Alexander S. Geha, Mark D. Siegel, and Lawrence S. Cohen, eds.
Cardiotext Publishing, ISBN: 978-1-935395-68-3.

✚ GENERAL PRINCIPLES

Figure 4.1 shows a typical defibrillator apparatus. The top portion is an EKG monitor, like those used at the bedside in all ICUs. This monitor displays the EKG on the oscilloscope screen and displays the pulse rate digitally; an EKG printout is available, and upper and lower pulse rate alarms can be set for monitoring. This EKG monitor is attached via a standard patient cable to EKG skin electrodes. The lower portion of the apparatus is the cardioverter/defibrillator proper. The charge is selected by dial, displayed digitally, and delivered via the patient paddles.

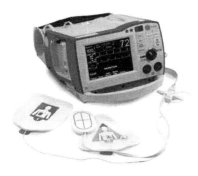

FIGURE 4.1

A typical defibrillator apparatus.

Because of their greater effectiveness and reliability,[1] direct current (DC) units have supplanted earlier alternating current models. When the unit is charged, the DC charge is stored in a capacitor. The amount of energy stored can be varied, usually from 0 to 200 watt-seconds, or joules (J). (Older units used to charge to 400 J, but newer units deliver a biphasic wave, and 200 J biphasic is as effective as 400 J monophasic.) When the unit is fired, the stored charge is delivered from the capacitor to the paddles. The delivery is completed in several milliseconds (Figure 4.2).[2] Delivery may be made asynchronously or in synchrony with the patient's EKG, at the discretion of the physician (see later). The delivered electrical

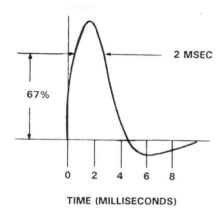

FIGURE 4.2

Pulse contour of delivered electric shock.

Source: Reproduced with the permission of Mennen Medical, Inc, Southampton, PA.

impulse depolarizes all or most of the muscle fascicles of the heart, interrupts the arrhythmia, and allows normal rhythms to emerge.[3]

Paddle Position

The cardinal principle regarding paddle position is that the current flowing between the paddles must encompass the heart. In the present era, pre-gelled pads that connect to the defibrillator are popular. This arrangement may use up critical time. More commonly, both paddles are held by hand (Figure 4.3), one to the right of the sternum just below the clavicle and the second below the left breast and back toward the scapula. This arrangement is convenient and effective.

Electrode paste must be used to obtain good electrical contact between paddles and patient; otherwise, skin burns will result. Gel pads have recently come into favor and serve the same purpose as the older electrode paste. Firm pressure against the patient helps to maximize current delivery. Personnel should step away from the bed to avoid inadvertent shocking. Likewise, electrode jelly should be kept from the paddle handles, as this can form a current path to the operator's hand. (In fact, one of the authors felt a "buzz"

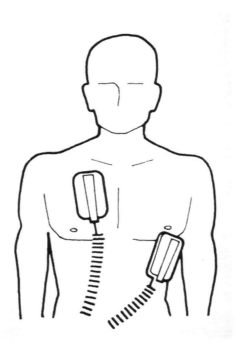

FIGURE 4.3

Standard paddle position. It is best to place the lateral paddle even more laterally than shown, if possible.

Source: Reproduced with the permission of Physio-Control Corp, Redmond, WA.

during an urgent defibrillation the day before this portion of the text was being written.) As mentioned above, a new type of flexible, self-adhesive, disposable paddle (Fast-Patch, R2 pads, and R2 Medical Systems, Niles, IL) is available; two such paddles can be left attached to the patient's chest and connected to the defibrillator—for high-risk patients, or those manifesting frequent arrhythmias.

If an elective cardioversion is performed in a conscious patient, analgesia and anesthesia must be effected. Intravenous midazolam is effective. An anesthesiologist can be extremely useful to administer propofol (or a similar drug), as in the operating room, to obtain complete, brief anesthesia. At the same time, the anesthesiologist can monitor and control respiration and airway. In critical situations, where vital signs and consciousness are lost, no anesthesia is necessary. Indeed, no time should be wasted in this setting in giving anesthetic medications. The house officer must not hesitate to defibrillate, as with each passing second of delay, the chances of effective restoration of rhythm and preservation of cerebral function diminish.

Energy Level

The greater the energy delivered, the greater the chance of achieving the desired conversion of rhythm. However, cardioversion does cause cardiac damage, and the extent of damage is directly related to the energy level used. The electrical energy is dissipated as heat, which injures myocardial cells in the path of the current.

Balancing chance for success against current-mediated cardiac muscle injury requires familiarity with conversion patterns of various rhythms. Certain rhythms are very sensitive to cardioversion, and low energy levels are likely to bring about conversion; such is the case for atrial flutter and ventricular tachycardia.[4] Other rhythms are relatively resistant to cardioversion and require higher energy levels; atrial and ventricular fibrillation fall in this category.[4] Further details are given in the discussion of cardioversion of particular arrhythmias.

The other factor that influences choice of energy level is the urgency of the situation. An elective cardioversion can be done at incremental energies until success is achieved. An emergency defibrillation, on the other hand, can justifiably be performed at a high energy level.

Most units in current use can provide up to 200 joules for external defibrillation. For internal defibrillation, much lower energies must be used. In fact, most units lock out all energy choices beyond 50 joules when connected to internal paddles.

◘ SYNCHRONIZED CARDIOVERSION OR ASYNCHRONOUS DEFIBRILLATION

The house officer should understand when to use synchronized cardioversion and when to use asynchronous defibrillation. The key principle in this decision is that a **so-called *vulnerable period*, corresponding to the T wave on EKG,** follows ventricular depolarization (Figure 4.4); **delivery of an impulse during the vulnerable period runs the risk of producing ventricular fibrillation.**

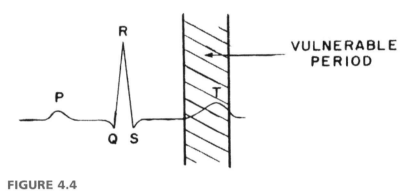

FIGURE 4.4

The vulnerable period of the cardiac cycle.
Source: Reproduced with the permission of Mennen Medical, Inc, Southampton, PA.

The cardioverter unit monitors the patient's EKG. When the "synchronized" mode is selected, an electrical circuit in the unit ensures that no impulse is fired during the vulnerable period; instead the impulse is timed to occur during the R wave. When the synchronized mode has been selected and the patient's EKG is being read well by the machine, the "sync" button or display will flash with each QRS complex detected. Furthermore, the oscilloscope will show a spike on each QRS complex where the machine would have delivered the depolarizing impulse if activated at that time (Figure 4.5).

Basically, synchronized cardioversion should be used for all rhythms (including atrial fibrillation, atrial flutter, paroxysmal atrial

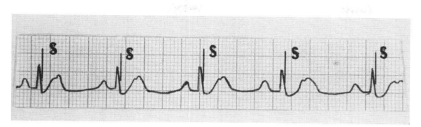

FIGURE 4.5

Synchronizer spike superimposed on the R wave of the EKG.

tachycardia, and ventricular tachycardia) except ventricular fibrillation, for which asynchronous defibrillation must be performed. The use of synchronized cardioversion will avoid the risk of precipitating ventricular fibrillation while treating a less serious arrhythmia. In ventricular fibrillation, this concern is not relevant. Furthermore, with the constant chaotic electrical and mechanical activity in ventricular fibrillation, no QRS or T waves exist or can be identified.

Now that this basic point regarding synchronous/asynchronous application has been made, some qualifications are in order:

- The risk of inducing ventricular fibrillation with asynchronous cardioversion, although real, is not great. It has been estimated at 2% to 5%.[1-3] For this reason, if an arrhythmia for which synchronization would normally be used causes major hemodynamic embarrassment, or if the "sync" apparatus cannot quickly be engaged, asynchronous delivery is justified.
- In ventricular tachycardia, it may not be possible for the physician or the machine to identify QRS and T waves, depending on the particular morphology. In this case, asynchronous delivery is acceptable.
- If a patient is discovered in extremis and precise cardiac rhythm cannot be determined rapidly, asynchronous cardioversion is acceptable.

- One practical matter deserves emphasis. When synchronized cardioversion is selected, the machine will not deliver the charge at the instant that the paddle controls are pressed; rather, delivery of the charge will be delayed until the appropriate time on the EKG. It is not uncommon to find a junior house officer letting up on the paddle pushbuttons when he or she doesn't see an immediate shock delivered. The house officer concludes the apparatus is not working and may repeat this cycle with continued failure to shock. In fact, the equipment is working appropriately. One must keep the pushbuttons depressed and wait a split second or more for synchronization and shock delivery.

✚ ELECTRICAL CONVERSION OF SPECIFIC RHYTHMS

The overall treatment patterns for specific arrhythmias are covered in Chapter 2 (Arrhythmias). Cardioversion and defibrillation are included in the recommended patterns for many of these rhythms. The particulars of application of cardioversion/defibrillation for specific rhythm disturbances will be covered here.

Cardiac Standstill

Defibrillation is of no use in cardiac standstill. Pacing is required in this circumstance. Occasionally, the question may arise of whether a nearly isoelectric EKG trace represents fine ventricular fibrillation. Defibrillation may be tried if this is considered a real possibility.

Atrial Fibrillation

As discussed in Chapter 2 (Arrhythmias), **cardioversion is indicated when acute-onset atrial fibrillation with rapid response causes major compromise of vital signs.** Synchronized cardioversion should be performed. Moderate energy levels may at times be required.

Cardioversion is often performed by cardiologists for chronic atrial fibrillation in hopes of improving cardiac output by restoring the atrial kick.

Atrial Flutter

Atrial flutter is often exquisitely sensitive to cardioversion. As little as 10 joules may suffice. Synchronized cardioversion is indicated.

Paroxysmal Atrial Tachycardia

Vagal or pharmacologic maneuvers usually are effective in paroxysmal atrial tachycardia. Synchronized cardioversion may be used if required.

Ventricular Tachycardia

Often ventricular tachycardia does not sustain vital signs. Cardioversion is indicated. Synchronization should be used if possible. If a bizarre configuration does not permit synchronization, asynchronous cardioversion is permissible. Very low energies, even 10 joules at times, often suffice.

Ventricular Fibrillation

The only treatment for ventricular fibrillation is defibrillation. Asynchronous delivery is imperative. High energies are required. There is no reason to use lower energies in such a serious circumstance. We recommend 200 joules as the initial energy. The house officer should remember to turn off the synchronizer circuit if ventricular fibrillation occurs following synchronized cardioversion of another rhythm.[5]

✚ COMPLICATIONS

As mentioned briefly earlier, cardioversion does cause myocardial damage. Myocardial enzyme release can be detected in 7% of patients.[6] This is the impetus for keeping energy levels as low as possible. In some cases, pulmonary edema or hypotension can be seen as a consequence of cardioversion[4]; these phenomena are thought to represent consequences of direct myocardial damage. The experience with extensive defibrillation for testing implantable defibrillators has taught the profession much more about the consequences of the procedures of defibrillation than was previously known.[7]

Pulmonary or systemic embolization can be seen when patients with chronic atrial fibrillation are converted electrically. This is the reason for anticoagulating these patients in preparation for cardioversion. **Embolization is not a serious risk in cases of acute-onset atrial fibrillation following cardiac or thoracic surgery.** A transesophageal echocardiogram is often obtained prior to cardioversion of chronic atrial fibrillation, to confirm that the atrial appendage is free of clot.

A number of abnormal rhythms may follow cardioversion/defibrillation. The risk of inducing ventricular fibrillation by asynchronous cardioversion has already been discussed. Even with properly synchronized cardioversion, ventricular fibrillation can occur. Ventricular fibrillation is especially likely when the overdigitalized patient is cardioverted.[2,4] The house officer should try to avoid cardioversion when digitalis toxicity may be present. Digitalis should be withheld, if possible, prior to cardioversion. If cardioversion must be performed in a patient maintained on digoxin, gradually increasing the energy level until conversion occurs may minimize the risk of precipitating ventricular fibrillation.[8,9]

Besides ventricular fibrillation, a number of other arrhythmias may appear following cardioversion/defibrillation. Atrial or ventricular premature beats, changing foci of rhythm, and nodal rhythm are commonly encountered and usually transient. **It is important for the house officer to recognize that asystole may occur following cardioversion.** This is especially common in patients with sick sinus syndrome,[10] who, as part of their rhythm disorder, normally manifest both fast and slow supraventricular rhythms. For this reason, **facilities for cardiac pacing should be available when cardioversion is performed.** As discussed in Chapter 3, Temporary Pacemakers, modern defibrillators usually are capable of transcutaneous cardiac pacing; cardiac surgical patients will already have temporary epicardial pacing wires in place. For the postsurgical cardiac patient, it is best to attach an external pacemaker to the epicardial pacing wires before cardioversion; the pacemaker can then be turned on following cardioversion if required. (See Chapter 3.)

REFERENCES

1. Resnekov L. Cardiac arrhythmias. 6. Present status of electroversion in the management of cardiac dysrhythmias. *Circulation.* 1973;47(6):1356-1363.
2. Mennen-Greatbatch Electronics, Inc. Operating manual: model 606/F mobile ECG monitor and defibrillator.
3. [No authors listed.] Standards for cardiopulmonary resuscitation (CPR) and emergency cardiac care. *JAMA.* 1974;227(7):Suppl: 837-868.
4. Lown B, DeSilva RA. The technique of cardioversion. In: Hurst JW, ed. *The Heart, Arteries, and Veins.* New York: McGraw-Hill; 1982:1752-1757.
5. Creed JD, Packard JM, Lambrew CT, Lewis AJ. Defibrillation and synchronized cardioversion. In: McIntyre KM, Lewis AJ, eds. *Textbook of Advanced Cardiac Life Support.* Dallas: American Heart Association, 1981:VII-l-VII-7.
6. Elefteriades JA, Handler A, Rosenfield LE, et al. Extensive defibrillation threshold testing for AICD placement does not produce myocardial necrosis. *Eur J Cardiol Pacing Electrophys.* 1992;2:A107.
7. Ehsani A, Ewy GA, Sobel BE. Effects of electric countershock on serum creatine phosphokinase (CPK) isoenzyme activity. *Am J Cardiol.* 1976;37(1):12-18.
8. Rubenstein E. *Intensive Medical Care.* New York: McGraw-Hill; 1971.
9. Mandel WJ. Cardiac arrhythmias. In: Berk JL, Sampliner JE, Artz JS, Vinocur B, eds. *Handbook of Critical Care.* Boston: Little, Brown; 1976:131-152.

10. Smith WM, Gallagher JJ. Management of arrhythmias and conduction abnormalities. In: Hurst JW, ed. *The Heart, Arteries and Veins.* New York: McGraw-Hill; 1982:557-575.

SUGGESTIONS FOR FURTHER READING

Sucu M, Davutoglu V, Ozer O. Electrical cardioversion. *Ann Saudi Med.* 2009;29(3):201-206.
A comprehensive review of the history and practice of electric conversion of cardiac arrhythmias.

HEMODYNAMIC MONITORING AND THE SWAN-GANZ CATHETER

Because ventricular performance in cardiac patients is often abnormal to start with and may be acutely worsened after cardiopulmonary bypass for cardiac surgery, precise hemodynamic monitoring is essential in both the coronary care and post cardiac surgical intensive care units. Monitoring includes assessment of volume status[1] and cardiac output. Traditional hemodynamic assessment criteria useful in less critically ill patients (such as evaluation of mucous membrane moisture, auscultation of the chest, auscultation of the heart, and examination for peripheral edema) may not suffice for the post infarct patient or the patient who has undergone open heart surgery; these techniques are notoriously unreliable, so more precise assessment may be required. Techniques and concepts for this precise hemodynamic assessment are the subject of this chapter.

The following principles apply equally well in the coronary care setting and in the post cardiac surgical intensive care unit.

The House Officer's Guide to ICU Care: Fundamentals of Management of the Heart and Lungs, 3rd ed. © 2013 John A. Elefteriades, Curtis Tribble, Alexander S. Geha, Mark D. Siegel, and Lawrence S. Cohen, eds. Cardiotext Publishing, ISBN: 978-1-935395-68-3.

✚ MONITORING OF VOLUME STATUS

Ideally, for volume status assessment, one would like to know *left ventricular end-diastolic pressure* (LVEDP). LVEDP is the ultimate volume status criterion. It conveys the "state of fullness" of the left ventricle before its contraction begins. In volume depletion, LVEDP will be low. In hypervolemia, LVEDP will be high.

A normal ventricle can pump well without being overfilled. Most normal hearts show an LVEDP of 5 to 15 mm Hg. Ventricles that require filling pressures of 15 to 20 mm Hg to pump are beginning to show dysfunction. A ventricle that requires a filling pressure greater than 20 mm Hg in order to pump is severely dysfunctional.

Unfortunately, left ventricular pressure, for practical purposes, cannot be monitored at the bedside. To gain access to the left ventricle requires either cardiac catheterization, with retrograde crossing of the aortic valve under fluoroscopic guidance, or thoracotomy for direct access.

After LVEDP, left atrial mean pressure (LA mean) is the next most accurate index of volume status. It is the mean left atrial pressure that is transmitted to the left ventricle through the open mitral valve in diastole. Unfortunately, the left atrium is likewise relatively inaccessible. In a very sick heart, the surgeon may leave a catheter (an "LA line") indwelling in the left atrium following cardiac surgery. In pediatric cardiac surery, a left atrial line is often left in place for ICU monitoring. This provides an excellent guide for volume management. Normal LA mean pressures, like normal LVEDP pressures, range between 5 and 15 mm Hg. LA lines, however, pose a number of serious hazards. Air or particulate embolism to the left side of the circulation (especially to the head or the coronary arteries) may occur while the catheter is in place; also, the LA catheter is removed percutaneously, and bleeding can occur from the atrial site. For these reasons, we usually restrict our use of left atrial lines to specific settings (eg, pediatric heart surgery, inability to float a Swan-Ganz catheter, pulmonary hypertension).

Thus direct bedside monitoring of the left side of the heart is not commonly used at present. The right side, however, is easily accessible: the great veins (subclavian and jugular) can be cannulated and lead directly to the right heart. Normal diastolic pressures in the right ventricle range from 5 to 10 mm Hg, slightly lower than in the left. Systolic pressures in the right ventricle, of course, are considerably lower than in the left: 25 to 35 mm Hg, as opposed to systemic pressures of about 120 mm Hg. **It is, however, the diastolic pressures that reflect volume state, or "preload."** Right atrial mean pressures range normally from 5 to 10 mm Hg. The RA mean pressure is identical to the well-known CVP (central venous pressure).

Thus left heart pressure is what we need to know, but the left heart is inaccessible. The right heart is accessible. It is well known, however, that right heart pressures, especially in the face of serious illness, do not accurately reflect left heart pressures[2-5]; compliance, contractility, and afterload may differ significantly between the right and left sides of the circulation. Figure 5.1 demonstrates the scatter between CVP and left heart pressures.

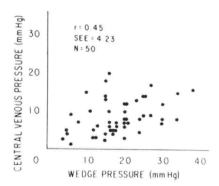

FIGURE 5.1

Discrepancy between right and left heart pressures. Wedge pressure represents left heart function (see text). Pressures represented here were measured in patients with acute myocardial infarction.

Source: Forrester JS, Diamond G, McHugh TJ, Swan, HJ. Filling pressures in the right and left sides of the heart in acute myocardial infarction. A reappraisal of central-venous-pressure monitoring. *N Engl J Med.* 1971;285(4):190-193.

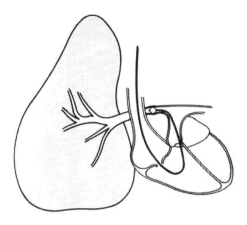

FIGURE 5.2

Schematic representation of the Swan-Ganz catheter in the pulmonary artery.

An indwelling pulmonary arterial (Swan-Ganz) catheter solves this dilemma. It allows us to assess left-sided pressures by right heart catheterization (Figure 5.2). The Swan-Ganz catheter is introduced through a great vein into the cavity of the right heart, passes through the chambers of the right heart, and is carried by blood flow through the pulmonic valve into the pulmonary artery. The catheter carries an inflatable balloon near its tip. With the catheter tip in the pulmonary artery, the balloon can be inflated. With the balloon inflated, the bloodstream carries the catheter tip distally along the pulmonary artery until the balloon impacts in a branch of the pulmonary artery. This is referred to as *wedging*. Herein lies the key. With the catheter wedged (Figure 5.3), the tip is no longer exposed to pressure from the right heart: the inflated balloon blocks forward transmission of pressure. The tip is exposed to the blood beyond the balloon in the distal radicles of the pulmonary artery. Through the capillaries of the pulmonary artery, these radicles communicate with the originating radicles of the pulmonary veins, which in turn communicate directly, without valves, with the left atrium. Thus with the catheter wedged, the pressure seen at the tip,

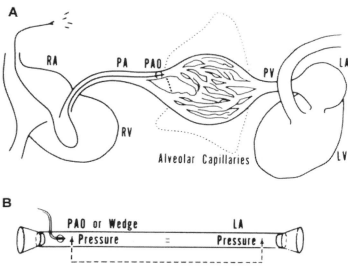

FIGURE 5.3

Schematic representation of the principle by which the Swan-Ganz catheter provides left heart information. When the balloon is inflated (**A**), the tip is isolated from forward pressure from the right ventricle. As in the "closed pipe" analogy (**B**), reading of the transmitted left atrial pressure is possible.

Source: Sprung CL. Direct measurements and derived calculations using the pulmonary artery catheter. *The Pulmonary Artery Catheter: Methodology and Clinical Applications.* Baltimore, MD: University Park Press; 1983.

the so-called pulmonary capillary wedge pressure (PCWP), approximates the LA mean pressure.

Wedging the catheter carries some risk (see later) and is somewhat temperamental: a given catheter may not wedge at all times desired. When not wedged, the catheter can be used to read pulmonary artery diastolic pressure (PADP). Although pulmonary arterial pressure is somewhat influenced by right heart function, toward the end of diastole the pressure in the pulmonary artery equilibrates fairly well with the pressure in the pulmonary veins and left atrium. **PADP can be used to approximate PCWP when necessary. PADP approximates PCWP much better than does CVP.** PADP is most discrepant with PCWP in the presence of lung disease with pulmonary vascular changes. In this case, right-sided pressures, including CVP and PADP, may be severely elevated, whereas PCWP is normal.

To recap: LVEDP is what we need to know. LA mean pressure accurately approximates LVEDP. The Swan-Ganz catheter is helpful because PCWP, which it measures, approximates LA mean. PADP approximates PCWP. CVP and RA mean, which approximate right ventricular end-diastolic pressure (RVEDP), may not accurately reflect left heart filling pressures in the seriously ill patient. This may be summarized as follows:

CVP ~ RA mean ~ RVEDP ~ PADP ~ PCWP ~ LA mean ~ LVEDP.

The correlation between left- and right-sided pressures is lost in cardiac and/or pulmonary disease, and the pulmonary artery catheter becomes essential for measuring left-sided pressures.

Furthermore, it should be pointed out that PADP approximates PCWP but is usually 2 to 5 mm Hg higher (after all, blood must flow forward into the lung). PCWP approximates LA mean pressure, but it also is usually 2 to 5 mm Hg higher (after all, blood must flow forward out of the lung).

Thus the pulmonary arterial indwelling catheter provides the best available index of the volume status of the left ventricle, short of cardiac catheterization or direct exposure. Figure 5.4 summarizes normal pressures in the various heart chambers.

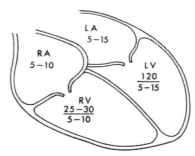

FIGURE 5.4

Normal pressures in the various cardiac chambers.

It is worth adding that, as bedside cardiac echocardiography proliferates, especially with the advent of miniaturized units, direct bedside echo can also be used to assess volume status in various chambers, including the left ventricle. This type of assessment, at the present time at least, is not expected to fall in the skill set of the junior house officer.

✚ USE OF THE SWAN-GANZ CATHETER

Particular aspects regarding use of the Swan-Ganz catheter will be addressed next.

Pressure Tracings at Different Catheter Positions

The house officer who places or uses the Swan-Ganz catheter must be familiar with the pressure wave forms in the different chambers of the heart (Figure 5.5). It is instructive to consider the tracings that one will see as the catheter is advanced through the chambers of the heart during placement.

In the great vein (jugular or subclavian), a typical CVP trace is seen. This is a low-amplitude, uneven sawtooth wave form. The house officer will recall from physiology that this wave form actually includes the a, c, and v waves of the venous pulse. The a wave corresponds to atrial contraction; c, to ventricular contraction with bulging of the atrioventricular valve; and v, to entry of blood into the atrium during late systole.[6] As the catheter passes to the right atrium, the same low-amplitude, uneven, sawtooth wave form continues to be seen. (There are no valves between the great veins and the right atrium.)

As the catheter is advanced through the tricuspid valve to the right ventricle, a marked change in the wave form occurs. One now sees a high-amplitude, smooth, regular wave form representing ventricular contraction. Important characteristics are that there is no dicrotic notch and that, at its lowest, the wave nears baseline (0 mm Hg).

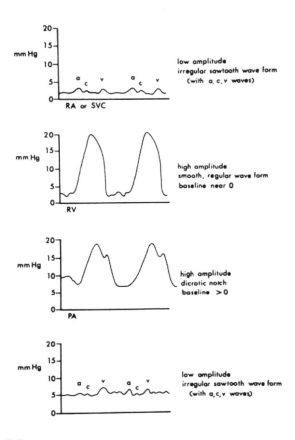

FIGURE 5.5

Wave forms displayed as the Swan-Ganz catheter advances.

As the catheter is advanced through the pulmonary valve into the pulmonary artery, two significant changes in wave form occur: (1) there is now a dicrotic notch, representing pulmonary valve closure, after the peak of systole; and (2) the baseline no longer comes close to zero, because the pulmonary valve serves to maintain diastolic pressure in the pulmonary arterial tree.

As the catheter is advanced further, into the wedge position, one sees again a low-amplitude, irregular, sawtooth wave form representing the wedge tracing. Again, a, c, and v waves can be discerned on close inspection. The mean pressure in this position is the one that best approximates LA mean pressure.

The house officer must become thoroughly familiar with these characteristic tracings. This is important initially in placing the catheter and subsequently in interpreting the tracings. The house officer should become familiar with the pulmonary arterial and wedge pressure tracings of each patient under his care. A change in trace should raise suspicion of dislodgement. It is not uncommon for the nurse to report a very low PADP that in fact represents RVEDP, after a Swan-Ganz catheter has been inadvertently withdrawn to the right ventricle. This mistake can lead to serious overtransfusion.

Physical Characteristics of the Swan-Ganz Catheter

Figure 5.6 illustrates the construction of the Swan-Ganz catheter. Figure 5.6A presents an overall schematic diagram of the catheter. The distal lumen leads to the opening at the tip (in the pulmonary artery). The proximal lumen leads to an opening 30 cm back from the tip (corresponding to the right atrium). The balloon inflation lumen leads to the balloon near the tip of the catheter (this lumen does not connect to the bloodstream). The particular catheter depicted is thermodilution-equipped to allow measurement of cardiac output (see below); for this purpose, an electrical connector leads via a wire to a thermistor 4 cm from the tip of the catheter.[7] Figure 5.6B shows a cross-section of a cut catheter. Figure 5.6C shows the distal opening at the tip of the catheter and the inflated balloon.

In general, the distal opening and lumen are used for pressure monitoring (PADP or PCWP). The proximal opening, which lies in the right atrium, can be used for CVP monitoring, for infusion of fluids or drips, or for rapid injection during cardiac output determination. The balloon lumen transmits air to and from the balloon for inflation and deflation.

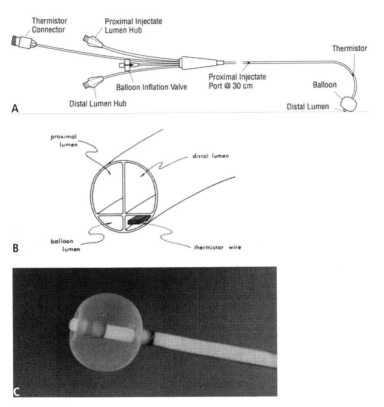

FIGURE 5.6

Physical characteristics of the Swan-Ganz catheter. (**A**) Schematic representation.

Source: Reproduced by permission of Edwards Lifesciences, Irvine, CA.

(**B**) Cross-section. (**C**) Tip with balloon inflated.

Source: Sprung CL. Complications of pulmonary artery catheterization. *The Pulmonary Artery Catheter: Methodology and Clinical Applications.* Baltimore, MD: University Park Press; 1983.

It should be noted that Swan-Ganz catheters are made with an additional proximal lumen (making four lumens overall), which may be used for continuous CVP monitoring or fluid or drug administration.

✚ INSTRUMENTATION: TRANSDUCERS, MONITORS, AND TECHNIQUES

The transducer translates the pressure wave form into an electrical signal that is amplified by the monitor and displayed on the oscilloscope screen. A digital read-out system selects and displays systolic, diastolic, or mean pressures from the graphic signal. The house officer should become familiar with the method of zeroing and calibrating the transducer and monitor system. This technique varies from system to system. In general, the system is "zeroed" (or "balanced") by opening the transducer to air and adjusting the monitor to read atmospheric pressure as zero. The system is calibrated by supplying a known signal and adjusting the gain until exactly the appropriate reading is obtained. This may be done electrically on the basis of a predetermined "calibration factor" for each transducer, or even more accurately by mechanical means—by applying a known pressure from an ordinary blood pressure cuff to the transducer and adjusting gain until the desired reading is obtained. Exact zeroing and balancing practices vary from unit to unit. Some disposable systems are so accurately produced that only zeroing need be done. (Calibration is unnecessary because of very close electrical tolerances in manufacture.) This is now almost invariably the case, so that only zeroing, and not calibration, is currently necessary. **Before taking important readings, the house officer and nurse should confirm zero and calibration together** according to local practice.

The system must give a crisp, accurate trace. Figure 5.7 indicates sites where leaks, bubbles, or occlusions can impair trace quality and accuracy.[8]

The patient must be placed supine for pressure measurements. Without this standardization, it will not be possible to interpret pressures consistently.

TROUBLE SHOOTING THE PRESSURE MONITORING SYSTEM

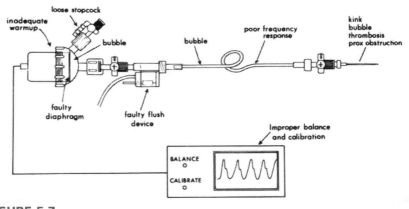

FIGURE 5.7

Sites of possible malfunction in pressure monitoring system.

Source: Reproduced with permission from Karp R, Kouchoukos N. Postoperative care of the cardiovascular surgical patient. In: Glenn WWL, Baue AE, Geha AS, Hammond GL, Laks H, eds. *Thoracic and Cardiovascular Surgery.* 4th ed. New York: Appleton-Century-Crofts; 1983:1120-1132.

The transducer must be located at approximately left atrial level. In some ICUs, this is done by placing the transducer on a box on the patient's mattress. Alternatively, the transducer may be taped to the upper surface of the patient's upper arm, which, in the supine position, closely approximates left atrial level. In other units, the transducer is firmly secured on a pole at the side of the bed. Left atrial level can be approximated at mid chest. For every centimeter that the transducer level is off the appropriate height, measured filling pressures will be off accordingly. **Too high a transducer will lead to falsely low pressures; too low a transducer, to falsely high pressures.**[2]

It is not at all uncommon for the house officer to make decisions on the basis of filling pressures that are recorded with poorly balanced transducers, with the patient not squarely supine, with the transducer inappropriately positioned, or with the catheter not in the pulmonary artery at all. If a decision regarding intervention is to be made, the house officer should not accept filling pressures as reported by phone or as listed on the day sheet, but must go to the bedside, evaluate the trace, assess patient and transducer position, confirm calibration, and only then read pressures and act on them.

The house officer should recall that electronic systems read pressures in mm Hg. Multiplying by 1.36 will give the equivalent in cm H_2O. Water, which used to be used for CVP monitoring, of course, is read in cm H_2O.

Abnormalities of the Swan-Ganz Trace

Three abnormalities in the pulmonary artery trace may confuse the house officer (Figure 5.8). A damped trace lacks the crisp contours of the properly functioning system. Readings cannot be relied upon in this setting. Eliminating a bubble, flushing the catheter, or correcting a kinked tubing may improve the trace and allow accurate readings.

Occasionally, physical characteristics of the system produce an overcrisp tracing with so-called "whip artifact" (see Figure 5.8). In such a case, unfavorable interaction of system components exaggerates pressure fluctuations, impairing parameter measurement. It may be necessary to replace the catheter to remedy this situation. (Sometimes deliberately placing a tiny bubble in the line or in the transducer can lessen or eliminate this "whip" in the trace.)

In some cases, with balloon inflation, an "overwedged" trace occurs (see Figure 5.8). In such a case, an initially proper wedge trace rises steadily to very high pressure levels. The exact mechanism is not known,[6] but the phenomenon is thought to be related to occlusion of the distal lumen opening by the balloon. Repeating balloon inflation slowly with very small volumes of air may rectify the trace. Alternatively, the Swan-Ganz catheter can be withdrawn slightly, with the balloon down, and then the wedging maneuver tried again.

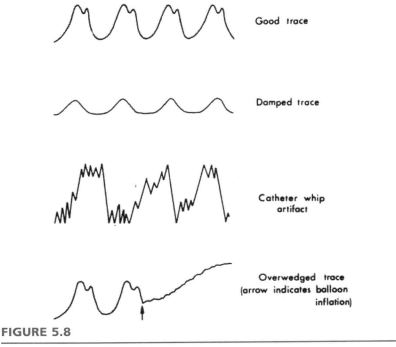

Good trace

Damped trace

Catheter whip
artifact

Overwedged trace
(arrow indicates balloon
inflation)

FIGURE 5.8

Common abnormalities of the pulmonary artery trace.

Complications of the Swan-Ganz Catheter

The most dreaded complication of Swan-Ganz catheterization is pulmonary artery perforation.[9] Fortunately, this frequently lethal complication is uncommon; its occurrence can be minimized by inflating the balloon with no more than 1.5 cc and terminating inflation as soon as the transition to a wedge trace occurs. (The Swan-Ganz catheter now comes with a special 3-cc syringe that has a deliberate perforation in the wall at the 1.5-cc mark, thus preventing inflation with more than 1.5 cc.) **Inflation should always be done gently. Overinflating can tear the pulmonary artery. Special care must be used in patients with pulmonary artery hypertension, who are more vulnerable to pulmonary rupture.** It is important as well never to leave the balloon inflated long term. Even with the balloon deflated, a continuous wedge trace may appear. This is thought to represent distal migration of the catheter tip as a result of expansion from body heat. **Whenever a continuous wedge trace is seen, the catheter should be withdrawn until a pulmonary artery trace reappears.** Some centers limit wedging to just once or several times daily because of the danger of perforation. (In fact, because of the danger of catastrophic pulmonary artery performation, some centers restrict wedging even further, permitting the wedge maneuver only by experienced physicians.) With even occasional wedging, the correlation between PADP and PCWP can be determined and PCWP predicted accurately from PADP in the interim.

Arrhythmias are seen commonly during placement of the Swan-Ganz catheter. PVCs are seen almost universally when the tip traverses the right ventricle. Ectopy usually quiets down when the pulmonary arterial position is reached. As discussed in Chapter 2, **a catheter that lies just beyond the pulmonary valve and flips in and out of the right ventricle may cause paroxysms of severe ventricular ectopy.** Occasionally, even with the tip of the catheter located well distally in the pulmonary artery, the loop in the ventricle may cause ectopy; it may on occasion be necessary to remove the catheter in such an instance.

Pulmonary infarction at the site of the catheter tip may be seen radiographically with some frequency (Figure 5.9). As the catheter is only 2 mm in diameter, the occluded or thrombosed pulmonary arterial radicle is usually small; any infarction is usually not of clinical significance. If the balloon were inadvertently left inflated, its 13-mm diameter could occlude a major pulmonary arterial branch and cause significant parenchymal injury.

Very frequently, the catheter quickly becomes coated with a thin layer of fibrin. Clot commonly forms in the great vein through which the catheter passes, but significant related clinical problems are rare. (Heparin-coated catheters can prevent these problems, but heparin is currently a feared medication, because of the recognized frequency of heparin allergy and associated heparin-induced

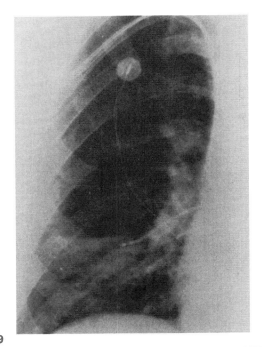

FIGURE 5.9

Radiographic appearance of pulmonary infarction distal to a Swan-Ganz catheter.

Source: Foot GA, Schabel SI, Hodges M. Pulmonary complications of the flow-directed balloon-tipped catheter. *N Engl J Med*. 1974;290(17):927-931.

thrombosis and thrombolism [HITT]. Thus, many units proscribe heparin-coated catheters.)

On occasion, the balloon at the tip of the catheter may rupture from overdistension or overuse. This may manifest as loss of resistance to syringe inflation or as blood return into the balloon lumen. In this instance, care must be taken to avoid continued instillation of air into the pulmonary artery.

✚ INFLUENCE OF RESPIRATION

Filling pressures can be read most accurately in a patient who is not breathing spontaneously—that is, in a patient on a ventilator who is sedated or paralyzed. This is the state of affairs in the critical first few hours after cardiac surgery. In fact, it has been suggested that temporary paralysis and mechanical ventilation be induced whenever filling pressures must be known unequivocally and with complete accuracy.[10]

With mechanical ventilation, the measured filling pressures, either PADP or PCWP, vary with the respiratory cycle (Figure 5.10). Pressures will increase during inspiration, as some of the positive endobronchial pressure is distributed intrathoracically. The correct pressures are those between inspirations.

Likewise, high values of positive end-expiratory pressure (PEEP) can affect pressure readings. **Approximately one-third of endobronchial pressure is distributed intrathoracically.**[11,12] The house officer can confirm this at the bedside in several of his patients. **Thus, as an approximation, one can subtract one-third of the PEEP value from the observed pressures.** That is, a

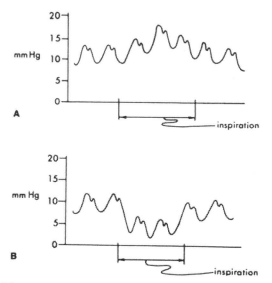

FIGURE 5.10

Influence of respiration on the Swan-Ganz trace. (**A**) Positive pressure ventilation. (**B**) Spontaneous (negative pressure) ventilation.

patient on 15 cm H_2O PEEP whose monitor records a PADP of 15 mm Hg has a real PADP of approximately 15 mm Hg minus one-third of 15 cm H_2O, or 10 mm Hg. A more precise true filling pressure can be read by taking the patient off the ventilator for a few seconds.[2,11,12] This maneuver can be reserved for patients on high amounts of PEEP. The 5 cm H_2O PEEP used routinely has very little effect on observed filling pressures.

If the patient is breathing spontaneously, the filling pressure trace will again vary cyclically with respiration (see Figure 5.10). In this case, intrathoracic pressure and observed filling pressure will fall with inspiration. This effect can bring observed filling pressures abnormally low. For this reason, we usually read filling pressures just before inspiration in spontaneously breathing patients.

Thus for either the positive pressure-ventilated or the spontaneously respiring patient, filling pressures are best read just before inspiration.[2,10] In the positive pressure-ventilated patient, inspiration will falsely raise pressures, and in the spontaneously respiring patient, inspiration will falsely lower pressures. With practice, the house officer can learn to correlate the continuously updated digital readout on the monitor with the phasic variation of the graphic pressure display.

✚ INFLUENCE OF STATE OF SEDATION

With very rare exceptions, the filling pressures may vary from hour to hour but do not change significantly from minute to minute. An acute rise in PADP or PCWP is often mistaken by the house officer for a significant alteration in myocardial performance, when really it represents the patient's beginning to awaken. **As a patient emerges from sedation, vasomotor tone increases and observed PADP may increase dramatically in seconds or minutes.** This does not represent myocardial dysfunction. Once it is confirmed that the patient's CNS function is intact, the best treatment may be to sedate the patient again. Diuretics or vasodilators are not indicated for changes in pressures seen upon awakening.

Obtaining, transducing, recording, and interpreting pulmonary artery pressures thus involve a complex process with many potential sites of error. Only through thorough understanding and practical experience can house officers ensure that they are obtaining accurate information on which to base therapeutic decisions.

✛ USE OF THE SWAN-GANZ CATHETER FOR SPECIFIC HEMODYNAMIC PROBLEMS

The Swan-Ganz catheter can diagnose and differentiate between acute mitral regurgitation and acute ventricular septal defect. Patients in the coronary care unit following myocardial infarction who demonstrate low cardiac output or cardiogenic shock may have isolated left ventricular myocardial insufficiency. On the other hand, these patients may have sufficient myocardial reserve but suffer from one of two serious acute mechanical defects: mitral regurgitation or ventricular septal rupture.[13] In acute mitral regurgitation from ischemic rupture or dysfunction of the mitral papillary apparatus, regurgitation from the left ventricle into the left atrium impairs left ventricular output and causes pulmonary vascular congestion. In ventricular septal rupture from ischemic transmural septal necrosis, regurgitation from the left to the right ventricle impairs left ventricular output and overwhelms the right heart. Each of these conditions causes a systolic murmur. Each condition is very poorly tolerated, and each requires urgent diagnosis and surgical treatment.

The Swan-Ganz catheter allows diagnosis of and discrimination between these two acutely life-threatening complications of myocardial infarction. In acute mitral regurgitation, the wedge trace shows a "v wave" representing the regurgitant flow into the left

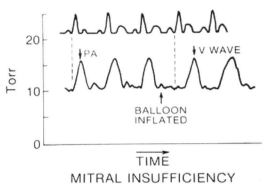

FIGURE 5.11

Pulmonary artery (PA) trace in a patient with mitral insufficiency. The v wave can be distinguished from an ordinary PA systolic wave by the fact that it occurs later with regard to the QRS complex.

Source: Sprung CL. Pulmonary artery catheter insertion. *The Pulmonary Artery Catheter: Methodology and Clinical Applications.* Baltimore, MD: University Park Press; 1983.

atrium (Figure 5.11). The height of the v wave can be read from the monitor and to some extent reflects the severity of the regurgitation.

In acute ventricular septal rupture, an oxygen step-up is seen between the right atrium and the pulmonary artery. Blood sampled from the distal port (in the pulmonary artery) shows an oxygen saturation level significantly higher than that of blood sampled from the proximal part (in the right atrium). This is diagnostic of an abnormal communication between the right and left heart chambers.

The Swan-Ganz catheter is also useful in the diagnosis of hemodynamically significant pulmonary embolus.[4] (See also Chapter 18, Management of Acute Pulmonary Disease.) Minor embolus insufficient to cause circulatory changes will not be detected. With major embolus, mechanical obstruction of the pulmonary arterial system and especially vasoactive amine-mediated constriction of the pulmonary arteries result in an acute elevation in pulmonary vascular resistance. As a consequence, all right heart pressures, including CVP and pulmonary artery systolic and diastolic pressures, rise,

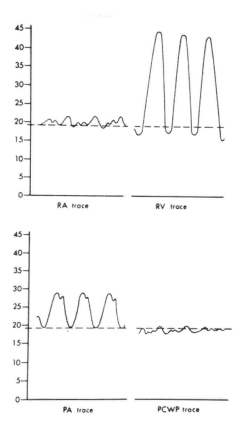

FIGURE 5.12

Characteristic pressures in cardiac tamponade. Note the equalization of RA mean, RVEDP, PADP, and PCWP near 20 mm Hg.

reflecting the strain on the right heart; PCWP, reflecting left heart function, remains unchanged. It is fair to state that **acute pulmonary embolus is not the cause of new-onset hypotension unless a rise is seen in CVP and pulmonary artery systolic and diastolic pressures.**

The Swan-Ganz catheter is useful as well in the diagnosis of cardiac tamponade. In tamponade, one sees equilibration of all pressures—RA mean, RVEDP, PADP, and PCWP—to a high value, usually near 20 mm Hg (Figure 5.12).

Limitations of the Swan-Ganz Catheter

Finally, recent evidence points out that even the PCWP may not accurately reflect LA mean in the postoperative cardiac patient or other critically ill patients.[11] Chronic obstructive pulmonary disease, with pulmonary hypertension, can render even the PCWP discrepant from LA mean. Likewise, pulmonary venous spasm, postulated to occur in acute respiratory distress syndrome (ARDS), may interrupt the continuity of the vascular channel between pulmonary artery and left atrium; estimation of left-sided pressures by pulmonary artery wedging is predicated on this continuity. It is likely that use of direct LA lines for postoperative patients with critically sick hearts will continue.

Evidence has shown as well[14] that another limitation of the Swan-Ganz catheter is that filling pressures do not correlate well with left ventricular end-diastolic volume (LVEDV), especially in critically ill and postoperative patients. LVEDV is probably the ultimate measure of preload state. ECHO measurements are being used increasingly to provide direct information regarding LVEDV.

◘ MONITORING OF CARDIAC OUTPUT

The experienced clinician combines multiple pieces of information into a gestalt that reflects adequacy of cardiac output (CO). We will discuss now the factors that enter into this assessment.

Clinical Criteria

The operating surgeon can tell much about myocardial performance from the look and feel of the heart after coming off cardiopulmonary bypass. The surgeon can tell a sluggishly contractile heart from one beating strongly and effortlessly. He or she can tell by watching the ventricles and feeling the pulmonary artery whether the heart is functioning at normal filling pressures or whether it is beginning to fail and to distend. In addition, in the modern era, transesophageal echocardiography (TEE) is performed routinely during essentially all cardiac surgery, providing to the team another very accurate means of assessment of the function and volume state of the heart. Thus by the time the chest is closed, the surgeon and the surgical team have a good idea of the state of cardiac function. All of this clinical and echocardiographic information should be conveyed to the house officer who will be caring for the patient in the ICU. Along with this information should be conveyed the measured details at the completion of the procedure before transfer from the operating room. The BP, CO, PADP, PCWP, and LA mean (if measured) at completion should be relayed. The type and rate of continuous infusions should be conveyed as well. This information will give the house officer a baseline for evaluation of hemodynamics in the ICU.

We will consider now the means available to the house officer in the ICU cardiac output assessment.

Blood pressure is, of course, an important parameter. If BP is low (say, less than 90 mm Hg systolic), it is likely, though not entirely certain, that CO is low. If BP is well maintained, it is likely that CO is satisfactory, though again, not always so. BP does not directly reflect CO because resistance of the systemic circuit (systemic vascular resistance, SVR) may vary. As will be recalled from physiology, the counterpart of Ohm's law is the familiar relation **BP = CO × SVR.** BP may be maintained by adequacy of CO or by high SVR. In fact, it is possible after cardiac surgery to have a very high BP from a marked elevation in resistance with very little effective CO.

Urine output is another excellent parameter. By and large, a urine output of 30 mL/h or more implies adequate renal perfusion and, by consequence, adequate CO. Several conditions in the postoperative cardiac patient may, however, invalidate this criterion. Most heart-lung machine perfusion regimens include mannitol or furosemide (Lasix) and may artificially produce a high urine flow even in the face of a low CO. The same holds true for osmotic diuresis from hyperglycemia, which is seen commonly after cardiac operations. These effects may linger for hours after return of the patient to the ICU. In the absence of the effects of diuretic agents, urine output is a good indicator of adequacy of CO.

Extremity perfusion is another important criterion. By and large, warm extremities indicate an adequate CO. It does, however, take time for the extremities to warm after the systemic hypothermia and vasoconstriction of cardiopulmonary bypass. In addition, vascular disease of the lower extremities, so common in cardiac surgical patients, can preclude warming of the feet and legs, even if CO is good.

Pulse volume on palpation of the radial, femoral, or dorsal pedal pulse can provide the experienced clinician a good assessment of stroke volume and, indirectly, of cardiac output. Feel your patients' pulses; with a modicum of experience, you too will learn to assess cardiac output by simple pulse palpation.

Level of consciousness is another useful criterion. A patient who is awake and alert is perfusing the brain adequately and is therefore likely to have satisfactory CO. Obtundation and restlessness are usually seen in low-output states. However, following cardiac surgery, several hours are usually required for full emergence from anesthesia; thus this criterion is not usually useful in the immediate postoperative period.

Arterial pulse volume on the arterial line tracing is a valuable criterion. We mentioned above that the experienced clinician can assess the strength of cardiac contraction by feeling a peripheral pulse. In the postoperative cardiac patient, who will have an indwelling arterial line, the strength of the peripheral pulse corresponds to the area under the arterial pressure curve (Figure 5.13). The area under this curve indicates, roughly, the effectiveness of stroke volume, and thus CO. In fact, numerous formulas have been devised to allow precise estimation of CO from the arterial pressure curve.[15] A narrow pulse curve or one with a low peak subtends a small area and indicates a low stroke volume; a brisk, wide pressure

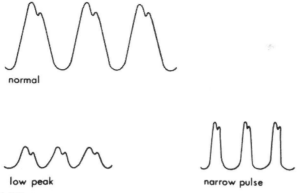

normal

low peak   narrow pulse

FIGURE 5.13

Characteristic arterial trace curves.

trace reflects an effective stroke volume. (In fact, it is this basic relationship that is used by the commercial FloTrac device to calculate cardiac output from the peripheral arterial trace.[16])

Objective Criteria

The experienced clinician, by taking all such factors into account, gets a reasonable idea of the CO of the patient. It has been demonstrated that such clinical criteria do correlate with objectively measured CO.[17] With some experience, the house officer as well will begin to formulate his or her own impression of CO. Even the most experienced clinician, however, needs to confirm this impression by objective measurements. **The Swan-Ganz catheter allows quantitative measurement of CO via two means: mixed venous oxygen determination and thermodilution.**

By providing access to the pulmonary artery, the Swan-Ganz catheter permits sampling of mixed venous blood for measurement of mixed venous pO_2 (pvO_2). Blood returning to the right atrium comes in streams that have varying O_2 content. Blood currents from the superior and inferior venae cavae and the coronary sinus usually have had different amounts of oxygen extracted. Coronary sinus blood is always quite desaturated. For this reason, to sample venous blood from the right atrium does not accurately reflect over-all oxygen extraction by the body as a whole. These different currents of venous blood mix in the right atrium, are further mixed in the right ventricle, and are then ejected into the pulmonary artery. Blood in the pulmonary artery is generally quite uniform in its O_2 saturation and is generally considered to represent true "mixed venous blood." This blood can be sampled by aspirating from the distal port of the Swan-Ganz catheter.

When arterial blood is adequately oxygenated, pvO_2 allows indirect assessment of CO. **If CO is poor, tissues extract more oxygen from each cycle of passing blood, and pvO_2 is low.** If CO is good, the tissues extract less oxygen per cycle, and pvO_2 is high. (This is the basis of CO estimation by the Fick principle.) Thus pvO_2 is directly related to CO. Table 5.1 is a rough guide for the assessment of cardiac output from pvO_2.[11,18,19] We rarely see a pvO_2 of 40 in postoperative cardiac surgical patients. **We are pleased by a pvO_2 in the high 30s, whereas pvO_2s in the 20s imply that something is seriously amiss** and must be rectified.

TABLE 5.1   Assessment of CO from pvO_2

pvO_2 (mmHg)	CO	pvO_2 sat
35-40	Excellent	75%
30-35	Good	60%
25-30	Fair	50%
20-25	Poor	40%
20 or below	Non-life-supporting	<40%

Modern Swan-Ganz catheters incorporate a fiberoptic oximetry system in the catheter itself,[20] allowing continuous bedside monitoring of mixed venous oxygen saturation. The information that was previously available by periodic sampling of mixed venous blood is now available continuously, "on line," in "real time," without withdrawal of blood. The normal range for saturation of the mixed venous blood is 60% to 80% (corresponding to vpO_2 of

30 to 50 mm Hg). Many hospitals have not yet bought into this technology, as it is not clear that continuous mixed venous saturation monitoring is clinically superior to conventional periodic sampling of mixed venous blood for blood gas analysis (and the catheters themselves are expensive.).

The Swan-Ganz catheter also allows calculation of cardiac output by thermodilution (Figure 5.14). Not all Swan-Ganz catheters are designed for measurement of CO; those designed for this purpose are appropriately labeled. CO measurement is done by thermodilution; the Stewart-Hamilton principle is applied, with a cold solution being the indicator measured.[21] Cold saline is injected into one of the proximal ports (emptying into the right atrium). A thermistor near the tip of the catheter (in the pulmonary artery) monitors the blood temperature curve as the cold bolus is ejected by the right heart. It is assumed that right and left heart CO values are the same—that is, that there are no right-to-left intracardiac communications. The faster the decay of the cold bolus seen at the thermistor,

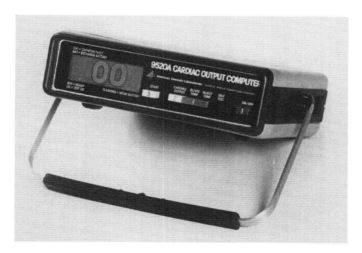

FIGURE 5.14

Thermodilution cardiac output computer. (These computers are being phased out as free-standing units, being incorporated into the main monitors used at the bedside in intensive care units.)

the better the CO. A computer connected electrically to the thermistor does the calculus involved and digitally displays a CO in liters per minute.

Modern thermodilution systems actually display the thermodilution curve, the graph of temperature over time (Figure 5.15). This can be helpful in evaluating the accuracy of a given measurement. "Bad curves" may have a double hump, or no hump, or an exaggerated undulation. **The cardiac output is inversely proportional to the area under the curve.** Tricuspid insufficiency characteristically gives a low, flat curve and underestimates the cardiac output due to reverse flow of some of the "cold" indicator backward into the right atrium.[22] Tricuspid insufficiency is quite common in critically ill patients, who often have volume overload with resultant dilatation of the tricuspid annulus.

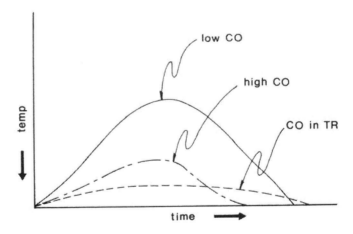

FIGURE 5.15

Thermodilution cardiac output (CO) curves (temperature vs. time, as "read" by the thermistor at the tip of the catheter). Cardiac output is inversely proportional to the area under the curve (Stewart-Hamilton equation). Curves shown are low CO; high CO; and flat curve of tricuspid insufficiency (which underestimates actual CO).

The house officer should be aware that these thermodilution CO readings, though displayed digitally to two decimal places, are of limited accuracy. They are very susceptible to error through changes in speed of injection of the bolus, insufficient cooling of the injectate, and many other factors.[5,23,24] It is quite common to see a wide scatter among different runs. Three runs should be averaged whenever a CO reading is required.

At times, pvO_2 proves more consistently reliable than thermodilution CO. Furthermore, pvO_2 reflects not only the mechanical pumping effectiveness of the heart, but also the adequacy of CO in meeting the metabolic requirements of the body. Many surgical patients have greatly increased CO needs. If CO meets metabolic requirements, pvO_2 will be normal; if CO falls behind metabolic requirements, pvO_2 will fall, as more oxygen is extracted peripherally by the tissues.

Thermodilution provides an assessment of CO in liters per minute. For purposes of comparison, **the cardiac index is obtained by dividing CO by body surface area** (average areas range from 1.4 to 2.0 m²), giving a value in liters per minute per square meter. For a postoperative cardiac patient, an index of 3.0 represents excellent CO. Mild reduction in CO is associated with an index in the range of 2.2 to 3.0. Moderately severe reduction is reflected by an index between 1.5 and 2.2. Extremely severe depression of CO is present when the index falls below 1.5. For postoperative cardiac patients, outputs in this range correlate with a high probability of cardiac death. **As a rule of thumb, maintain an index above 2.2, and you and the patient will be OK.**

The house officer should keep in mind that the objective criteria of CO are not totally accurate. By integrating the clinical criteria described earlier with the objective measures of CO, the clinician can gain a well-substantiated assessment of cardiac performance.

REFERENCES

1. Frank Peacock W, Soto KM. Current technique of fluid assessment. *Congest Heart Fail.* 2010;16 (Suppl 1):S45-51.

2. O'Quin R, Marini JJ. Pulmonary artery occlusion pressure: clinical physiology, measurement, and interpretation. *Am Rev Respir Dis.* 1983;128(2):319-326.

3. Samii K, Conseiller C, Viars P. Central venous pressure and pulmonary wedge pressure: a comparative study in anesthetized surgical patients. *Arch Surg.* 1976;111(1):1122-1125.

4. Buchbinder N, Ganz W. Hemodynamic monitoring: invasive techniques. *Anesthesiology.* 1976;45(2):146-155.

5. Civetta J. Pulmonary artery catheter insertion. In: Sprung CL, ed. *The Pulmonary Artery Catheter: Methodology and Clinical Applications.* Baltimore: University Park Press; 1983:21-72.

6. Sedlock S. Interpretation of hemodynamic pressures and recognition of complications. *Crit Care Nurse.* 1980;1(1):39-54.

7. Edwards Laboratories. The Swan-Ganz flow-directed thermodilution catheter (package insert). Santa Ana, CA: Edwards Laboratories.

8. Barash P, Kopriva C. Anesthesia for cardiac surgery. In: Glenn WWL, Baue AE, Geha AS, Hammond GL, Laks H, eds. *Thoracic and Cardiovascular Surgery.* 4th ed. New York: Appleton-Century-Crofts; 1983:1076-1090.

9. Barash PG, Nardi D, Hammond G, et al. Catheter-induced pulmonary artery perforation: mechanisms, management and modifications. *J Thorac Cardiovasc Surg.* 1981;82(1):5-12.

10. Schuster DP, Seeman MD. Temporary muscle paralysis for accurate measurement of pulmonary artery occlusion pressure. *Chest.* 1983;84(5):593-597.

11. Eaton RJ, Taxman RM, Avioli LV. Cardiovascular evaluation of patients treated with PEEP. *Arch Intern Med.* 1983;143(10):1958-1961.

12. Gershan JA. Effect of positive end-expiratory pressure on pulmonary capillary wedge pressure. *Heart Lung.* 1983;12(2):143-148.

13. Kopf GS, Meshkov A, Laks H, Hammond GL, Geha AS. Changing patterns in the surgical management of ventricular septal rupture after myocardial infarction. *Am J Surg.* 1982;143(4):465-472.

14. Hansen RM, Viquerat CE, Matthay MA, et al. Poor correlation between pulmonary arterial wedge pressure and left ventricular end-diastolic volume after coronary artery bypass graft surgery. *Anesthesiology*. 1986;64(6):764-770.

15. Alderman EL, Branzi A, Sanders W, Brown BW, Harrison DC. Evaluation of the pulse-contour method of determining stroke volume in man. *Circulation*. 1972;46(3):546-558.

16. Edwards Lifesciences. Minimally invasive hemodynamic monitoring. http://www.edwards.com/products/mininvasive/mininvasivehome.htm. Accessed August 8, 2010.

17. Karp R, Kouchoukos N. Postoperative care of the cardiovascular surgical patient. In: Glenn WWL, Baue AE, Geha AS, Hammond GL, Laks H, eds. *Thoracic and Cardiovascular Surgery*. 4th ed. New York: Appleton-Century-Crofts; 1983:1120-1132.

18. Sprung CL, Rackow EC, Civetta JM. Direct measurements and derived calculations using the pulmonary artery catheter. In: Sprung CL, ed. *The Pulmonary Artery Catheter: Methodology and Clinical Applications*. 1st ed. Baltimore, MD: University Park Press; 1983:105-140.

19. Weidemann HP, Matthay MA, and Matthay RA. Cardiovascular-pulmonary monitoring in the intensive care unit (part I). *Chest*. 1984;84(4):537-548.

20. Waller JL, Kaplan JA, Bauman DI, Craver JM. Clinical evaluation of a new fiberoptic catheter oximeter during cardiac surgery. *Anesth Analg*. 1982;61(8):676-679.

21. Geha AS. Postoperative low cardiac output. In: Glenn WWL, Baue AE, Geha AS, Hammond GL, Laks H., eds. *Thoracic and Cardiovascular Surgery*. 4th ed. New York: Appleton-Century-Crofts; 1983:1133-1146.

22. Boerboom LE, Kinney TE, Olinger GN, Hoffman RG. Validity of cardiac output measurement by the thermodilution method in the presence of acute tricuspid regurgitation. *J Thorac Cardiovasc Surg*. 1993;106(4):636-642.

23. van Grondelle A, Ditchey RV, Groves BM, Wagner WW Jr, Reeves JT. Thermodilution method overestimates low cardiac output in humans. *Am J Physiol*. 1983;245(4):H690-692.

24. Elkayam U, Berkley R, Azen S, Weber L, Geva B, Henry WL. Cardiac output by thermodilution technique. Effect of injectate's volume and temperature on accuracy and reproducibility in the critically ill patient. *Chest.* 1983;84(4):418-422.

SUGGESTED FURTHER READING

Edwards Lifesciences. Understanding continuous mixed venous oxygen saturation (SvO$_2$) monitoring with the Swan-Ganz oximetry TD system. 2nd ed. Irvine, CA: Edwards Lifesciences; 2002. http://www.edwards.com/products/pacatheters/svo2edbookpdf.htm. Accessed August 8, 2010.
A simply superb, masterfully illustrated review of cardiopulmonary physiology and its application in mixed venous saturation monitoring.

Buchbinder N, Ganz W. Hemodynamic monitoring: invasive techniques. *Anesthesiology* 1976;45(2):146-155.
A brief, succinct discussion of the utility of the Swan-Ganz catheter by one of its originators.

Sprung CL. *The Pulmonary Artery Catheter: Methodology and Clinical Applications.* 1st ed. Baltimore, MD: University Park Press; 1983.
A short text devoted to the Swan-Ganz catheter. Recommended for the reader with a special interest in ICU care.

HEMODYNAMIC MANAGEMENT

M any factors impair myocardial performance during critical cardiac illness or following cardiac surgery. Acute myocardial infarction obviously destroys cardiac muscle and, accordingly, diminishes pump function. Long-standing valvular or ischemic cardiac disease causes irreparable myocardial damage, irreversible by even the best surgical procedure. Cardiopulmonary bypass and valvular or coronary artery surgery are associated with significant postoperative myocardial depression. Myocardial function improves with every passing hour following cardiac surgery, but several days are usually required before optimization. A given operative procedure may leave certain cardiac defects untreated. For example, mild valvular lesions may be tolerated and valve replacement not performed during a cardiac procedure for another purpose, or a given area of myocardium may prove not amenable to revascularization. Also, metabolic abnormalities abound following cardiac surgery. For all these reasons, myocardial performance may suffer postoperatively. The house officer must be familiar in depth with the optimization of myocardial

The House Officer's Guide to ICU Care: Fundamentals of Management of the Heart and Lungs, 3rd ed. © 2013 John A. Elefteriades, Curtis Tribble, Alexander S. Geha, Mark D. Siegel, and Lawrence S. Cohen, eds. Cardiotext Publishing, ISBN: 978-1-935395-68-3.

performance in the setting of acute myocardial infarction and in the postoperative setting. Data obtained via the monitoring techniques discussed in the last chapter form the basis for hemodynamic decisions. Not only coronary care unit patients and postoperative cardiac surgical patients, but also those in the general surgical intensive care unit may show impaired myocardial performance, as following major abdominal or vascular surgery or from trauma or sepsis. The principles to be enumerated for the cardiac and postoperative cardiac patient apply equally well to optimizing myocardial performance in the acutely ill general surgical patient. As the house officer will see, there are 5 factors that we can manipulate to optimize cardiac output: the electrical state of the heart (rate, A-V synchrony, rhythm), preload, contractility, afterload, and, often neglected, compliance (or distensibility of the left ventricle).

✚ DETERMINANTS OF CARDIAC OUTPUT

Before addressing hemodynamic manipulation, it is useful to examine the clinical factors that influence cardiac output. These are as follows (Figure 6.1):

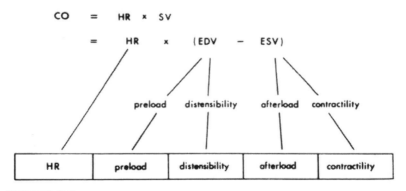

FIGURE 6.1

Determinants of cardiac output.

Cardiac output (CO) is the product of heart rate (HR) and stroke volume (SV). That is, if the heart beats 80 times per minute and ejects 60 mL with each beat, it will pump 80 x 60 mL, or 4800 mL of blood per minute.

Stroke volume is the difference between the ventricular volume at end-diastole (EDV) and the ventricular volume at end-systole (ESV)—that is, the difference between the volume in the ventricle before it beats and the volume remaining after the beat:

$$CO = HR \times SV = HR \times (EDV - ESV).$$

Two factors determine EDV and two factors determine ESV. Those determining EDV, or filling of the ventricle, are **preload** and **ventricular distensibility**. *Preload* represents the pressure driving blood into the ventricle in diastole. The greater the volume in the vascular tree, the greater the driving pressure. Also, an effective, coordinated, synchronized atrial contraction (as in normal sinus rhythm) helps considerably in preloading the left ventricle—just like a turbocharger increases the amount of air and fuel in the combustion chamber of a car. *Ventricular distensibility* refers to the degree to which the ventricle can stretch to accommodate volume. **A chronically hypertrophied or scarred ventricle may have poor distensibility. The higher the preload and the more distensible the ventricle, the greater will be the EDV.**

The factors that determine ESV are **ventricular contractility** and **afterload**. *Ventricular contractility* refers to the "in-shapeness" of the ventricle, **that is, the strength of its contraction compared to other conditions or other ventricles.** Afterload represents the resistance in the aorta against which the ventricle must pump. **A higher systemic blood pressure presents a higher afterload to the ventricle. The greater the contractility and the lower the afterload, the lower will be the ESV; the lower the ESV, the more blood ejected.**

Thus the 5 factors bearing on cardiac output are the following:

1. Heart rate.
2. Preload.
3. Ventricular distensibility.
4. Contractility.
5. Afterload.

These are the factors that the house officer needs to manipulate in order to optimize CO.[1]

The well-known Frank-Starling mechanism and ventricular function curves deserve mention (Figure 6.2). As the house officer will recall from physiology, the Frank-Starling law states that the larger the diastolic volume of the heart, the more blood the ventricle will pump. In technical terms, stroke volume rises with rising EDV. As will be recalled, this relationship reaches a plateau when ventricular filling becomes excessive. Beyond this point, further increase in filling does not increase CO. If the ventricle is filled significantly beyond the plateau, CO may fall as the ventricle is made to fail from volume overload. Thus for all states of contractility, there is a point on the plateau of the curve at which increasing filling pressure will no longer increase CO.

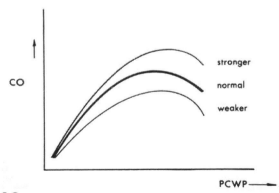

FIGURE 6.2

The Frank-Starling mechanism and ventricular function curves. Cardiac output is plotted against PCWP (*pulmonary capillary wedge pressure*).

A strong ventricle will have a curve above and to the left of normal on the CO-PCWP plot. That is, this ventricle will pump more, at lower filling pressures. A weak ventricle will have a curve below and to the right of normal on the CO-PCWP plot. That is, a weak ventricle will pump less, at higher filling pressures, than a normal one. Stated in another way, the function plateau is reached at a lower level of CO and at higher levels of filling pressure in the impaired than in the normal heart.

✚ CARDIAC OUTPUT MANIPULATION

If CO is found inadequate, remedial measures must be taken. We will now consider how CO can be optimized by adjusting the determinants discussed earlier. Although the major factors determining CO are intimately interrelated, we will examine each separately from the point of view of evaluation and intervention.

Heart Rate

In general, to optimize CO, heart rate must usually be adjusted to the range of 80 to 110/min. Slower rates are clearly deleterious for ICU patients because CO is determined by rate. We shall explain later why faster rates may be deleterious.

Treatment of bradycardias and of tachycardias has been covered in Chapters 2 and 3. The principles elucidated in those chapters can be applied to obtain rates in the optimal range.

Occasionally, a continuous infusion β-agonist will be selected to increase rate to the upper portion of the optimal range. Dopamine, dobutamine, and isoproterenol are often used for this purpose. Use of continuous infusion agents is covered in the next chapter.

One point deserves further elaboration. The house officer may wonder why rates higher than 110/min are not recommended for the ICU patient. Certainly a healthy athlete can continue to increase cardiac output at rates well above 110/min. Two factors compromise the sick or operated heart at higher rates: (1) the time for ventricular filling in diastole falls, and the poorly compliant heart may not fill adequately; and (2) myocardial perfusion suffers, because oxygen demand rises with increasing rate, but the length of diastole (when coronary flow occurs) decreases, leading to coronary blood flow insufficiency. For these reasons, higher rates are usually detrimental in the ICU patient. (The house officer may not be aware that **coronary artery blood flow occurs mainly during diastole; during systole, the heart muscle is contracting, thus squeezing on the coronary artery branches and impeding blood flow.** This physiological phenomenon is unique to the heart.)

Preload

Adjusting preload is the major intervention required most commonly of the house officer in the care of the patient with coronary ischemia or the postoperative cardiac surgical patient.

As discussed earlier, CO rises as preload is increased—until the optimal preload on the Starling curve is exceeded. By and large, **house officers may on their own initiative raise PCWP to 18 to 20 mm Hg to optimize CO.** Filling pressures in this range will not overdistend either a normally contractile or a severely diseased heart. An important point deserves emphasis: **It is not necessary to increase filling pressures to this range if a satisfactory CO is achieved at lower filling pressures.** Stated another way, the optimal volume status is that with the lowest filling pressures consistent with a good CO—output being judged not only by computer, but by all the criteria discussed in the previous chapter. An efficient heart—for example, that in a young patient without valvular heart disease or prior infarction who undergoes uncomplicated coronary bypass—may be able to pump very well at PCWPs of 10 to 15 mm Hg. The one very important advantage of running patients as "dry" as possible is that the lungs benefit. With lower filling pressures, the balance of forces across the pulmonary capillary membrane is more in favor of keeping fluid inside the capillary lumen and out of the interstitium, thus improving oxygenation. This is especially important because total body water is always increased after major cardiac surgery and nearly always increased in ICU patients in general.

If CO, as judged by all the preceding criteria, is still seriously inadequate despite achieving a reasonable heart rate and raising PCWP to 18 to 20 mm Hg, the house officer should seek consultation in further management. Other parameters may need to be manipulated. The experienced clinician will ensure that the other factors (rate, contractility, afterload) are optimized and then proceed further to optimize preload. For the sick heart—especially one that has withstood the insult of major prior infarctions or chronic valvular heart disease, or one that has undergone an especially complex, lengthy, or complicated open heart procedure—filling pressures higher than 18 to 20 mm Hg may be required. The preoperative hemodynamics serve as a good guide to postoperative management. The previously described "sick" heart may have functioned at a PCWP of 24 or 28 mm Hg preoperatively. Similarly high pressures may be required postoperatively. The filling pressures required to come off cardiopulmonary bypass during cardiac surgery provide an additional guide. If higher-than-normal pressures were required to come off bypass, chances are that high pressures will be required in the ICU as well.

The experienced clinician in such a setting will judiciously administer fluid to raise filling pressures slowly beyond 20 mm Hg. He or she will monitor cardiac performance closely at these higher pressures, in essence determining the Frank-Starling curve for that particular heart. The clinician will carefully avoid overdistending the heart by ceasing volume administration as soon as it becomes apparent that CO is not increasing with added volume. **Overdistention of the postoperative heart is very dangerous.** Laplace's law states that wall tension is proportional to pressure and diameter. Thus wall tension increases as the ventricle is filled further. Wall tension is known to be a major determinant of myocardial oxygen consumption. Thus as the ventricle is distended, myocardial oxygen demand increases. At the same time, however, myocardial oxygen supply decreases, because coronary blood flow is impeded by the elevated left ventricular end-diastolic pressure. The net result is a decrease in the oxygen supply-demand ratio, leading to myocardial ischemia, with its potent negative inotropic effect. The situation may become irretrievable when this occurs, and cardiac arrest may ensue. This is the reason the house officer must seek consultation before raising PCWP above 18 to 20 mm Hg.

If, under the guidance of an experienced clinician, PCWP is raised to 25 mm Hg and CO is still inadequate, this is a grave sign. Very few hearts require filling pressures higher than this. Chances of recovery from such a state are not great.

If volume excess occurs for any reason, with filling pressures higher than optimal, various pharmacologic vasodilators are available that can lower filling pressures acutely. These are discussed in the next chapter.

Ventricular Distensibility

Ventricular distensibility is the factor in the CO equation over which one has the least control. Distensibility is largely determined by the long-term history of the ventricle. Scarring or hypertrophy from chronic valvular heart disease or hypertension or ischemic infarction will make the ventricle stiff. Such a ventricle will not fill well at normal preload. There is usually no way this factor can be manipulated or ameliorated acutely or in the postoperative setting. (The one common exception is cardiac tamponade following open heart surgery; in this instance, relief of tamponade can restore ventricular distensibility.) Some amelioration in ventricular distensibility can be seen over weeks to months after correction of valvular heart disease, especially in aortic stenosis with left ventricular hypertrophy.

On rare occasions, the surgeons may choose to leave the chest open in a tenuous open heart patient; doing so decreases the external pressure on the ventricles, in essence improving their distensibility and their ability to fill with blood.

Contractility

If CO is inadequate at normal filling pressures, chances are the contractile strength of the heart is inadequate. Under these circumstances, it is appropriate to use an inotropic agent. Again, this is a determination that should not be made by the house officer alone; consultation should be obtained. Inotropic agents are all dangerous. The need to use an inotrope unexpectedly may indicate a major problem—such as cardiac tamponade, myocardial infarction, or valvular prosthetic malfunction—that only the experienced clinician may recognize. Details regarding selection and use of inotropic agents will be discussed in the next chapter.

Again, requirements for coming off bypass serve as a useful guide. If the surgeon finds it necessary to use inotropic support in coming off bypass, chances are that such support will need to be continued in the ICU.

One additional point deserves emphasis. **Acidosis severely depresses contractility, even in the normal heart.** Respiratory or metabolic acidosis must be corrected. Even the response to potent inotropes will be blunted in an acidotic milieu. Simply put, one might even say that inotropes do not work if the pH is less than 7.25.

Afterload

Afterload, or systemic vascular resistance, can be calculated from the Ohm's law relationship discussed in Chapter 5, Hemodynamic Monitoring and the Swan-Ganz Catheter:

$\Delta P = CO \times SVR$, or

$SVR = \Delta P/CO$, or

$SVR = [BP\ (mean) - RA\ (mean)]/CO$

Note: ΔP signifies the change in pressure across a vascular bed, in this case, the systemic vasculature. SVR is systemic vascular resistance. CO is cardiac output. BP (mean) is mean arterial blood pressure. RA (mean) is mean right arterial pressure.

Multiplying this value by 80 gives a result in dyne × sec × cm⁻⁵. The normal range for SVR is 900 to 1400.

Afterload manipulation is predicated on the principle that by decreasing arterial pressure in the aorta, it becomes easier for the left ventricle to eject blood, thereby increasing CO. This is not without its price, because if aortic pressure is dropped significantly, coronary or other end-organ perfusion (to the brain, intestine, or kidneys) may suffer, especially if the arterial bed to a particular end organ has a fixed stenotic lesion.

The house officer may on his or her own initiative adjust afterload to keep arterial blood pressure at 100 to 140 mm Hg systolic. Alternatively, mean blood pressure may be adjusted; 70 mm Hg represents the lower acceptable limit.[2] In the early postoperative period, one likes to keep arterial pressure below 140 mm Hg to prevent bleeding (see Chapter 15). This goes hand in hand with afterload reduction to improve cardiac function. By and large, house officers should not on their own initiative drop blood pressure below 100 mm Hg systolic for purposes of afterload reduction. This may be necessary in selected cases but should be carried out only after consultation with an experienced clinician. The clinician will carefully assess hemodynamics and risk of end-organ hypoperfusion for that particular patient.

Afterload reduction may be especially helpful in 3 particular lesions: aortic regurgitation, mitral regurgitation, and ventricular septal defect. In aortic regurgitation, lowering arterial pressure will decrease diastolic backflow across the abnormal valve into the ventricle. In mitral regurgitation, decreasing aortic pressure will decrease peak systolic ventricular pressure commensurately and decrease the fraction of blood regurgitating across the abnormal mitral valve into the left atrium. In ventricular septal defect, for the same reasons, left-to-right ventricular flow during systole is decreased. Ideally, major lesions of this type will be corrected surgically.

Vasodilator Therapy

Vasodilator therapy for cardiac pump failure has become very popular. The vasodilator agents discussed in the next chapter can be extremely useful in pump failure because of their synergistic effect on preload and afterload. The arterial vasodilator effect decreases afterload, allowing the heart to eject blood more easily. Although the venous vasodilator effect reduces preload by pooling blood in the capacitance vessels, this does not reduce CO appreciably in the failing heart, which is operating on a depressed and flat Frank-Starling relation. On the flat part of the Frank-Starling curve, preload can be reduced without fall in CO. Decreased preload and decreased afterload combine to minimize the actual workload on the heart. Because of this decreased workload, the myocardial oxygen supply-demand ratio improves myocardial oxygen supply-demand ratio. The improved relative oxygen supply leads to improved contractility, leading to a beneficial feedback loop.

These principles allow the house officer reliably to assess and to **optimize CO.** As has been seen, this is done largely **by manipulating rate, preload, contractility, and afterload.**

Mechanical assistance with the intra-aortic balloon pump represents another major modality available for augmentation of cardiac output and myocardial performance. Determining that balloon counterpulsation is required, and inserting the device, should be performed only by the experienced clinician. The intra-aortic balloon pump is covered specifically in Chapter 8.

✚ PATTERNS OF FLUID BALANCE

Cardiopulmonary bypass represents a controlled state of shock. Blood pressure during bypass is usually 40 to 70 mm Hg. Flow during bypass is nonpulsatile. Effective cardiac index during cardiopulmonary bypass is rarely more than 2.2 L/min/m^2. Studies have shown that cell membrane function is disturbed by shock states, so that cells swell diffusely throughout the body.[3-5] Under such circumstances, massive volume replacement is required to maintain intravascular volume. The house officer will notice the pattern that, **over the 24 hours during and after surgery, the cardiac surgical patient often will require several liters of fluid to maintain filling pressures.** Much of the house officer's attention during this period is devoted to keeping up with this volume requirement. This is compounded by the obligatory diuresis after cardiopulmonary bypass (see above) brought about by mannitol or Lasix in the heart-lung machine.

The house officer often needs assistance in deciding which fluid to give when volume is necessary. No definitive scientific evidence exists on many aspects of this controversial question. Practices vary from center to center. We practice the following:

- If the hematocrit is less than desired, we give blood, as packed cells. Previously, we kept hematocrit at 30% or greater. In recent years, to avoid transmission of infectious agents and the general negative prognostic impact of blood transfusion, we have allowed hematocrit to drift to 26% or even lower in young, healthy patients without end-organ vascular disease or low cardiac output. (In the presence of end-organ vascular disease or low cardiac output, we still transfuse to 30% hematocrit to maximize oxygen-carrying capacity.) Years of experience with hemodilution for cardiopulmonary bypass have shown that low hematocrits are well tolerated, probably because lowered viscosity improves flow and compensates for lowered oxygen-carrying capacity.[6,7]
- If the hematocrit is greater than the criterion level, we give non-blood fluid. We use 5% albumin in D5 1/2NS or hetastarch. Five hundred milliliters given over 1 to 2 hours is a safe volume and rate for an adult. We feel that the colloid of the albumin or hetastarch may help to keep the administered fluid in the vascular tree.[8,9] This has not been

demonstrated unequivocally by experimental data, and electrolyte solution alone may suffice, but the global experience of generations of cardiac surgeons would argue in favor of colloid. Among the 2 choices of collagen fluids—albumin and hetastarch, it is important to keep in mind the serious concerns about exacerbation of bleeding by hetastarch solutions. We prefer albumin, especially for major procedures like aortic replacement, cardiac transplantation, or LVAD placement, but the cost may be discouraging at some centers.

A common pattern is to give 1 or 2 liters of fluid quickly after arrival of the post cardiac surgical patient in the ICU, and 1 or 2 additional liters in 500-mL aliquots at intervals over the first night. **It is uncommon to need to transfuse fluid beyond 24 to 36 hours after surgery.** By that time, the "shock" effect has been controlled and myocardial function is improving. The extra fluid required perioperatively will usually be mobilized and excreted as urine over the next 5 to 7 days.

Urine output patterns deserve mention. Different centers use different regimens of pump fluids and drugs. It is quite common to give diuretics—either the osmotic diuretic mannitol or the loop diuretic furosemide (Lasix)—with the pump prime to keep urine flowing briskly through the tubules. **These agents often lead to a brisk obligatory diuresis in the first 4 to 6 hours after arrival in the ICU.** Osmotic diuresis from postoperative hyperglycemia may compound this obligatory loss. **The house officer usually needs to replace at least one-half to three-fourths of this obligatory urine loss to avoid falling behind on volume. Losses into chest tubes and vasodilation as the patient warms usually obligate even further volume replacement.** The house officer can presume that the patient was delivered by the surgical team in a euvolemic state to the ICU; thus, losses in urine, chest tubes, and vasodilation will need to be replenished just to avoid falling behind on volume.

By the first or second day after surgery, this obligatory loss has terminated and hormonal effects on urine are seen. The "stress" response to major cardiac surgery includes up to several days of high antidiuretic hormone and aldosterone secretion.[10] Urine volume may be low because of these hormonal factors. By and large, after the first 24 hours, unless cardiac function is obviously abnormal or volume status obviously and seriously low, oliguria is usually hormonally mediated, and diuretics are required to keep urine flowing and to mobilize excess total body salt and water. We usually use furosemide (Lasix), 40 mg, at intervals as required, usually once or twice daily. Valve patients, especially, often come to operation with chronic congestive heart failure and fluid retention and routinely require diuretics after the first night whenever urine output falls.

◼ COMMON PATTERNS IN VALVULAR HEART DISEASE

Each of the 4 common valvular lesions causes particular types of dysfunction with which the house officer needs to be familiar for proper postoperative management. (See Chapter 14, Acute Management of Valvular Heart Disease, for more detailed review.)

Aortic stenosis causes severe concentric ventricular hypertrophy. Usually, surgery is performed before irreversible ventricular dysfunction occurs. The hypertrophied ventricle is difficult for the surgeon to protect during the ischemic operative time, but if the operation proceeds smoothly, the ventricle usually functions very well postoperatively. With stenosis relieved, the ventricle functions much more effortlessly, but may still require higher filling pressures early on, as the ventricle is still relatively noncompliant.

Aortic regurgitation causes some hypertrophy, but predominantly dilatation results. Dilatation may be advanced by the time of surgery. The dilated, thin-walled ventricle may strain or fail after valve replacement.

Mitral stenosis floods the lungs but protects the ventricle. The left ventricle is neither volume nor pressure overloaded; ventricular function is often well preserved. After relief of mitral stenosis, the ventricle sees more volume load than it is used to, but usually the ventricle is capable of coping well.

Mitral regurgitation places a volume overload on the ventricle, leading to dilatation. This dilated ventricle is often weak. Valve replacement in mitral regurgitation takes a load off the lungs, as the regurgitation into the pulmonary venous system with each beat is immediately controlled. However, **valve replacement for mitral regurgitation is unique among the valvular lesions in placing a severe acute load on the left ventricle.** The dilated left ventricle is used to ejecting a good portion of its end-diastolic volume into the low-pressure left atrium during systole. When a competent prosthetic valve is placed, this low-pressure out-flow is immediately closed; the ventricle sees a much-increased afterload, as all stroke volume must be ejected into the high-pressure aorta. Under these circumstances, the dilated, weakened LV may not tolerate the acute strain brought on by valve replacement and may well fail. In recent years, it has become appreciated as well that the division of the papillary muscles inherent in conventional valve replacement weakens the support of the ventricular wall normally provided by the papillary apparatus, further potentiating the tendency to dilatation and left ventricular failure.[11] Attention to preservation of the subvalvular papillary apparatus has become a surgical priority in recent years (in both mitral repair and replacement), thus mitigating the potential adverse effects of papillary muscle division.

REFERENCES

1. Geha A. Postoperative low cardiac output. In: Glenn WWL, Baue AE, Geha AS, Hammond GL, Laks H, eds. *Thoracic and Cardiovascular Surgery*. 4th ed. New York: Appleton-Century-Crofts; 1983: 1133-1146.

2. Guyton AC. *Textbook of Medical Physiology.* 6th ed. Philadelphia: WB Saunders; 1981.

3. Matthews RE, Douglas GJ. Sulphur-35 measurements of functional and total extracellular fluid in dogs in hemorrhagic shock. *Surg Forum.* 1969;20:3-5.

4. Cunningham JN Jr, Shires GT, Wagner Y. Cellular transport defects in hemorrhagic shock. *Surgery.* 1971;70(2):215-222.

5. Rutherford RB. The pathophysiology of trauma and shock. In: Ballinger WF II, Rutherford RB, Zuidema GD, eds. *The Management of Trauma.* 2nd ed. Philadelphia: WB Saunders; 1973:24-69.

6. Thompson A, Farmer S, Hoffman A, Isbister J, Shander A. Patient blood management—a new paradigm for transfusion medicine? *ISBT Science Series.* 2009;4(2):423-435.

7. Lewis D. Resuscitation from shock and trauma—general principles. In: Condon RE, Nyhus LM, eds. *Manual of Surgical Therapeutics.* 4th ed. Boston: Little, Brown; 1978:1-11.

8. Virgilio RW, Rice CL, Smith DE, et al. Crystalloid vs. colloid resuscitation: is one better? A randomized clinical study. *Surgery.* 1979;85(2):129-139.

9. Cope JT, Banks D, Mauney MC, et al. Intraoperative hetastarch infusion impairs hemostasis after cardiac operations. *Ann Thorac Surg.* 1997;63(1):78-82; discussion 82-83.

10. Geha AS. Acute renal failure in cardiovascular and other surgical patients. *Surg Clin North Am.* 1980;60(5):1151-1166.

11. David TE, Komede M, Pollick C, Burns RJ. Mitral valve annuloplasty: The effect of the type on left ventricular function. *Ann Thorac Surg.* 1989;47:524-527; discussion 527-528.

SUGGESTED FURTHER READING

Thompson A, Farmer S, Hoffman A, Isbister J, Shander A. Patient blood management—a new paradigm for transfusion medicine? *ISBT Science Series.* 2009;4(2):423-435.

An excellent summary of meta-analytic information about the benefits and short- and long-term liabilities of blood transfusion. Should be required reading.

CONTINUOUS INFUSION AGENTS

This chapter focuses on those agents that, because of their potency, must be given by carefully controlled continuous infusion in critically ill patients. Each ICU has special drug delivery infusion pumps that are used for this purpose. These powerful agents fall into 2 general categories: (1) *inotropes*, which are used to increase the strength of cardiac contraction and often to raise blood pressure (BP); and (2) *afterload-reducing agents*, which are used to decrease systemic vascular resistance and to lower BP.

The House Officer's Guide to ICU Care: Fundamentals of Management of the Heart and Lungs, 3rd ed. © 2013 John A. Elefteriades, Curtis Tribble, Alexander S. Geha, Mark D. Siegel, and Lawrence S. Cohen, eds. Cardiotext Publishing, ISBN: 978-1-935395-68-3.

✚ INOTROPES

There are many settings in which the strength of cardiac contraction is inadequate; this inadequacy is manifested as low BP or inadequate cardiac output (CO) in the face of adequate preload (normal to high pulmonary capillary wedge pressure; see Chapter 6). This may occur in the coronary care unit following acute myocardial infarction with loss or impairment of significant portions of the left ventricle, in cases of decompensated valvular heart disease, or in the general surgical ICU in very sick patients whose overall septic or traumatic states impair myocardial function. Most commonly, inadequate strength of cardiac contraction is seen in the operating room or in the cardiac ICU following major cardiac surgery using cardiopulmonary bypass.

The heart subjected to major surgery on cardiopulmonary bypass is often very sick. Prior infarcts may have affected large portions of the left ventricle. Acute infarction or ischemia may impair additional muscle. Long-standing valvular heart disease, with pressure or volume overload of the left ventricle, may chronically impair myocardial contractility. In the present era, many operations are done in patients with advanced heart failure, with an eye toward avoiding a semipermanent mechanical assist device or a heart transplant; these patients are especially prone to intraoperative and early postoperative myocardial failure. Above and beyond the impairment that predates surgery, the operation itself further hampers myocardial function. Most procedures involve a period of time during which the aorta is cross-clamped. During this period, the myocardium is deprived of blood supply. Although modern cardioplegic techniques (especially retrograde delivery through the coronary sinus) have greatly improved myocardial preservation during this period, there is no doubt that **the heart that has just come off cardiopulmonary bypass suffers impaired contractility**. Myocardial function will improve minute by minute and hour by hour, especially if appropriate revascularization and valve repair or replacement procedures have been successfully carried out. By 1 or 2 days post-operatively, most of the myocardial depression of surgery will have resolved. From that point on, the heart can "enjoy" and benefit from its newfound blood supply or newly competent valves.

It is common for the heart to require inotropic support follow-ing major cardiac procedures on cardiopulmonary bypass. This may manifest in a number of ways. Myocardial function may be inade-quate to allow termination of cardiopulmonary bypass. In this case, blood pressure is inadequate despite adequate filling of the heart. In such a case, the surgeon will usually resume bypass, institute inotropic support, and attempt once again to terminate bypass. Of-ten, with inotropic support in effect, the heart can be weaned suc-cessfully from cardiopulmonary bypass. In other cases, the heart can be successfully weaned from cardiopulmonary bypass without ino-tropes, but cardiac action is sluggish or CO is low. Again, inotropic support is instituted in such circumstances. The house officer should be aware that **the surgeon generally prefers to institute inotropic support rather than to give volume to the point of overfilling and overdistending the heart that has just come off cardiopul-monary bypass.** The heart just off bypass is very vulnerable; disten-tion increases wall tension and myocardial workload and oxygen demand; the volume-overloaded heart may not be able to cope and may fail acutely or fibrillate.

In other patients, myocardial performance in the operating room may appear satisfactory; at some time following return to the ICU, however, CO may become inadequate. This may manifest as hypo-tension, poor peripheral perfusion, poor urine output, poor mixed venous O_2, poor measured CO, and so on, as discussed in Chapter 6.

In any of these circumstances, in the coronary care unit, the general surgical ICU, or the cardiac surgical ICU, a choice of inotropic agent must be made. **Five continuous infusion cate-cholamines are in common clinical use as inotropic agents: norepinephrine, epinephrine, isoproterenol, dopamine, and**

dobutamine (Table 7.1).[1-14] **One noncatecholamine—milrinone—is also commonly used for inotropic support.**

TABLE 7.1   Inotropic Agents in Common Use

Generic Name (Trade Name)	Activity	Dilution	Dose Range	Comments
Norepinephrine (Levophed)	$\alpha > \beta$	2 mg/250 mL (8 µg/mL)	0.02-0.2 µg/kg/min	Rarely useful—peripheral vasoconstriction overshadows positive inotropism
Epinephrine (Adrenalin)	α and β	1 mg/250 mL (4 µg/mL)	0.01-0.1 µg/kg/min	Useful agent
Dopamine (Inotropin)	α and β	200 mg/250 mL (800 µg/mL)	1-30 µg/kg/min	Useful agent Dose-related pattern of effect: 1-2 µg/kg/min—renal vasodilation 3-10 µg/kg/min—β-agonism 10-15 µg/kg/min—α- and β-agonism >15 µg/kg/min—α-agonism Compared to more potent agents: Less tachycardic effect Less arrhythmogenicity
Dobutamine (Dobutrex)	α and β	250 mg/250 mL (1000 µg/mL)	1-30 µg/kg/min	Useful agent No specific renal vasodilatory effect Little tachycardic effect
Isoproterenol (Isuprel)	β	1 mg/250 mL (1000 µg/mL)	0.01-0.1 µg/kg/min	Useful agent—the β-agonist
Milrinone (Primacor)	NA	1 mg/mL	0.375-0.75 µg/kg/min	Loading dose 25-50 µg/kg
Vasopressin (Pitressin)	NA	5g/250 mL	0.01-0.1 u/min (or 0.6-6 u/h)	Loading dose 1-2 u
Phenylephrine (Neosynephrine)	α	5mg/250 mL	0.5-9 µg/kg/min	2-5 mg

The catecholamine agents differ in the balance of α- and β-effects generated. Pure α-agonists cause predominantly peripheral vasoconstriction without primary cardiac enhancement; pure β-agonists increase heart rate and myocardial contractility, and they also often cause peripheral vasodilatation. Table 7.1 indicates the relative α- and β-activity of each agent. At one extreme is norepinephrine, which has predominantly α-activity as well as some mild β-agonism. At the other extreme is isoproterenol, which has almost exclusively β-activity; isoproterenol is the β-agonist. The other agents have mixed effects. Epinephrine has both α- and β-activity. For dopamine and dobutamine, α- and β-agonism varies with dosage range (see later). For a given patient, one of these drugs may provide the most appropriate balance of α- and β-activity. In general, α-agonists, although they raise blood pressure, are frowned upon, because the increased afterload increases myocardial workload and oxygen consumption and often decreases CO despite the increased BP.

The house officer will notice from Table 7.1 that the listed agents fall into 2 categories of potency. Norepinephrine, epinephrine, and isoproterenol are potent agents, active in doses on the order of hundredths of a microgram per kilogram per minute. Dopamine and dobutamine are less potent agents, requiring microgram-per-kilogram doses about 100 times greater than the more potent agents. At our center, **we prefer the potent agents for patients who have serious difficulties after cardiopulmonary bypass; the less potent agents are preferred for patients who merely require some inotropism in the ICU to optimize hemodynamics.** Usage patterns vary greatly from center to center. Many centers do use dopamine or dobutamine, in high-dosage ranges, for patients seriously ill in the operating room; this usage pattern can also be effective.

Table 7.1 includes recommended dilutions for these potent agents. These dilutions each represent "1 amp" (1 commercial ampule of drug) per 250-mL bag of solution. With these dilutions, infusion rates of 20 to 60 mL/h will give dosages in the middle of the recommended ranges for most adults. Standard dilutions vary from center to center; any dilution can be used, as long as the rate of administration is appropriately adjusted. In the present era, there is a tendency for standard solutions to be delivered to ICU from the pharmacy, rather than to prepare the solutions on-site. Thus, you will likely be provided a standard concentration of drug. The infusion pump should tell you the dose per kilogram per minute being delivered at any set rate.

The house officer should be aware that an individual patient may respond to one inotropic agent but not to another. If one agent, even a potent one, fails to maintain BP or CO, a switch to another agent should be made. All experienced cardiac surgeons can recall thinking all to be lost in a particular case, only to see a dramatic and sustained response with a change to another, "last-ditch" inotrope. On certain occasions, the experienced clinician will even administer concomitantly 2 or more different inotropic agents.

Norepinephrine (Levophed)

Norepinephrine is a potent catecholamine with both α- and β-activity. Because α-activity usually predominates, norepinephrine is not currently thought to be beneficial to most patients; its peripheral vasoconstriction overshadows its inotropism. Although blood pressure will increase, this is at the expense of increased afterload on the heart; cardiac output may actually decrease. Nevertheless, some patients whose blood pressure cannot be maintained by other drugs can be salvaged by the use of norepinephrine, and some cardiac surgeons use this medication commonly and to good effect. A recent study[8] actually shows norepinephrine to be an effective treatment for shock of various causes.

Norepinephrine can at times be useful to improve coronary perfusion by raising central aortic pressure. At times, this may interrupt a vicious cycle of inadequate cardiac function, hypotension, decreased coronary flow, and further impairment of cardiac function. This paradigm underlies the use of norepinephrine in cardiac tamponade (see Chapter 16, Chest Trauma) and after cardiac arrest (see Chapter 11, Cardiac Arrest and Near Arrest). See the discussion of the "vasoplegia syndrome," below.

Norepinephrine is specifically indicated in those patients with hypotension from decreased systemic vascular resistance (with preserved CO). This can be seen in sepsis and following severe neurologic events. The dysfunction is not primarily cardiac in such a setting.

Some surgeons use a so-called Canadian cocktail for patients who cannot be weaned from cardiopulmonary bypass. This cocktail is made by combining norepinephrine with the potent vasodilator phentolamine (Regitine) in a 4:5 ratio by milligram. The phentolamine completely counteracts norepinephrine's peripheral vasoconstriction, leaving strong, unopposed inotropism. This cocktail is indeed a potent and effective inotrope.

Epinephrine (Adrenalin)

Epinephrine is a potent catecholamine with both α- and β-activity. Unlike the vasoconstriction resulting from norepinephrine, that from epinephrine does not outshine the inotropism. The balance of actions is more suitable with this drug for primary cardiac dysfunction, especially when any of the afterload-reducing agents discussed later is administered concomitantly. Epinephrine is often the first agent selected for the patient who needs help coming off cardiopulmonary bypass or who shows severely inadequate CO in the ICU.

Isoproterenol (Isuprel)

Isoproterenol has almost pure β-activity.[1] For this reason, it is considered by many the inotrope of choice for patients who cannot be weaned from cardiopulmonary bypass or who manifest severely low CO. Because it has almost no α-activity, isoproterenol may actually lower BP, while increasing CO; this may occur because the unopposed β-agonism produces peripheral vasodilatation in addition to inotropism.

Isoproterenol is intensely arrhythmogenic. Serious ventricular arrhythmias are commonly seen with moderate-to-high dose administration.

One major advantage of isoproterenol is that it is the only one of the potent inotropes that decreases pulmonary vascular resistance. This aspect of the action of isoproterenol is particularly useful in patients with chronic pulmonary hypertension (especially mitral valve patients) and in patients with acute right ventricular failure.

Isoproterenol is especially useful and commonly applied in heart transplantation, where all of its properties are helpful: the induced tachycardia is helpful to the new heart; the β-agonism helps the new heart to recover from the hours of preservation; and the β-agonism dilates pulmonary vasculature, counteracting the commonly elevated high PVR (pulmonary vascular resistance) that can be the Achilles' heel of the transplant procedure. This is probably the most common setting in which isoproterenol is used in the present era.

Dopamine (Inotropin)

Dopamine is a potentially useful agent from the category of less potent inotropes. The difference in potency is partially compensated by a hundredfold increase in concentration of the solution prepared (see Table 7.1).

The balance of α- and β-effects with dopamine varies with the rate of administration. At infusion rates of 1 to 2 µg/kg/min, specific renal vasodilatation predominates. At 2 to 10 µg/kg/min, β-activity predominates above α-activity. At greater than 10 µg/kg/min, α-activity increases, and above 15 µg/kg/min, α-activity predominates.

Many surgeons find dopamine a nearly ideal agent in the 5- to 10-µg/k/min range of administration. This agent provides significant augmentation of contractility. Less tachycardia and less arrhythmogenicity are seen than with more potent agents (although a recent study[8] questions this). For these reasons, at some centers dopamine is the agent of choice for low-output states or even for weaning from cardiopulmonary bypass. Nonetheless, in certain cases, despite higher drug concentrations, dopamine just does not provide the strength of effect that epinephrine or isoproterenol does.

Although dopamine is known to dilate the renal vasculature, the house officer often overestimates the significance of this effect. Dopamine has not convincingly been shown to alter the course of acute tubular necrosis in humans.[7] This hope from the past has simply not been realized.

Dobutamine (Dobutrex)

Dobutamine is another useful agent from the category of less potent inotropes. Overall dosages are similar to those for dopamine. Unlike dopamine, dobutamine has no specific renal vasodilating effect. In its favor, dobutamine causes even less tachycardia (5 to 15 beats per minute) and is less arrhythmogenic than dopamine. Dobutamine produces a fall in systemic vascular resistance, even in the high-dosage range. Dobutamine is a gentle drug especially suitable for support of chronic heart failure patients.

Milrinone (Primacor)

Milrinone is a relatively recently introduced inotropic agent that belongs to a completely different category of drugs than the agents discussed up to this point. The other agents discussed earlier all stimulate α- and/or β-receptors in cardiac muscle and blood vessels. Milrinone belongs to a class of agents that inhibit phosphodiesterase (thus the name of the category, phosphodiesterase inhibitors, or PDE inhibitors). Phosphodiesterase inhibition increases cyclic AMP (adenosine monophosphate) levels, improving the contractile mechanism of cardiac muscle. It is important to emphasize that this mechanism of action is entirely different from that of the catecholamines. (The loading dose is 25 to 50 µg/kg; the maintenance dose is 0.375 to 0.75 µg/kg/min.)

Milrinone has been found to be a useful agent for congestive heart failure and for postoperative low cardiac output. The house officer will find this agent useful in both the coronary care unit and the postoperative cardiac intensive care unit. Milrinone increases cardiac output. Because the mechanism of increase in cardiac output does not involve catecholamine stimulation, the cardiac output increases without increase in heart rate. Because the heart rate does not increase, myocardial oxygen demand does not increase. For similar reasons, milrinone is not arrhythmogenic. Also, unlike most catecholamines, milrinone decreases systemic vascular resistance. This effect further helps to increase cardiac output and to decrease myocardial oxygen demand. Thus milrinone has the advantages of increasing cardiac output without increasing heart rate or myocardial oxygen demand.

An additional advantage of milrinone is its ability to decrease pulmonary vascular resistance. This can be of particular importance in patients with mitral valve disease and increased pulmonary vascular resistance on that basis. The ability to decrease pulmonary vascular resistance makes milrinone specifically useful in patients with right ventricular failure, as after right ventricular infarction or pulmonary embolism. This drug is commonly employed intraoperatively and postoperatively for right ventricular dysfunction after open heart surgery.

Yet an additional advantage of milrinone is a synergistic effect when combined with catecholamine treatment. By virtue of their different mechanisms of action, milrinone and catecholamines, when used together, produce an improvement in cardiac performance greater than that of either drug used alone. It is very common, in the setting of seriously low cardiac output following cardiac surgery, for the house officer to find the patient on both milrinone and a powerful catecholamine.

Because of the unique advantages described above, milrinone has, in a short time, become a very widely used myocardial stimulant. Some authors have even advocated prophylactic treatment with a bolus of milrinone before initiating cardiopulmonary bypass in high-risk candidates, so that a level of drug will already be on board by the completion of the open heart procedure.

The main caution for the house officer is induction of hypotension during loading with milrinone, or even during maintenance treatment. The loading dose should be administered over at least 10 minutes.

Vasopressin (Pitressin)

The group at Columbia University popularized the use of vasopressin (Pitressin) for hypotension seen after cardiac surgery.[12] Vasopressin is not an inotrope, but rather a noncardiac drug that raises blood pressure.

Vasopressin is the same drug as DDAVP (desmopressin) and antidiuretic hormone. This is a natural hormone synthesized in the hypothalamus and released after shock and trauma to increase renal water retention. In terms of hemodynamics, vasopressin acts as a pure vasoconstrictor and, because of its intense vasoconstricting properties, has been used for decades to treat gastrointestinal bleeding by constricting gastric and intestinal vessels. More recently, this drug has found favor for pure vasoconstriction in cardiac patients with good cardiac function and hypotension from low peripheral vascular resistance.

Vasopressin is given by continuous infusion at 0.01 to 0.1 units per minute (or 0.6 to 6 units per hour). We find this drug to cause less troublesome generalized vasoconstriction (limb ischemia or other ischemic complications) than other agents such as norepinephrine. It is our agent of choice for postoperative hypotension due to vasoconstriction. Vasopressin (1 to 2 units) of can be given as an IV push for severe hypotension, while the infusion is prepared. (Vasopressin has also been used in asystolic cardiac arrest, in which case a massive dose—40 units—is given, to raise BP and encourage cardiac perfusion.)

Phenylephrine

Phenylephrine (Neosynephrine) is another direct vasoconstrictor that can be used by continuous infusion in the ICU to raise the blood pressure in hypotensive patients. This agent has nearly pure α-effects and thus does not provide inotropy for the heart. Phenylephrine can be given as a bolus of 2 to 5 mg for initial treatment of hypotension, followed by an infusion of 0.5 to 9 µg/kg/min.

✚ CHOICE OF INOTROPES

The house officer may be intimidated by the broad range of choices of inotropic and vasoconstrictive agents at his disposal. It behooves the house officer to become familiar with a small number of drugs representing the various categories of effect and mechanism.

Institutions tend to have their own patterns and protocols. In such a case, the house officer will quickly gather the routines in his own ICU.

The practices of the authors are fairly standard and suitable until the house officer becomes familiar with the local routines and develops his own usage patterns.

The ICU use of inotropic and vasoactive medications tends to parallel the use in the operating room for weaning from cardiopulmonary bypass, where drugs are usually started in cardiac surgical patients.

Dobutamine use intraoperatively and perioperatively for cardiac surgery is not generally a good choice, as this has been associated with adverse patient outcomes. This drug is useful in other settings (as in the coronary care unit), but should not be started by the house officer in the cardiac surgical unit unless under direct instruction from senior personnel.

We use epinephrine as our first-line agent for weaning from cardiopulmonary bypass. We like the potency of this drug. We like the combination of positive inotropy with a component of vasoconstriction as well. The institution of epinephrine is usually effective in producing satisfactory hemodynamics after cardiac surgery.

In case epinephrine is insufficient, especially if there is a component of right ventricular failure (often the case if epinephrine does not suffice), we add milrinone in addition to epinephrine.

Milrinone and epinephrine act by different mechanisms and thus are mutually synergistic.

In case both epinephrine and milrinone are insufficient, that usually means that pharmacologic support will not suffice to wean that patient from cardiopulmonary bypass. In such a case, mechanical support with the intra-aortic balloon pump (IABP; see Chapter 8, The Intra-aortic Balloon Pump) will likely be necessary. (See Table 7.2)

For a patient who needs inotropic support instituted after his arrival in the ICU, epinephrine is nearly always a reasonable choice. Milrinone is a good choice if dysfunction seems to be limited to the right heart (as after a transplant, for example; see Chapter 10, Heart Transplantation). If the situation is a mild one, in which the patient is not hypotensive but has mildly decreased cardiac output, dopamine is a satisfactory choice. This guidance—epinephrine for serious cardiac support and dopamine for "just a touch"—will give the house officer a starting point from which to work, until senior consultation is available. It is a good general rule that the chief resident and/or attending physician should be notified if inotropic medications need to be started in the ICU. In the case of a postoperative cardiac surgical patient, the unanticipated need for inotropic support after arrival in the ICU may indicate a new, surgical problem—like graft closure, valve dysfunction, or cardiac tamponade. The chief resident and surgical attending will evaluate for such issues. In the coronary care unit, new need for inotropic support may indicate progression of ischemia, incremental myocardial infarction, or mechanical complications of myocardial infarction (such as papillary muscle rupture or postinfarction ventricular septal defect). The

TABLE 7.2   Sequence for Failure to Wean from Cardiopulmonary Bypass (or Inotropic Support Early After Cardiac Surgery)

Epinephrine
↓
Milrinone
↓
IAPB

senior medical resident or attending cardiologist will be tuned in to the potential for such adverse developments. That is to say, after starting treatment, one must determine why the need for new inotropic support has developed.

We recommend to the house officer what we call the "Barash" rule: Once epinephrine or other inotrope is started in the OR, it is not discontinued in the OR or in the early hours after arrival in the ICU. There is much wisdom in this recommendation. Whatever the initial reason for the need for inotropic support, this reason (be it inadequate myocardial protection, ischemia, vasodilation, or other cause) can recur, so hypotension and low CO may return as well. It is safer to keep some baseline epinephrine on board (say, at 0.02 or 0.03 μg/kg/min) to prevent such deterioration. If BP is too high, it is better to add an afterload-reducing drug rather than to eliminate epinephrine completely. By the following morning, after a good night, it is unlikely that hypotensive issues will recur, and the epinephrine can be weaned safely.

For acute episodes of hypotension, the house officer should be prepared to treat immediately while he assesses the situation. Calcium chloride (1 ampule, equal to 1 g) is a good first choice. Calcium raises blood pressure but does not usually overshoot to very high pressures. Calcium does not produce undue tachycardia. Calcium is not arrhythmogenic.

Other bolus agents that can be used include a small dose of epinephrine (1 cc, equal to 0.1 mg), which will raise the pressure

TABLE 7.3   Bolus Agents for the House Officer's "Bag of Tricks" for Initial Response to Hypotensive Bouts

Calcium Chloride	1 amp	1 g
Epinephrine	1 cc	0.1 mg (of 1:10,000 sol'n)
Pitressin	1-2 u	
Phenylephrine	2-5 mg	

substantially. NOTE: *Do not administer an entire 10-cc ampule of epinephrine (10 cc), which has a high likelihood of inducing ventricular fibrillation.* Epinephrine does induce tachycardia and is arrhythmogenic, but the effect of a bolus usually dissipates within several minutes.

Other useful agents for bolus administration for hypotension include vasopression (1 to 2 u) and phenylephrine (2 to 5 mg).

◘ VASOPLEGIC SYNDROME

The vasoplegic syndrome[10] is a fairly recently recognized clinical scenario in which the SVR (systemic vascular resistance) is low during attempted weaning of cardiopulmonary bypass, or in the early postoperative period. Cardiac performance and cardiac output are fine, but blood pressure is low. This syndrome has been found to be quite common, affecting as many as 10% of open heart patients. A high percentage of open heart patients in the present era are on ACE inhibitors or calcium channel blockers preoperatively; these drugs cause vasodilatation and have been found to increase the risk of vasoplegic syndrome. Preoperative treatment with heparin is also thought to predispose to vasoplegic syndrome.

Standard vasoconstricting drugs described in the section above may be used to treat the vasoplegic syndrome. Vasopressin is thought to be especially well suited for this purpose. Norepinephrine or epinephrine can be used as well.

To treat the vasoplegic syndrome, one can also employ an old-time medication, methylene blue, at 2 mg/kg given over 20 minutes. Methylene blue[10] is believed to act by competing with NO (nitric oxide), one of the body's own potent vasodilators. Methylene blue is generally given in case of failure of conventional vasoconstrictors; nonetheless, some authors suggest considering using methylene blue as first-line therapy, but this is not yet generally accepted. Remember that the urine will turn blue and the skin may take on a bluish hue as well, which can be disturbing to the patient and family and warrants strong reassurance. Remember also that the circulating methylene blue throws off the cutaneous O_2 saturation monitor, producing falsely low readings.

✚ AFTERLOAD-REDUCING AGENTS[15-19]

Pharmacologic intervention to reduce afterload is required most commonly for the severe hypertension that so often follows cardiac surgery. Many factors may enter into producing this postoperative hypertension. Catecholamine and renin-angiotensin excess may be involved. Generalized hypothermia and concomitant vasoconstriction increase afterload and cause hypertension.[20] Whatever the cause, hypertension promotes bleeding (see Chapter 15, Postoperative Bleeding) and reduces CO (see Chapter 5, Hemodynamic Monitoring and the Swan-Ganz Catheter). Postoperative hypertension must always be corrected, and it is the afterload-reducing agents discussed in this section that are used for that purpose.

As discussed in Chapter 6, afterload reduction is also used, even in normotensive patients, to increase CO in low-output states associated with congestive failure and to minimize the impact of the mechanical lesions of acute ventricular septal defect and acute mitral regurgitation. The agents to be discussed are useful in these settings as well.

Two drugs are used commonly by continuous infusion in the intensive care setting to reduce blood pressure and afterload: sodium nitroprusside and nitroglycerine (Table 7.4). These agents are so potent that beat-to-beat monitoring of arterial pressure by arterial line is a necessity for their use.

TABLE 7.4   Afterload-reducing Agents Used by Continuous Infusion

Generic Name (Trade Name)	Arterial or Venous Predominance	Dilution	Dose Range	Toxicity	Comments
Sodium nitroprusside (Nipride)	Arterial	100 mg/250 mL	1-10 µg/kg/min	Cyanide intoxication Increased intrapulmonary shunting	Mainstay agent degraded by light
Nitroglycerine (TNG)	Venous	200 µg/mL	1-5 µg/kg/min	None	Special beneficial effects on myocardial O_2 supply/demand balance

Sodium Nitroprusside (Nipride)

Nitroprusside is an extremely effective afterload-reducing agent. Almost all patients respond. Nitroprusside acts by a direct effect on both capacitance (venous) and resistance (arterial) vessels. Venodilatation reduces blood pressure by way of decreased venous return and decreased CO. This can be compensated by volume repletion. Arteriolar dilatation reduces blood pressure by way of afterload reduction, often with an increase in CO.

Nitroprusside will lower blood pressure within seconds to minutes of administration. Likewise, nitroprusside's effect will dissipate within seconds to minutes of discontinuance. This immediacy of response and predictability make nitroprusside especially appropriate for the postoperative cardiac patient, in whom conditions may change very quickly.

Nitroprusside may be prepared as 100 mg in 250 mL of solution. Accepted chronic infusion rates up to 8 µg/kg/min are safe. In our unit, we use up to 10 µg/kg/min overnight following cardiac surgery, without problems. This translates to an infusion rate of 100 mL/h for the 70-kg male at the dilution stated. This maximum safe rate of 100 mL/h is easy for the house officer to recall. Nitroprusside is degraded by light exposure, so infusion bags are commonly wrapped in foil or other opaque coverings. The dissolved drug is normally pale brown and turns blue when degraded by light.

The major serious toxicity of nitroprusside is cyanide intoxication.[15] The chemical makeup of nitroprusside includes 5 cyanide radicals. These can be liberated by metabolism of nitroprusside. It is interesting to note that metabolism is believed to occur mainly with hemoglobin rather than in the liver. Excess dosage must be used for a prolonged period for toxicity to develop. This occurs only rarely. Caution in dosage should be exercised when a patient develops tachyphylaxis—that is, when a patient who previously responded requires more and more drug for an effect to be seen. When toxicity does occur, it may manifest via acidosis (from anaerobic tissue metabolism resulting from the poisoning of the aerobic cycle by cyanide) and via elevated mixed venous O_2 (from interference in oxygen extraction). Treatment regimens for toxicity have been described.[4] Treatment kits with "antidotes" and instructions are generally available in hospital pharmacies. **It is important for the house officer to keep an index for suspicion for cyanide toxicity in patients not doing well for unclear reasons, especially with acidosis and high mixed venous pO_2.** Without a high index of suspicion, mortality may quickly ensue.

Another possible toxic effect of nitroprusside is an increase in right-to-left shunting with resultant hypoxia. This is not commonly problematic in clinical practice.

Nitroprusside will become a close friend to the house officer who spends some time in a cardiac intensive care unit.

Nitroprusside is also the gold standard for treatment of acute aortic dissection (see Chapter 20, Aortic Emergencies), in which "anti-impulse" therapy is required, with iatrogenic decrease in both blood pressure and contractility.

Nitroprusside is used somewhat less frequently than in the prior era, largely because so many cardiac patients are on afterload-reducing drugs chronically at home; these ACE (angiotensin converting enzyme) inhibitors and ARBs (angiotensin receptor blockers) have effects that linger through a cardiac procedure and into the postoperative recovery phase. With those drugs on board, the powerful agent nitroprusside is not required as frequently as previously.

Nitroglycerin (TNG)

Nitroglycerin has been used for more than 100 years as the mainstay of treatment for angina. Intravenous nitroglycerin is a useful vasodilator for the postoperative open heart patient, especially following coronary artery bypass grafting, and for the patient in coronary care with active myocardial ischemia (see Chapter 13).

Nitroglycerin has more predominant capacitance (venous) vessel effects than does nitroprusside. At doses of nitroglycerin of less than 1 µg/kg/min, venodilatation predominates. At higher doses, some arterial dilatation occurs. As might be expected from this balance of effects, **nitroglycerin is a more effective reducer of preload than of afterload. Nonetheless, some measure of blood pressure control can be achieved with nitroglycerin** in the postoperative setting.

If nitroglycerin is not as effective in blood pressure control as nitroprusside, why is it used after cardiac surgery? In very basic terms, **nitroglycerin is good for the heart with coronary disease.** Nitroglycerin exerts a beneficial effect on the oxygen demand-supply ratio by influencing both sets of factors in this ratio. **Oxygen demand is decreased, largely by way of reduction in preload,** with concomitant reduction in left ventricular wall tension and energy requirements. This can be accomplished as well by nitroprusside. **Unlike nitroprusside, however, nitroglycerin can increase oxygen supply. Nitroglycerin is known to dilate coronary arteries;** this effect is demonstrated routinely during coronary angiography. Both large and small coronary arteries, including collateral vessels, are dilated by nitroglycerin. This may increase flow to the vulnerable subendocardial myocardium. Although it is true that fixed anatomic coronary lesions cannot respond to nitroglycerin,

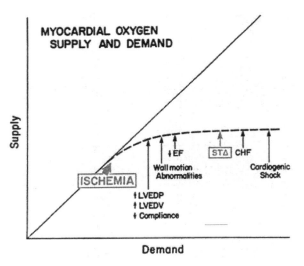

FIGURE 7.1

Relationship of myocardial oxygen supply and demand under ischemic burden.

Source: Reproduced with permission from Barash, PG. Monitoring myocardial oxygen balance: physiologic basis and clinical application. *American Society of Anesthesiologists Annual Refresher Course Lectures.* 1985:13;21-32.

the spasm that often superimposes on fixed anatomic lesions may respond dramatically. Collateral flow around a fixed anatomic lesion may be improved as well. Nitroglycerin has been shown to improve ischemic EKG changes during coronary artery bypass surgery.

Figure 7.1 illustrates schematically the adverse events, and their clinical evidence, consequent upon imbalance of oxygen supply and demand. Demand is illustrated on *x*-axis, and supply on the *y*-axis. When supply falls short of demand (by definition, an ischemic state), left ventricular end-diastolic pressure starts to rise as the heart strains, left ventricular end-diastolic volume rises as the heart swells, and myocardial compliance falls. As ischemia becomes more severe, regional wall motion abnormalities become discernible on echocardiography, and a bit later, ejection fraction (EF) falls. As ischemia worsens, ST-segment changes appear on the EKG. Ultimately, congestive heart failure and cardiogenic shock supervene.

This schematic is important for the house officer, demonstrating both the clinical sequence of events and the discernible clinical signs of decompensation.

Now why would a postoperative patient still be at risk for ischemia following coronary artery bypass grafting? First, coronary artery spasm can occur following bypass—at times to a severe extent. Second, it is unusual to achieve total coronary revascularization—that is, to make the patient's coronaries entirely normal. More often than not, small diseased vessels remain. Vessels less than 1.5 mm in diameter are usually not grafted. Also, some milder disease usually persists beyond the major lesions bypassed. Distal disease is especially common in diabetics. The initial period following coronary artery surgery is a critical one (see Chapter 6). The heart needs all the help it can get during this time. Nitroglycerin may provide just that increased margin of coronary blood flow required to keep even the adequately revascularized patient out of trouble during the vulnerable early postoperative phase.

Concentrations of nitroglycerin in commercial preparations vary. In our unit, the nitroglycerin comes as 200 μg/mL. **Nitroglycerin has no known serious toxicity.** Headaches do occur but are not of importance in the heavily sedated patient emerging from cardiac surgery. Accordingly, there is no definite known maximum tolerable dose. Common ranges are 1 to 4 μg/kg/min. It is unusual to see much additional benefit at doses beyond 4 μg/kg/min. In fact, blood pressure reduction effect is already maximal at 2 μg/kg/min.

In our postcardiac surgical unit, we use both nitroglycerin and nitroprusside in many patients. Nitroglycerin is started initially, to gain some measure of blood pressure control and to benefit from its coronary vasodilating properties. The rate of infusion of nitroglycerin is increased to maintain control of hypertension. Once medium-dose ranges of nitroglycerin are reached, nitroprusside is added if required for blood pressure control. In this way, the coronary benefits of nitroglycerin are combined with the potent afterload-reducing properties of nitroprusside. These agents are usually tapered (not abruptly discontinued) the day following surgery, when blood pressure control can safely be liberalized (see Chapter 15).

It is important to remember that both TNG and nitroprusside can have significant antiplatelet effects; this can contribute to post-operative bleeding after cardiac surgery.

Other Intravenous Afterload-Reducing Agents

Nicardipine (Cardene) is another useful, more recent, intravenous continuous infusion hypotensive agent. Some studies indicate that nicardipine works more quickly than nitroprusside, requires fewer adjustments, and has fewer adverse events. Nicardipine is begun at 5 mg/h and increased gradually up to a maximum of 15 mg/h to obtain the desired effect.

Some studies show similar advantages for a very new drug, clevidipine (Cleviprex). Clevidipine is begun at 1 to 2 mg/min and increased gradually up to 4 to 6 mg/h.

Neither nicardipine nor clevidipine have adverse effects on platelets or produce cyanide toxicity.

The house officer may become familiar with these newer drugs, especially if they are in fashion at his center, but nitroprusside is the gold standard. Also, both TNG and nitroprusside are orders of magnitude cheaper than nicardipine or Cleviprex.

Bolus Agents

Unlike the afterload-reducing agents discussed thus far, hydralazine (Apresoline) is usually given by bolus injection rather than by continuous infusion. These additional agents may be useful to the house officer in controlling postoperative hypertension.

Hydralazine can be used by the house officer to effect a transition from continuous infusion agents to bolus agents—to "get the patient off drips," in effect. By the first or second day after surgery, vasoconstriction and severe hypertension usually resolve. BP control can be liberalized, as bleeding is no longer likely and the heart is no longer as vulnerable to increased afterload. BP that was maintained at 110 to 120 mm Hg early after surgery can be liberalized to 140 to 160 mm Hg. Hydralazine given by bolus can provide this measure of blood pressure control and allow the continuous infusion of nitroprusside to be stopped.

Hydralazine is a potent direct arterial vasodilator. It must be used with caution. Common doses are 10 to 50 mg IV every 4 to 6 hours. The house officer is advised to start with low doses and to increase them gradually. The drug can be given in about the same doses orally when the patient begins oral intake. If tachycardia is seen during hydralazine treatment, or as a general response to the postoperative state (see Chapter 2), it is convenient to add a β-blocker (like metroprolol). The β-blocker will further facilitate BP control.

Nifedipine, given sublingually at 10 to 20 mg every 4 to 6 hours, is also an effective bolus agent for blood pressure control.

Care should be taken with all bolus antihypertensive agents, starting with only a small dose, until the individual patient's response can be gauged. Also, greater care must be taken with IV compared to PO doses of hydralizine.

As the patient enters his first, second, or third postoperative day, a gradual resumption of preoperative antihypertensive medications is begun.

REFERENCES

1. Innes IR, Nickerson M. Drugs acting on postganglionic adrenergic nerve endings and structures innervated by them (sympathomimetic drugs). In: Goodman LS, Gilman A, eds. *The Pharmacologic Basis of Therapeutics.* New York: Macmillan; 1970:478-523.
2. White R. Cardiovascular pharmacology. Part I. In: McIntyre K, Lewis AJ, eds. *Textbook of Advanced Cardiac Life Support.* Dallas: American Heart Association; 1981:VIII-1-VIII-16.
3. McIntyre K. cardiovascular pharmacology. Part II. In: McIntyre K, Lewis AJ, eds. *Textbook of Advanced Cardiac Life Support.* Dallas: American Heart Association; 1981:IX-1-IX-16.

4. Glass D. Cardiovascular drugs. In: Civetta J, ed. *Intensive Care Therapeutics.* New York: Appleton-Century-Crofts; 1980:197-261.

5. Zito R. Cardiovascular clinical pharmacology. In: Glenn WWL, Baue AE, Geha AS, Hammond GL, Laks H, eds. *Thoracic and Cardiovascular Surgery.* 4th ed. New York: Appleton-Century-Crofts; 1983:1063-1075.

6. Behrendt DM, Austen WG. *Patient Care in Cardiac Surgery.* Boston: Little Brown; 1985.

7. Raijifer S, Golberg L. Sympathomimetic amines in the treatment of shock. In: Shoemaker WC, Thompson WL, Holbrook PR, eds. *Textbook of Critical Care.* Philadelphia: WB Saunders; 1984.

8. De Backer D, Biston P, Devriendt J, et al; for SOAP II Investigators. Comparison of dopamine and norepinephrine in the treatment of shock. *N Engl J Med.* 2010;362(9):779-789.

9. Jones DR, Lee HT. Perioperative renal protection. *Best Pract Res Clin Anesthesiol.* 2008;22(1):193-208.

10. Shanmugam G. Vasoplegic syndrome—the role of methylene blue. *Eur J Cardiothorac Surg.* 2005;28(5):705-710.

11. Lehmann A, Boldt J. New pharmacologic approaches for the perioperative treatment of ischemic cardiogenic shock. *J Cardiothorac Vasc Anesth.* 2005;19(1):97-108.

12. Argenziano M, Chen JM, Choudhri AF, et al. Management of vasodilatory shock after cardiac surgery: identification of predisposing factors and use of a novel pressor agent. *J Thorac Cardiovasc Surg.* 1998;116(6):973-980.

13. Masetti P, Murphy SF, Kouchoukos NT. Vasopressin therapy for vasoplegic syndrome following cardiopulmonary bypass. *J Card Surg.* 2002;17(6):485-489.

14. Butterworth J. Dobutamine: too dangerous for "routine" administration? *Anesthesiology.* 2008;108(6):973-974.

15. Robin ED, McCauley ME. Nitroprusside-related cyanide toxicity. Time (long past due) for urgent, effective interventions. *Chest.* 1992;102(6):1842-1845.

16. Harris SN, Rinder CS, Rinder HM, Tracy JB, Smith BR, Hines R. Nitroprusside inhibition of platelet function is transient and reversible by catecholamine priming. *Anesthesiology.* 1995;83(6):1145-1152.

17. Halpern NA, Goldberg M, Neely C, et al. Postoperative hypertension: a multicenter, prospective, randomized comparison between intravenous nicardipine and sodium nitroprusside. *Crit Care Med.* 1992;20(12):1637-1643.

18. Levy JH, Mancao MY, Gitter R, et al. Clevidipine effectively and rapidly controls blood pressure preoperatively in cardiac surgery patients: the results of the randomized, placebo-controlled efficacy study of clevidipine assessing its preoperative antihypertensive effect in cardiac surgery. *Anesth Analg.* 2007;105(4):918-925.

19. Aronson S, Dyke CM, Stierer KA, et al. The ECLIPSE trials: comparative studies of clevidipine to nitroglycerin, sodium nitroprusside, and nicardipine for acute hypertension treatment in cardiac surgery patients. *Anesth Analg.* 2008;107(4):1110-1121.

20. Hoar PF, Stone JG, Faltas AN, Bendixen HH, Head RJ, Berkowitz BA. Hemodynamic and adrenergic responses to anesthesia and operation for myocardial revascularization. *J Thorac Cardiovasc Surg.* 1980;80(2):242-248.

SUGGESTED FURTHER READING

Robin ED, McCauley ME. Nitroprusside-related cyanide toxicity. Time (long past due) for urgent, effective interventions. *Chest.* 1992;102(6):1842-1845.

A "must-read" on this life-threatening syndrome.

Butterworth J. Dobutamine: too dangerous for "routine" administration? *Anesthesiology.* 2008;108(6):973-974.

An important cautionary tale.

Management of surgical low cardiac output syndrome. Levy JH, Wynands JE, eds. *J Cardiothorac Anesth.* 1990;4(Suppl 5):1-41.

A lucid monograph by experts like Dr. Hines, although weighted in favor of the PDE inhibitors.

Appreciation is expressed to Dr. Paul Barash, of Yale University Section of Cardiac Anesthesia, for his valuable insights incorporated into this chapter.

THE INTRA-AORTIC BALLOON PUMP

The house officer is often frightened at the prospect of caring for a patient with an intra-aortic balloon pump (IABP). Yet more and more patients are becoming candidates for intra-aortic balloon counterpulsation.[1-10] This chapter will review important basic concepts regarding the balloon pump with which the house officer should be familiar.

The House Officer's Guide to ICU Care: Fundamentals of Management of the Heart and Lungs, 3rd ed. © 2013 John A. Elefteriades, Curtis Tribble, Alexander S. Geha, Mark D. Siegel, and Lawrence S. Cohen, eds. Cardiotext Publishing, ISBN: 978-1-935395-68-3.

✚ PHYSICAL CHARACTERISTICS

The balloon itself is an inflatable plastic device that is positioned in the descending aorta, usually via the common femoral artery (Figure 8.1). The balloon is attached to a console, which monitors either EKG or arterial pressure (or both). The console triggers the balloon in concert with the EKG or arterial pressure. **The balloon is deflated in systole and inflated in diastole.** (The volume in adults is usually 40 mL.) **This provides systolic unloading and diastolic augmentation** (Figure 8.2). This is a difficult concept to grasp and requires further elaboration.

FIGURE 8.1

(Left) The intra-aortic balloon pump.

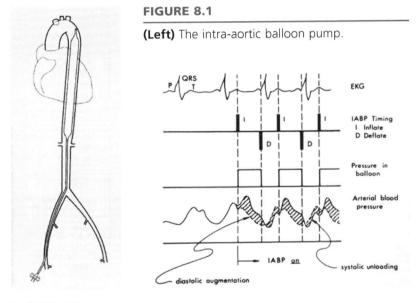

FIGURE 8.2

(Right) Timing of the IABP. The top trace shows EKG. The second trace marks balloon inflation and deflation. The third trace shows pressure in the balloon itself. The final trace represents intra-arterial blood pressure. (The dotted line represents the arterial pressure curve that would be obtained without the IABP; the solid line indicates the curve with the IABP.) The cross-hatched areas represent lowering of blood pressure in systole (systolic unloading) and raising of blood pressure in diastole (diastolic augmentation).

⊞ PHYSIOLOGIC EFFECTS

Consider the events of the cardiac cycle, starting in diastole just after aortic valve closure, with the IABP functioning. The balloon inflates in the thoracic aorta. This raises the diastolic pressure in the aorta and displaces an additional volume of blood, equal to that of the balloon, from the aorta into runoff organs—a sort of augmentation of cardiac output. One of the organs that benefits most is the heart, as some of the displaced volume passes down the coronary arteries. The increased diastolic pressure in the aorta is especially beneficial because it is during diastole that most coronary flow occurs. During systole, the myocardium is contracting, and the pressure exerted on the coronary arteries by the surrounding myocardium prevents significant coronary flow.

The balloon is maintained inflated by the console until just before systole, when balloon deflation occurs. This lowers systolic pressure in the aorta and makes it easier for the left ventricle to eject its stroke volume. The workload of the left ventricle is diminished.

Thus the IABP is beneficial to the heart because (1) diastolic augmentation improves coronary flow and myocardial oxygen supply and (2) systolic unloading decreases the workload of the left ventricle and myocardial oxygen demand. The combination of greater coronary flow with less load on the heart can produce a dramatic improvement in myocardial performance.

This is an appropriate point to introduce the house officer to the concept of myocardial perfusion pressure. Myocardial perfusion pressure is the difference between the diastolic aortic pressure (the "driving force" for coronary perfusion) and the right atrial pressure (the "back pressure" faced by the blood flowing through the coronary arterial system. A normal individual—yourself, for example—has a diastolic aortic pressure of about 80 mm Hg and a right atrial pressure of about 10 mm Hg. That makes for a robust 70 mm Hg perfusion pressure. A hypotensive patient with a struggling heart may have a diastolic pressure of only 40 or so, and a right atrial pressure of 20 or so, leaving only a paltry net 20 mm Hg myocardial perfusion pressure. This patient would be in trouble, his myocardium ischemic and dysfunctional. The IABP can improve this situation, by increasing the pressure in diastole. (Also, the IABP is likely to decrease the right atrial pressure, again beneficially.) Some experts use the myocardial perfusion gradient as an indicator that the IABP is needed after cardiac surgery; if the perfusion gradient is less than 25 mm Hg, an IABP is placed.

It is instructive to compare the use of IABP for hypotension and low cardiac output to conventional medical intervention. β-agonists can increase cardiac output, but at the expense of increased myocardial oxygen consumption. α-agonists can raise BP, but at the expense of increased afterload and, again, increased myocardial oxygen consumption. Only the IABP can effect amelioration of this circulatory state without increased oxygen consumption. As myocardial ischemia is so commonly the cause of the low-output state, this advantage of the IABP may be truly critical.

✚ APPLICATIONS

The IABP is used most commonly in 3 situations (see Table 8.1): (1) It can be used following open heart surgery to assist a weak heart in sustaining the circulation after coming off cardiopulmonary bypass. Along these lines, it is becoming increasingly advocated to place the IABP prophylactically before high-risk cardiac surgery. In this way, the IABP is already in place and providing support for patients with marginal myocardial reserve. See below. (2) Another setting of common use is in the preoperative patient in the coronary care unit who continues to have angina despite full treatment with β-blockers, calcium antagonists, and nitrates (usually intravenous nitroglycerin), as well as anticoagulants (usually including heparin and a platelet inhibitor). Because the IABP decreases cardiac workload and increases flow through the diseased coronary vessels, the IABP almost always eliminates even refractory anginal pain. (3) In addition, the IABP may be used to support the failing heart in post myocardial infarction (cardiogenic) shock.

TABLE 8.1   Settings in Which the IABP Is Used

1. Inability to wean from CPB after open heart surgery.
2. Unstable angina refractory to conventional management.
3. Post myocardial infarction cardiogenic shock.

There are other, less common settings in which the IABP may be used. The mechanical defects of ventricular septal rupture and papillary muscle rupture with acute mitral regurgitation may follow myocardial infarction. Both of these life-threatening complications can be ameliorated by the IABP. The systolic unloading decreases peak left ventricular pressures; this, in turn, decreases left-to-right shunting in acute ventricular septal defect and decreases regurgitation into the atrium in acute mitral valve dysfunction. In these settings, the IABP is usually used as an adjunct in the preparation of the patient for surgery for correction of the mechanical defect. In addition, the IABP may be used to protect coronary disease patients with especially precarious anatomy during induction of anesthesia and the precardiopulmonary bypass period of the coronary bypass operation.[1,3,9] Patients with severe left main coronary lesions may require this protection (especially if the right coronary artery has severe disease as well). Use of the IABP for left main disease is becoming less common as monitoring and anesthetic techniques improve. In rare cases, the IABP may be useful in controlling refractory, life-threatening ventricular arrhythmias in the coronary care unit.

As patients with more advanced left ventricular dysfunction and more complex cardiac disease are submitted to corrective open heart procedures, an important role is emerging for the IABP for prophylactic perioperative (pre- and postoperative) support electively around the time of cardiac surgery.[1,3,9] It used to be felt that the IABP could be applied in case of inadequate pump function in the operating room at the completion of the open heart repair. Our group has found the IABP extremely useful as a *prophylactic* measure, especially for coronary bypass in patients with severe preexisting damage[9] and for left ventricular aneurysmectomy (especially aneurysmectomy combined with directed arrhythmia surgery).[8]

One major contraindication to use of the IABP is aortic regurgitation. The principles of operation of the IABP enumerated earlier presume a competent aortic valve. Without aortic valve competence, inflation of the balloon in diastole may exacerbate the regurgitation from the aorta to the left ventricle, possibly overwhelming the ventricle.

POSITIONING AND REMOVAL

In its early use, the IABP was placed by a surgical procedure to expose the common femoral artery and anastomose a diverticulum of Dacron to the side of the vessel. The balloon was then passed through the diverticulum. Subsequently, the Seldinger technique for passing the IABP has been popularized. With this technique, the IABP, which has a central lumen, is passed over a guidewire through a sheath placed into the common femoral artery. The guidewire and sheath can be placed percutaneously. IABP removal can be done closed (with pressure to control the arterial site) or open (with direct repair of the arterial site). A sheathless model of the IABP (which has a tapered, firm tip) is also available (Datascope, Montvale, New Jersey); this model is placed directly through the skin over a guidewire into the femoral artery, eliminating the sheath and thus decreasing the overall diameter of the apparatus.

The house officer is often responsible for removal of the IABP. This is a serious procedure, as the corresponding opening in the femoral artery is large and the vessel is under arterial pressure. Firm pressure must be held for at least 30 minutes, with careful evaluation of the groin for bleeding and assessment of distal pulses after IABP removal. (An automated pressure-holding device may be used to supplement the manual physician pressure.) Most important is to remember that pressure should be held proximal to the skin puncture site, because the original needle-stick of the femoral artery is done with the needle angling cephalad. Holding pressure on the needle site itself may permit continued internal bleeding; the opening of the artery will be higher up the femoral artery than the skin site, and that is where pressure must be maintained. (See Figure 8.2.)

Keep in mind as well that particles of thrombus may embolize to the distal vessel, so that confirmation of good pedal pulses after IABP removal is vital. Much of the responsibility for IABP removal and post-removal assessment falls to the house officer. Remember also that continued bleeding from the IABP site in the femoral artery may enter the retroperitoneal space, and thus not produce local swelling at the groin site itself.

✚ CARE AND COMPLICATIONS

The IABP can result in aortic dissection or vascular perforation during its introduction, especially in a patient with aortoiliac disease. The incidence of these serious, and often fatal, complications has been markedly reduced by the use of a wire-guided central lumen balloon.

The IABP can impair blood flow to the extremity supplied by the femoral artery through which it is introduced.[10] This is especially likely when there is associated aortoiliac or femoropopliteal occlusive disease, when the IABP is inadvertently introduced through the superficial femoral artery rather than through the common femoral, or when cardiac output is very low. **The house officer must closely monitor lower-extremity perfusion in the patient with the IABP,** using all traditional criteria (pulses, warmth, color, sensation, motor strength, etc). Assessment must be made at the time of placement of the IABP and at regular intervals thereafter, as thrombus around the IABP may form late after placement.

The IABP is traumatic to formed blood elements, especially platelets. The house officer must follow platelet counts closely, especially when the IABP has been in place more than 12 or 24 hours.[11] Falling counts or counts below 40,000 should be called to the attention of senior staff.

The IABP can provide a nidus for intra-arterial thrombosis and embolization. Clot forms on the inflating/deflating balloon membrane itself. Clot is less likely to form when the balloon is firing frequently. If the balloon were not to fire for a significant period of time, thrombosis would be almost certain. For this reason, **we never run the IABP at a rate of less than 1:3** (ie, one IABP inflation for every 3 heartbeats) **for any significant period of time.** (Recent device modifications on the Datascope balloon do not permit rates less than 1:3 for this reason.)

The question of anticoagulation of patients with the IABP deserves elaboration. There is much variation in operating principles from center to center. Our operating protocols will be described to serve as a baseline for the house officer.

We do anticoagulate patients who have the IABP placed preoperatively. We do this with heparin by continuous infusion (usually 800 to 1000 units/h IV). We stop the heparin several hours preoperatively. We aim for a PTT of 50 to 70.

We do not anticoagulate patients who have the IABP in place postoperatively. After cardiac surgery, blood coagulation mechanisms are disturbed. Furthermore, with fresh incisions and suture lines, anticoagulation would not be safe. The IABP is usually withdrawn by the time coagulation normalizes and anticoagulation would be safe. If the IABP were required for a prolonged period of time—say, beyond the second preoperative day—some form of anticoagulation would be considered.

The house officer should understand the process of "timing" the IABP (see Figure 8.2). Adjustments of timing are necessary with changes in rhythm or rate and can be done by the house officer with an understanding of the process. As mentioned, the IABP may be triggered by the EKG or by the arterial trace; likewise, it can be set according to the electrical events of the EKG or the mechanical events of the arterial pressure monitor. We shall discuss both techniques of setting timing.

The initial setting is done by EKG. **The IABP should be set to inflate at the peak of the T wave;** by this point in the EKG, systole is certain to be complete. **The IABP is set to deflate just before the beginning of the QRS;** in this manner, it will be deflated before any significant mechanical contraction of the ventricle occurs with the next systole. The reader should follow the EKG timing in Figure 8.2.

Fine-tuning can be done by observing the arterial trace. The IABP-augmented pressure should begin where the dicrotic notch would start. Inflation is moved forward or backward to achieve this. The presystolic dip in pressure should be as low as possible. Deflation can be moved forward or backward to achieve this.

One usually finds that tuning by the dicrotic notch on the arterial trace sets IABP inflation a little more accurately than the peak of the T wave by EKG. On the other hand, setting deflation at the beginning of the QRS rarely requires adjustment based on the arterial trace. To summarize, then

- Set inflation to occur at the dicrotic notch of the A-line.
- Set deflation to occur just before the QRS of the EKG.

These adjustments of **the IABP timing should achieve a "double-hump" arterial trace,** as discussed below. This can be seen also in Figure 8.3. In this figure, the IABP is set at 1:3. The double hump of the augmented beat is visible, in contrast to the single-hump native arterial beats.

The modern Datascope IABP performs much of this adjustment automatically and independently.

As rate changes or as rhythm varies, the inflate/deflate timing will need to be adjusted. If a paced rhythm becomes necessary, major readjustment of inflation/deflation will be required. In this circumstance, the arterial trace is the best guide. It must be remembered that an improperly timed IABP may well impair cardiac function. This would be the case, for example, if the balloon inflated during any part of systole. Again, the modern Datascope IABP detects and

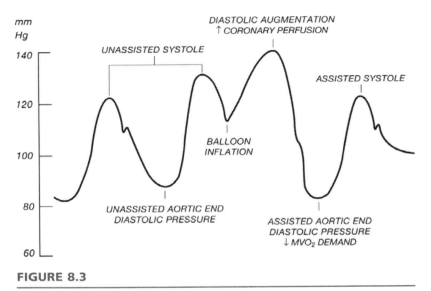

FIGURE 8.3

Arterial trace showing comparison between unassisted and assisted beats.

Source: Reproduced by permission from MAQUET Cardiovascular, Mahwah, NJ.

compensates for such changes automatically. The house officer should make certain that the double-hump arterial trace is maintained under all circumstances. This constitutes a physician double-check of the machine algorithms.

One additional question often troubles the house officer, namely, the evaluation of the arterial trace during IABP support (Figure 8.4). On the arterial trace in the patient without the IABP, the pressure spike representing left ventricular systole is followed by a small dicrotic notch (Figure 8.4, top). In the patient with the IABP functioning, a second major spike follows the left ventricular systolic spike (Figure 8.4, middle). This represents inflation of the balloon, with the expected rise in aortic diastolic pressure. This IABP spike is often higher than the left ventricular systolic spike. The automatic pressure monitor that reads the patient's arterial pressure at the bedside reads the highest spike as "systolic" pressure. However, **with the IABP functioning, "systolic" (peak) pressure is transferred to diastole.**

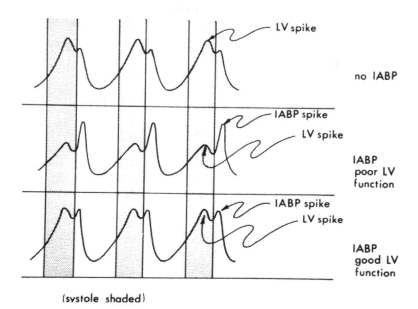

(systole shaded)

FIGURE 8.4

Common patterns in arterial pressure trace with the IABP. **Top:** No IABP. **Middle:** IABP operating in a patient with poor LV function. **Bottom:** IABP functioning in a patient with good function. Shading marks mechanical systole.

In patients with good or adequate cardiac output, the IABP spike will not always exceed or reach that of left ventricular systole (Figure 8.4, bottom). This is seen at times in patients who have had the IABP placed for angina rather than for cardiogenic shock. Failure of the IABP spike to exceed that of native systole need not, in and of itself, be cause for concern and may be entirely consistent with good IABP function and excellent augmentation. Note again that this second pressure spike, the IABP spike, represents pressure generated in diastole by the balloon at no expense to the heart. This will raise mean aortic pressure significantly, with consequently improved organ perfusion.

In fact, comparing the IABP spike to the native left ventricular spike has been used to calculate cardiac output.[12,13] Because the volume of balloon inflation is precisely known, left ventricular stroke volume can be inferred. Calculation of cardiac output by this method has been shown to be very accurate. A small native spike with a tall IABP spike (Figure 8.4, middle) implies a native stroke volume considerably below the 40 cc of the IABP—that is, poor left ventricular function.

The IABP is usually used for a few days only, since prolonged use frequently leads to major complications. Limb ischemia, blood element destruction, thrombosis with embolization, and sepsis become increasing concerns. (In rare cases, the IABP has been left in place for a month or more.) In cases of postoperative low cardiac output, recovery is usually complete within 72 hours.

IABP support should not be withdrawn abruptly. Rather, the patient is gradually weaned from the IABP. Usually, this is done by reducing the pumping rate from 1:1 to 1:2 and then 1:3 (augmentation with every third heartbeat). Another approach to weaning reduces the volume of balloon inflation progressively (from 40 to 30 to 20 mL). Cardiac function is assessed carefully at each stage, including determinations of pulmonary capillary wedge pressure, cardiac output, and mixed venous pO_2. Weaning proceeds if cardiac function remains satisfactory. The IABP is removed if function is satisfactory on 1:3 or at inflation to 20 mL.

Experience is required before the house officer will be comfortable with the IABP. Bearing in mind the principles enumerated above should allow easier familiarity. Study of the operator's manual for each IABP console type is also essential.

REFERENCES

1. Dyub AM, Whitlock RP, Abouzahr LL, Cinà CS. Preoperative intra-aortic balloon pump in patients undergoing coronary bypass surgery: a systematic review and meta-analysis. *J Card Surg.* 2008;23(1): 79-86.
2. Kantrowitz A, Tjonneland S, Freed PS, Phillips SJ, Butner AN, Sherman JL Jr. Initial clinical experience with intra-aortic balloon pumping. *JAMA.* 1968;203(2):113-118.
3. Lorusso R, Gelsomino S, Carella R, et al. Impact of prophylactic intra-aortic balloon counter-pulsation on postoperative outcome in high-risk cardiac surgery patients: a multicentre, propensity-score analysis. *Eur J Cardiothorac Surg.* 2010;38(5):585-589.
4. Berger R. Circulatory assistance with intra-aortic balloon counterpulsation. In: Berk J, Sampliner S, Artz J, Vinocur B, eds. *Handbook of Critical Care.* Boston: Little, Brown; 1976.
5. Bregman D, Hawbert S, Self M. Intra-aortic balloon counterpulsation: a primer. *J Cardiovasc Med.* 1984;607-615.
6. Mueller H. Intra-aortic balloon pumping at the community hospital: a matter of qualifications and communications. *Cardiac Assists.* 1984; 1-6.
7. Reemtsma K, Bregman D, Cohen S. Mechanical circulatory support. In: Shoemaker W, Thompson C, Holbook P, eds. *Textbook of Critical Care.* Philadelphia: WB Saunders; 1984:482-489.
8. Elefteriades JA, Solomon LW, Salazar AM, Batsford WP, Baldwin JC, Kopf GS. Linear left ventricular aneurysmectomy: modern imaging studies reveal improved morphology and function. *Ann Thorac Surg.* 1993;56(2):242-250; discussion 251-252.
9. Elefteriades JA, Tollis G Jr, Levi E, Mills LK, Zaret BL. Coronary artery bypass surgery in severe left ventricular dysfunction: excellent survival with improved ejection fraction and functional state. *J Am Coll Cardiol.* 1993;22(5):1411-1417.
10. Beckman CB, Geha AS, Hammond GL, Baue AE. Results and complications of intra-aortic balloon counterpulsation. *Ann Thorac Surg.* 1977;24(6):550-559.
11. Lundell DC, Hammond GL, Geha AS, Laks H, Wolfson S. Randomized comparison of the modified wire-guided and standard intra-aortic balloon catheters. *J Thorac Cardiovasc Surg.* 1981;81(2):297-301.

12. Roche Medical Electronics. Intra-aortic Balloon Pump: Model 10, Operator's Manual.

13. Herzlinger GA. Absolute determination of cardiac output in intra-aortic balloon pumped patients using the radial arterial pressure trace. *Circulation.* 1976;53(3):417-421.

SUGGESTED FURTHER READING

Kantrowitz A, Wasfie T, Freed PS, Rubenfire M, Wajszczuk W, Schork MA. Intra-aortic balloon pumping 1967 through 1982: analysis of complications in 733 patients. *Am J Cardiol.* 1986;57(11):976-983.
Dr. Kantrowitz, one of the early pioneers of cardiac surgery, invented the IABP, and this is his account of the early clinical experience.

Pre-Inservice Self-Study Guide to Intra-Aortic Balloon Counterpulsation. Available at: http://www.datascope.com/ca/pdf/preinservice_self_study_guide.pdf. Accessed July 19, 2012.
A valuable reference.

Bolooki H. *Clinical Application of Intra-aortic Balloon Pump.* 2nd ed. Mount Kisco, NY: Futura Publishing; 1984.
A comprehensive and clearly written text, with much important general information on care of critically ill patients.

CARDIAC ASSIST DEVICES

I n past years, if a post infarction or post cardiac surgery patient demonstrated inadequate cardiac pump function despite inotropic and intra-aortic balloon pump support, all was lost. Currently, however, a variety of advanced cardiac assist devices are available that can take over the workload of the circulation temporarily (until improvement is realized or cardiac transplantation is performed) or even permanently (as a permanent left heart replacement).[1-3] The devices in current use are all designed to replace a single ventricle only—usually the left. The early worldwide experience (and subsequent efforts) with totally implanted cardiac replacements—left as well as right ventricles—by an artificial heart has been fraught with difficulties, especially infection and stroke. Accordingly, government and medicine have shifted the focus largely to univentricular assist devices. The present chapter provides an overview for the house officer of the settings in which application of cardiac assist devices is appropriate and the technological devices that are available.

The House Officer's Guide to ICU Care: Fundamentals of Management of the Heart and Lungs, 3rd ed. © 2013 John A. Elefteriades, Curtis Tribble, Alexander S. Geha, Mark D. Siegel, and Lawrence S. Cohen, eds. Cardiotext Publishing, ISBN: 978-1-935395-68-3.

✚ TEMPORARY CARDIAC ASSISTANCE

A massive myocardial infarction can produce cardiogenic shock, especially if more than 40% of the left ventricular muscle is destroyed. Shock is quite common as well after open heart surgery—so-called *postcardiotomy shock*—which is seen historically in about one of every 25 cases (perhaps less in the present era). This phenomenon may occur unexpectedly, even in patients without underlying left ventricular dysfunction, even when the conduct of the operation has not been troublesome in any way. It is postulated that inadequacy of myocardial protection (cardioplegia), uncorrected ischemia, coronary artery spasm, air or particulate embolization to the coronary arteries, and myocardial edema and/or hemorrhage may be important factors. Experience has shown that dysfunction in such cases is often reversible if cardiac performance can be augmented temporarily. In fact, in most cases where recovery occurs, this recovery is complete, with restoration of normal or near-normal left ventricular function. Cardiac performance is most commonly supported temporarily by inotropic medication. (See Chapter 7, Continuous Infusion Agents.) If this is inadequate, then the intra-aortic balloon pump is applied. (See Chapter 8, The Intra-aortic Balloon Pump.) This remarkably efficacious device salvages nearly one-half of patients with postcardiotomy shock.

When inotropic medications and the intra-aortic balloon pump do not suffice to restore life-supporting vital signs, cardiac assist devices need to be considered. Without the application of these devices, the outcome is lethal. The cardiac assist device serves 2 general purposes: (1) to supply the systemic circulation to vital organs during the period that myocardial performance is inadequate; and (2) to unload the left ventricle, decreasing its oxygen requirements, so that recovery of dysfunctional but viable myocardium is permitted or enhanced.

Similar circumstances necessitating the application of cardiac assist device support may arise not only in the cardiac operating room, but also in the coronary care unit, with refractory postmyocardial infarction shock or shock from end-stage chronic heart failure of any cause (such as ischemic heart disease, valvular heart disease, viral cardiomyopathy, postpartum cardiomyopathy, or familial cardiomyopathy).

The criteria for application of left ventricular assistance are quite specific: BP < 90 mm Hg systolic and CI (cardiac index) < 1.8 L/min/m² despite a left atrial pressure of 25 mm Hg on maximal inotropic and intra-aortic balloon pump support. The left atrial pressure criterion indicates inadequate pump function despite maximum volume repletion. The pulmonary capillary wedge pressure is used to approximate left atrial pressure (see Chapter 5, Hemodynamic Monitoring and the Swan-Ganz Catheter).

Of course, certain patients are not suitable candidates for such aggressive support measures, including the elderly (over age 70 or 75), those with a limited life expectancy (due to malignancy or other severe illness), those with uncontrollable hemorrhage as the major cause of intraoperative instability, those whose underlying cardiac condition is nonremediable in the long term, and those with irreversible dysfunction of noncardiac organs (especially lungs, brain, liver, and kidneys).

In some patients, not only *left*, but also *right* ventricular function is inadequate after cardiopulmonary bypass. Biventricular support with both a left and a right ventricular device may be necessary. **Criteria for right ventricular assistance parallel those for left ventricular assistance: a cardiac index of less than 1.8 L/min/m² despite a right atrial pressure of 20 mm Hg.**

Several general types of mechanical devices are available for cardiac assistance. Some are geared more toward short-term support and some toward long-term support. There are multiple makes and models. We will discuss a few representative examples, which we use at our center and which are widely utilized globally. Many individual models from multiple manufacturers are in use throughout the world. See Figures 9.1 to 9.6.

Temporary Cardiac Support

Roller-type pumps. These are essentially the pump heads of the heart-lung machine. They can be used as assist devices to propel blood, usually from the left atrium to the aorta. This means of temporary cardiac support involves using the ordinary roller pump from the heart-lung machine to propel blood from the left atrium to the aorta, thus supporting (or bypassing) the left ventricle. This will perfuse the body organs well, while unloading the left ventricle to permit its recovery (Figure 9.1).

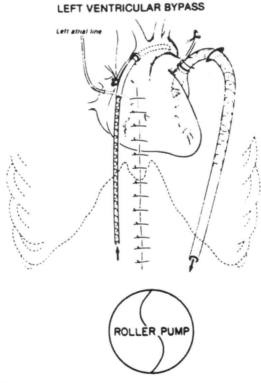

FIGURE 9.1

Roller-pump left heart assist (left atrium to aorta).

Source: Kesselbrenner M, Bregman D, Sack J. Mechanical support of the failing heart. In: Casthely PA, Bregman D, eds. *Cardiopulmonary Bypass: Physiology Related Complications and Pharmacology.* Mount Kisco, NY: Futura Publishing; 1991. With permission from Wiley-Blackwell.

Centrifugal pumps. Also, other pumps can be used for this purpose. A centrifugal pump can be used (Figure 9.2). The Biomedicus pump is the prime example. These pumps are more favorable to the formed elements of the blood (compared to roller pumps) in long-term application.

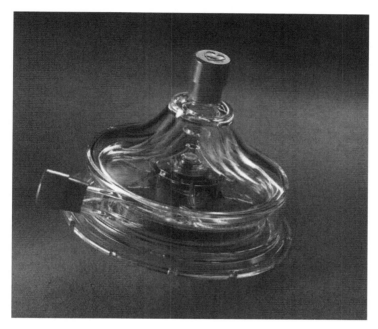

FIGURE 9.2

The Biomedicus pump.

Source: Reproduced by permission from Medtronic, Inc, Minneapolis, MN.

Accessory ventricles. These "partial artificial hearts" are actually implanted inside the body (or just outside the body) and driven by pressure lines or electrical connections that pass through the body wall to a console outside the body. Some cardiac assist devices are designed specifically for such a support role. One popular device is the Abiomed AB5000. Tubes bring the blood out of the body, as with the other temporary devices, and this pneumatic-driven device provides powerful pulsatile blood flow (Figure 9.3).

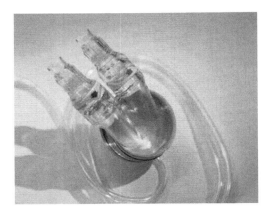

FIGURE 9.3

The Abiomed AB5000 Ventricle.

Source: Reproduced by permission from Abiomed Inc, Danvers, MA.

ECMO (extracorporeal membrane oxygenation). Another means of temporary support is ECMO, or extracorporeal membrane oxygenation[4-7] (Figure 9.4). This method of support is essentially equivalent to having the patient on a miniature cardiopulmonary bypass machine. The blood is removed from the right atrium, passes through an oxygenator, and is delivered—oxygenated and pressurized—to the aorta to perfuse the body. This method of support not only compensates for left ventricular dysfunction, but also supports the right ventricle and the lungs. This is used to substantial benefit in children after open heart surgery, but in adults, patient salvage is marginal.

Certain complications regularly accompany use of ventricular assist devices. Hemolysis and thrombocytopenia from destruction of the formed elements of the blood by the mechanical action are common. Postoperative bleeding is very common, especially originating where the cannulas attach to the heart or the aorta. The bleeding tendency reflects the adverse effects on hemostasis of the prolonged period on cardiopulmonary bypass that usually precedes placement of an assist device. Sepsis and multiple organ failure are common, reflecting the very critical status of the patients. The

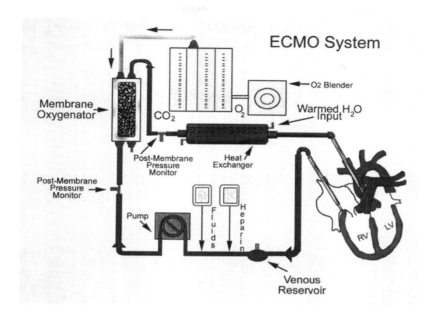

FIGURE 9.4

Schematic representation of ECMO system.

Source: Reproduced with permission from Pandemic Ventilator Project. Available at: http://panvent.blogspot.com/2009/09/using-dialysis-machine-to-do-ecmo.html. Accessed July 19, 2012.

potential for thrombus formation in the devices—which can produce systemic embolization—leads most surgical teams to use anticoagulation of some type when the patient's coagulation profile returns to normal postoperatively. Anticoagulation may take the form of dextran, subcutaneous or intravenous heparin, antiplatelet agents like aspirin or Plavix, or Coumadin, depending on the patient and the device. **In patients with mechanical assist devices, there is always a conflict in the mind of the team between concern about bleeding but fear of stroke. The concern about bleeding discourages early or aggressive anticoagulation. The fear of stroke encourages early anticoagulation.** Local and device-specific protocols will be available to guide the house officer on local customs and practices in his particular unit.

With cardiac assistance in progress, cardiac recovery usually occurs within 3 to 5 days. The device is gradually weaned and then removed.

About 1 in 2 supported postcardiotomy patients is successfully weaned from cardiac assistance, and about one-half of those weaned survive to be discharged from the hospital. There is an overall sentiment emerging that **mechanical circulatory assistance is generally instituted too late in postcardiotomy shock.** Late institution carries the penalties of prolonged cardiopulmonary bypass (myocardial and pulmonary edema, multiple organ failure, bleeding diathesis, sepsis). If available, **a cardiac assist device should be placed promptly—within 1 hour after completion of the cardiac procedure**—if the patient cannot be weaned from cardiopulmonary bypass by conventional means.

The house officer will have guidance in his care of patients on ventricular assist devices. Nonetheless, he will often be the doctor on the front lines, even for these complex patients. So, it is important that he be familiar with the general principles and common complications enumerated above.

✚ PERMANENT CARDIAC ASSISTANCE

In the past, patients supported on a left ventricular assist device who could not be weaned from cardiac assistance died or, if appropriate, candidates were listed for cardiac transplantation. An exciting new option has emerged—permanent mechanical assistance of the left heart.

For the last 2 decades, large, pulsatile devices held sway, with the Novacor and the HeartMate I competing like Ford and Chevrolet for global position in this market. Both devices proved valuable. The HeartMate was stroke-resistant, and the Novacor was extremely durable.[8] Each made an important contribution.

Because of frequent infections due to the sheer size of these 2 devices, efforts toward miniaturization have been made. Smaller devices now commonly utilize miniature, continuously rotating high-speed impellers instead of the large pulsatile pumping chambers of the past.[9] These newer devices require minimal or no subcutaneous pockets and are more infection-resistant. Only an electrical power cord exits the body, leading to an external electric drive unit. While the miniature profile is advantageous, the drawback of the rotating impeller pumps is that the blood flow is nonpulsatile, and the patient often has no palpable pulse. This can be off-putting to the house officer as well as the nursing and ER staff. **It was originally thought that the body could not thrive without pulsatile blood flow, but enough experience has accumulated to indicate that the body can do perfectly well with blood flow without a pulse. The brain, kidneys, and heart muscle, along with the other organs, are perfectly happy despite lack of a pulse.** Also on a positive note, the hemolysis that was originally feared from the blood's passing through a high-speed impeller has not materialized; amazingly, the "Waring blender" phenomenon has not been a frequent problem.

Recent evidence indicates that survival with these new devices can be excellent if an early decision is made to implant the device— before nutritional, infectious, and end-organ complications of advanced heart failure develop.

In Figures 9.5 and 9.6, we illustrate 2 of the modern impeller-type, nonpulsatile left ventricular assist devices—the HeartMate II and the Jarvik 2000. These devices can support the patient until a heart becomes available for transplantation (so-called "bridge to transplantation") or indefinitely, if needed (so-called "destination therapy").

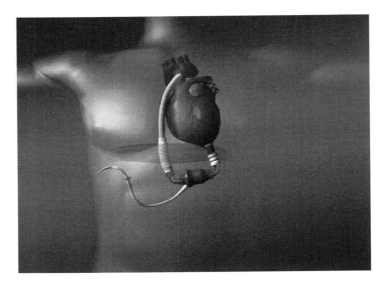

FIGURE 9.5

The HeartMate II left ventricular assist device.

Source: Reprinted with the permission of Thoratec Corporation, Pleasanton, CA.

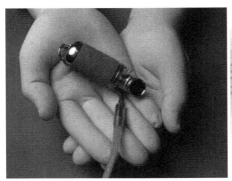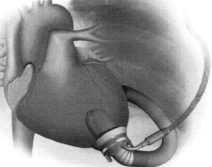

FIGURE 9.6

The Jarvik 2000 ventricular assist device. **Left:** Close-up of the device. Note small size. **Right:** The device as connected to the left ventricle and the descending aorta.

Source: Reproduced with permission from Jarvik Heart, New York, NY.

REFERENCES

1. Bojar RM. *Adult Cardiac Surgery*. Boston: Blackwell Scientific Publications; 1992.
2. Elefteriades JA. Cardiac assist devices. *Cardiol Clin*. 1988;6(3):449-459.
3. Elefteriades JA, Botta DM Jr. Left ventricular assist devices. Preface. *Cardiol Clin*. 2011;29:xiii-xiv.
4. Betit P. Extracorporeal membrane oxygenation: quo vadis? *Respir Care*. 2009;54(7):948-957.
5. Sidebotham D, McGeorge A, McGuinness S, Edwards M, Willcox T, Beca J. Extracorporeal membrane oxygenation for treating severe cardiac and respiratory disease in adults: Part 1—overview of extracorporeal membrane oxygenation. *J Cardiothorac Vasc Anesth*. 2009; 23(6):886-892.
6. Sidebotham D, McGeorge A, McGuinness S, Edwards M, Willcox T, Beca J. Extracorporeal membrane oxygenation for treating severe cardiac and respiratory failure in adults: Part 2—technical considerations. *J Cardiothorac Vasc Anesth*. 2010;24(1):164-172.
7. Farkas EA, Elefteriades JA. Assisted circulation: experience with the Novacor Left Ventricular Assist System. *Expert Rev Med Devices*. 2007;4(6):769-774.
8. Siegenthaler MP, Frazier OH, Beyersdorf F, et al. Mechanical reliability of the Jarvik 2000 Heart. *Ann Thorac Surg*. 2006;81(5):1752-1758; discussion 1758-1759.
9. Lietz K, Long JW, Kfoury AG, et al. Outcomes of left ventricular assist device implantation as destination therapy in the post-REMATCH era: implications for patient selection. *Circulation*. 2007;116(5):497-505.

SUGGESTED FURTHER READING

Elefteriades JA, Botta DM Jr. Left ventricular assist devices. *Cardiol Clin*. 2011;29(4).
A complete, up-to-date review of this important topic.

Cooley EG. *University of Michigan Health System Family Guide to Adult ECMO*. Ann Arbor, MI: University of Michigan Regents; 2001. Available at: www.med.umich.edu/ECMO/patient/AdultECMO.pdf. Accessed July 19, 2012.
A very informative, commonsense information manual.

10

HEART TRANSPLANTATION

This chapter focuses on hemodynamic issues following heart transplantation. There are differences of the transplanted heart that profoundly affect management—and the house officer must be familiar with these.

General care of the transplant patient—in terms of immunosuppression, infection prevention, and the like—are beyond the scope of this book and will not be covered in this chapter.

The House Officer's Guide to ICU Care: Fundamentals of Management of the Heart and Lungs, 3rd ed. © 2013 John A. Elefteriades, Curtis Tribble, Alexander S. Geha, Mark D. Siegel, and Lawrence S. Cohen, eds. Cardiotext Publishing, ISBN: 978-1-935395-68-3.

✚ PULMONARY HYPERTENSION AND THE PARADOX OF HEART TRANSPLANTATION

Pulmonary hypertension remains the Achilles' heel of clinical heart transplantation. Right heart failure after transplantation remains the predominant cause of the nearly 10% early mortality still seen after transplantation, even in the current era.[1-5] We will examine now how a paradox in heart transplantation related to right heart failure impacts early posttransplant care by the house officer—making proper decision making essential for good patient outcome.

The donor left ventricle, of course, is much stronger than the recipient left ventricle; this is the reason for the transplantation procedure being performed. Regarding the right ventricles, however, the paradox arises.

Consider first the hemodynamics in the recipient. In the patient with long-standing heart failure, the lungs become water-logged—chronically so. Consequently, the pulmonary artery pressures are high. This means that the right heart faces, and copes with, this pulmonary hypertension. After all, the patient, albeit in heart failure, is alive; this means that his native right ventricle is coping. **The recipient right ventricle has, over time, acclimated itself against the increased afterload of high pulmonary artery pressures resulting from the failing left ventricle.** This right ventricle is thick, muscle-bound, and able to tolerate high pulmonary artery pressure. (See Figure 10.1.)

Consider now the hemodynamics in the donor. The donor has a normal heart. The donor right ventricle, paradoxically, is accustomed only to normal pulmonary artery pressures and can fail easily after transplantation. It is thin walled, relatively weak, and has never had an opportunity to accustom to high pulmonary artery pressures.

With regard to the ability to cope with elevated recipient pulmonary artery pressures, the discarded recipient right ventricle is often

The lethal paradox of clinical heart transplantation

Recipient RV: STRONG

Discarded

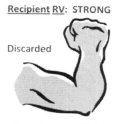

•Accustomed to high PVR
•Hypertrophic

Donor RV: WEAKER

Installed

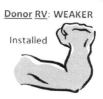

•Accustomed to low PVR
•Thin-walled

FIGURE 10.1

The lethal paradox of clinical heart transplantation, accounting for the majority of early postoperative deaths after transplantation. (See text.)

much stronger than the transplanted donor right ventricle. Even with β-agonist or phosphodiesterase inhibitor support of the transplanted donor right ventricle and with vasodilatation of the pulmonary arteries via nitrates, nitroprusside, prostaglandins, and inhaled nitric oxide, right heart failure after transplantation can still be irremediable and, frequently, lethal. When mechanical support of the right ventricle needs to be implemented, mortality may approach 50%.

So, this paradox—that the donor right ventricle is weaker than the recipient's original right heart—means that the house officer must be on constant guard to prevent and/or detect right heart failure.

Right heart failure after transplantation usually occurs in the operating room or in the early postoperative phase (immediately upon ICU arrival or within 48 to 72 hours). After that time, 2 factors come into play that obviate right heart failure: (1) the lungs "dry up," as they are no longer exposed to high left atrial pressures of a failing left ventricle; and (2) the donor right ventricle adapts, and hypertrophies, quite quickly in the new, challenging milieu. So, if the house officer steers the heart transplant recipient safely through the first day or two, the patient will be "home free" with respect to hemodynamic function of the new heart.

In fact, the adverse impact of preexisting pulmonary hypertension on function of the new heart is so powerful that the level of preexisting pulmonary hypertension is a deciding factor in the decision to perform heart transplantation. For this purpose, we calculate the *pulmonary vascular resistance* (PVR). The PVR is expressed by the following equation:

PVR = (PA mean − PCWP)/CO

The house officer should not be intimidated by this equation. It is simply a version of the familiar Ohm's law, or V = I × R, from electricity (where V is voltage, I is current, and R is resistance). In that electrical equation, R = V/I; in other words, the resistance of a circuit equals the voltage drop across the circuit divided by the current flow. (See Figure 10.2).

In the case of the PVR equation above, the pulmonary vascular resistance is the pressure drop across the lungs (more on this in a moment) divided by the flow (cardiac output)—exactly analogous to the familiar equation from physics. Now, the pulmonary vascular

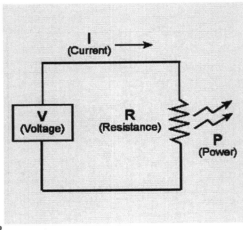

FIGURE 10.2

Ohm's law. This concept of pressure drop across the lungs is applied to the calculation of pulmonary vascular resistance.

resistance represents the resistance of the pulmonary vasculature. The pressure in front of the pulmonary vasculature is the PA pressure, characterized by the PA mean. The pressure in back of the pulmonary vasculature is the PCWP. So, the pressure drop across the pulmonary vasculature is the PA mean minus the PCWP. (See Chapter 5, Hemodynamic Monitoring and the Swan-Ganz Catheter and Figure 5.3 for a review of these pressures and anatomic connections.)

Thus arises the important equation for PVR. Please note that a larger pressure drop across the lungs means a higher PVR. A lower CO also means a higher PVR. The PVR is measured in the cath lab or whenever a PA catheter (Swan-Ganz) is in place.

The level of PVR determines the patient's candidacy for heart transplantation. We express PVR in Wood units. The number obtained by the above equation is already in Wood units and requires no conversion factors.

Your PVR, and ours, is normally 1 to 2 Wood units. Patients with pulmonary artery resistance in the range of 1 to 3 Wood units are optimal candidates for heart transplantation. With pulmonary vascular resistance between 3 and 6 Wood units, patients become high risk. Several studies have shown that patients in this high-risk group have an early mortality of 17% to 60% after transplantation. Above 6 Wood units, most authorities believe that heart transplantation is contraindicated (Table 10.1).

TABLE 10.1   Impact of PVR (Pulmonary Vascular Resistance) on Candidacy for Heart Transplantation. (HTx: heart transplantation)

PVR < 3 Wood units	OK
PVR 3-6 Wood units	High risk
PVR > 6 Wood units	HTx contraindicated

Now, PVR is not a completely static phenomenon—it can vary from time to time and under different ambient circumstances. In fact, in the cath lab, if the PVR is seen to be high, testing is done

to determine if the elevated PVR is "fixed." Finding of fixed elevation is bad, indicating that pharmacologic intervention will not
ameliorate the situation, either preoperatively, intraoperatively, or
postoperatively. **To test the reversibility of the PVR, we give
nitroprusside intravenously—the so-called "nipride test."** If the
PVR comes down with nitroprusside, that tells us that the PVR is,
to some extent, reversible. In such a circumstance, it can be expected that vasodilating drugs would favorably influence the PVR
and that the PVR would be expected to normalize upon transplantation of a new heart, with a normal left ventricle. In fact, the exact
mortality risk of transplantation can be predicted from the results of
the nipride test (Table 10.2).

TABLE 10.2 Impact of Pulmonary Hypertension, as Assessed by the
Nipride Test, on Early Mortality of Heart Transplantation

	3-month mortality p HTx
PVR < 2.5 u	6.9%
PVR > 2.5 u	17.9% (p < 0.02)

Source: Costard-Jackle A, Fowler MB. Influence of preoperative pulmonary artery
pressure on mortality after heart transplantation: testing of potential reversibility
of pulmonary hypertension with nitroprusside is useful in defining a high risk
group. *J Am Coll Cardiol.* 1992;19(1):48-54.

**So, how does the house officer recognize right heart failure
after transplantation?** In the early postoperative phase in the ICU,
hypotension would be the main indicator. Hypotension could
arise from many causes, but in the absence of arrhythmia, bleeding,
or tamponade, right heart failure should be suspected. **Another
indicator would be rising CVP.** As the right heart fails, the back
pressure behind the right ventricle—the CVP—rises. We do not like
to see CVP above 15 mm Hg in a transplant patient.

How Should Right Heart Failure Be Treated?

There are 2 main avenues at the house officer's disposal to treat heart failure after heart transplantation: decreasing PVR and stimulating right heart function.

The first way to decrease the PVR is to eliminate physiologic factors that exacerbate pulmonary hypertension. **Hypoxia and hypercarbia are potent pulmonary vasoconstrictors.** So, you must ensure that you are oxygenating and ventilating your transplant patient very well. Also, PEEP increases PVR by virtue of "squeezing" the pulmonary capillaries; you should decrease PEEP as much as possible to decrease PVR.

Another means to decrease PVR is to administrate pulmonary vasodilators. The problem is that most agents that decrease PVR also decrease systemic vascular resistance (SVR) and exacerbate hypotension. Usually, if you have right heart failure after heart transplantation, the blood pressure will be low, and you may not have much blood pressure "room" for vasodilators. Nitroglycerine is a gentle vasodilator and is an appropriate first choice. Nitroprusside is an appropriate next agent. Prostacyclines are somewhat pulmonary selective and may be used as well, but only in consultation with senior staff.

An excellent pharmacologic approach to decreasing PVR is the use of inhaled nitric oxide. Nitric oxide given via the endotracheal tube powerfully dilates the pulmonary vessels, without much impact on the SVR and the systemic blood pressure. The effect is nearly immediate and powerful. We usually start with 5 to 10 ppm and increase in increments to 40 ppm or even 80 ppm in select cases. The administration is continued until pulmonary hypertension resolves; usually, in 24 to 48 hours, the problem of pulmonary hypertension and right heart failure improves or dissipates, and administration of nitric oxide can be tapered and discontinued. Administration requires an endotracheal tube, so the drug must be weaned in order for the patient to be extubated and mobilized.

The second avenue of treatment for right heart failure posttransplantation is pharmacologic support of the right ventricle. See Chapter 7 (Continuous Infusion Agents) for a full discussion of inotropic agents. **Suffice it to say here that isoproterenol and milrinone are uniquely suited to posttransplant right heart failure. Both drugs stimulate the right ventricle powerfully and both dilate the pulmonary arteries—leading to a beneficial synergy of effects.**

If the above measures are insufficient, mechanical support of the right heart can be instituted (via a right ventricular assist device, or RVAD). See Chapter 9 on mechanical cardiac assistance. Some patients may be salvaged, but the risk of adverse outcome is high if mechanical support proves necessary.

Perhaps the most important point to be made about right heart failure posttransplant is that the house officer must be alert in its recognition. Early detection and treatment in the incipient stages is much more fruitful than treatment of the full-fledged syndrome; once the right heart becomes strained, swollen, and dilated, it is difficult, if not impossible, to reverse the process. Hypotension and rising CVP are the key indicators. The house officer must take immediate measures, as described above, and inform and involve senior staff immediately.

Inotropic Support Posttransplant

The house officer should be aware that the standard heart transplant patient will come to ICU on multiple inotropic agents. Just consider what the transplanted heart has been through. It has undergone the challenge of the original injury to the donor, be it trauma or a brain event, both of which tax the heart. During harvest, the heart is separated from its blood supply. It is ischemic, sitting in a cold bucket, usually for several hours, if not more. It is edematous. Then, it is handled and sutured into place. And, finally, we ask it to turn on instantly and beat strongly, often in a milieu of pulmonary hypertension and immunologic hostility. It is not surprising that the transplanted heart needs some pharmacologic support.

Different institutions have specific protocols; we usually use low doses of isoproterenol, epinephrine, and milrinone to achieve the desired heart rate and blood pressures. In contradistinction to an ordinary, nontransplant open heart patient, in a transplant patient, the drips are usually continued for 1 to 3 days, while the new heart recovers and compensates for its milieu; even then, the inotropic drugs are weaned only slowly.

The EKG Posttransplant

Remember that you will likely have 2 P waves in the posttransplant EKG, one from the new atria and one from the remnants of the original atria. This can lead to an initially confusing EKG. Just remember to be on the lookout for 2 sets of P waves, one correlating with the QRS, and the other following its own rhythm, out of sync with the QRS.

Cardiac Denervation

Remember that the new heart is permanently denervated.[6] It is no longer connected to the sympathetic and parasympathetic neural networks that control heart rate. So, the new heart will not be capable of instantaneous heart rate response. You and we can respond immediately with tachycardia to a threat or to hypotension or bleeding. The transplanted heart, denervated as it is, can respond only more slowly, when catecholamine hormones have been secreted and reached the heart to enact a bloodborne stimulation of the heart rate and contractility. On a similar note, remember that drugs that act through the parasympathetic nervous input to the heart will be ineffective on the transplanted heart (eg, atropine, digoxin). **Atropine is nearly useless for bradycardia in a heart transplant recipient.**

The denervation of the heart also implies that transplant patients are largely incapable of feeling angina; you need not be concerned that any complaints of chest pain in the ICU transplant patient are anginal in origin.

Heart Rate

We customarily keep the heart rate high in the ICU patient posttransplant (usually 100 to 120 bpm). This helps to maintain cardiac output. Also, the donor heart is usually young and free of coronary artery disease and thus quite able to tolerate a tachycardia. This is in contradistinction to many of the other ICU patients. We keep the transplant heart rate high using isoproterenol and/or atrial pacing. The sinus node is often dysfunctional for hours to days after heart transplantation, and pharmacologic or pacing support of heart rate overcomes this factor as well.

Tamponade and Pericardial Effusion Posttransplant

Keep in mind that there are at least 4 major suture lines constructed in heart transplantation. Also, the patients often do not generate clotting factors well due to severe, preexisting hepatic congestion and dysfunction. Bleeding and tamponade are not uncommon, and the house officer must be vigilant.

Later on, when the patient is well and recovering on the step-down unit, if an echo is done, a pericardial effusion will always be seen. Remember that the pericardial space of the dilated, excised heart will have been very large. Then, a small donor heart is implanted in that space. The residual, unoccupied space must obligatorily fill with fluid. Do not be alarmed to see pericardial fluid, often a generous amount; in the patient who is clinically well, it is of no consequence. The cardiac silhouette will still be large on CXR, reflecting the original size of the pericardium and the contained fluid. Over weeks to months, the fluid will be reabsorbed, and the cardiac silhouette on CXR will normalize.

REFERENCES

1. Elefteriades JA, Lovoulos CJ, Tellides G, et al. Right ventricle-sparing heart transplant: promising new technique for recipients with pulmonary hypertension. *Ann Thorac Surg.* 2000;69(6):1858-1864.

2. Costard-Jackle A, Fowler MB. Influence of preoperative pulmonary artery pressure on mortality after heart transplantation: testing of potential reversibility of pulmonary hypertension with nitroprusside is useful in defining a high risk group. *J Am Coll Cardiol.* 1992;1(1)9: 48-54.

3. Haj RM, Cinco JE, Mazer CD. Treatment of pulmonary hypertension with selective pulmonary vasodilators. *Curr Opin Anesthaesiol.* 2006;19(1):88-95.

4. Blaise G, Langleben D, Hubert B. Pulmonary arterial hypertension: pathophysiology and anesthetic approach. *Anesthesiology.* 2003; 99(6):1415-1432.

5. Stobierska-Dzierzek B, Awad H, Michler RE. The evolving management of acute right-sided heart failure in cardiac transplant recipients. *J Am Coll Cardiol.* 2001;38(4):923-931.

6. Young JB. Physiology and pharmacology of the transplanted heart. In: Cooper DKC, Miller LW, Patterson GA, eds. *The Transplantation and Replacement of Thoracic Organs.* 2nd ed. Dordrecht/Boston/London: Kluwer; 1997:299-337.

SUGGESTED FURTHER READING

Elefteriades JA, Lovoulos CJ, Tellides G, et al. Right ventricle-sparing heart transplant: promising new technique for recipients with pulmonary hypertension. *Ann Thorac Surg.* 2000;69(6):1858-1864.

This reference reviews the impact of pulmonary hypertension on transplantation quite fully and presents an innovative potential solution—in the form of a novel anatomic approach to the transplant operation itself.

Young JB. Physiology and pharmacology of the transplanted heart. In: Cooper DKC, Miller LW, Patterson GA, eds. *The Transplantation and Replacement of Thoracic Organs.* 2nd ed. Dordrecht/Boston/London: Kluwer; 1997:299-337.

11

CARDIAC ARREST AND NEAR ARREST

Much of the pertinent information for management of cardiac arrest is covered elsewhere in this guide. Respiratory management is discussed in Chapter 1. Arrhythmias are covered in Chapter 2. Temporary pacemakers and the defibrillator are covered in Chapters 3 and 4, respectively. Hemodynamic management is discussed in Chapter 6. Inotropes are covered in Chapter 7. Bleeding following cardiac surgery and particular problems that may follow thoracic surgery are discussed in Chapters 15 and 19, respectively. Thus what remains for this chapter is mainly to synthesize material covered elsewhere with particular reference to the setting of cardiac arrest.

The present chapter reviews fundamentals in management of cardiac arrest and touches on some controversies and up-to-date trends and recommendations.[1-4]

The House Officer's Guide to ICU Care: Fundamentals of Management of the Heart and Lungs, 3rd ed. © 2013 John A. Elefteriades, Curtis Tribble, Alexander S. Geha, Mark D. Siegel, and Lawrence S. Cohen, eds. Cardiotext Publishing, ISBN: 978-1-935395-68-3.

✚ NEAR ARREST

The "near arrest" is very common in a postoperative cardiothoracic ICU and not uncommon in a CCU. Blood pressure (BP) may fall precipitously for many reasons, even in patients who are doing well generally. Intravascular volume may abruptly fall short of the minimum that maintains compensation. Bleeding may occur and lower intravascular volume quickly. A brady- or tachyarrhythmia may develop. Myocardial performance may become sluggish because of acidosis or other factors. Iatrogenic interventions, such as administration of intravenous narcotics or afterload-reducing agents, may abruptly lower vascular tone and cause hypotension. An inadvertent bolus of an afterload-reducing agent may be given as a line is flushed. In any of these settings, the house officer may be called urgently to the bedside because of hypotension. It is not uncommon to be called for BP of 80 mm Hg, 60 mm Hg, or even lower.

The house officer must react instinctively to prevent further deterioration. The general response should be as follows:

1. **Confirm that BP is low.** Many times the arterial line is reading spuriously low. The trace may be obviously dampened; a power flush of the line may remedy the problem.

   With time, the house officer will come to be able to assess BP very accurately by feeling the femoral pulse. One gets to know the "feel" of 80 mm Hg and that of 60 mm Hg. This may save critical time by making cuff BP confirmation unnecessary in the immediate response interval.

   Quick assessment of the level of consciousness will help. The patient who is wide awake is perfusing the cerebrum adequately, and BP must be acceptable. If the patient has lost consciousness, it is likely that BP has fallen to a critically low level.

2. **Ascertain that cardiac rhythm and rate are adequate.** A glance at the monitor usually suffices. If a profound bradycardia or a serious tachycardia is seen, appropriate remedial measures must be taken immediately.

    Likewise, a rhythm that cannot support vital signs—a rapid ventricular tachycardia or ventricular fibrillation— must be treated immediately. Often rhythm and rate will be adequate, with some other factor causing the hypotension.

3. **Take measures to raise BP. Calcium chloride is the inotrope par excellence.** Other inotropes act via their effect on intracellular calcium flux. **Intravenous administration of calcium chloride will stimulate myocardial contractility and raise BP no matter what the cause of hypotension.** Calcium chloride comes as 1 g/10 mL in rapid-inject syringes. One-quarter ampule (2.5 mL) can be given for mild hypotension; one-half ampule (5 mL) can be given for moderate hypotension; and a full ampule (10 mL) can be given for severe hypotension. This drug must be given by central line. Once again, **calcium should be the house officer's instinctive response to hypotension.** If calcium is not effective by itself, epinephrine can be given by injection, as discussed later. Once BP is restored, a thorough assessment can be undertaken to determine the cause of near arrest and to effect a remedy.

✚ MECHANICS OF RESUSCITATION

It is not uncommon to find house officers at an arrest concentrating heavily on the EKG machine and on drug administration yet neglecting artificial respiration and circulation. **Resuscitation is primarily a mechanical intervention: respiration and circulation must be maintained artificially.**

In the ICU, ventilation is best provided by quick intubation and respiration by bag using supplemental oxygen. (This is in distinction to resuscitation in the community, where mouth-to-mouth resuscitation may be required, although non-respiration CPR is currently fashionable for out-of-hospital arrest.) Every house officer must be capable of intubating quickly and reliably. This skill comes only through experience; a rotation on the anesthesia service can concentrate this experience. **One hundred percent O_2 should be administered.** Oxygen toxicity is not a relevant danger in this acute setting. The house officer should be cautioned that in urgent situations it is not uncommon for staff to forget to connect the ventilating bag to the O_2 supply. Vigorous ventilation should be performed. The aim is to provide a minute volume much greater than normal, so that preexisting CO_2 retention and hypoxia can be corrected.

Many ineffective resuscitations owe their lack of success to mistaken intubation of the esophagus instead of the trachea. It is essential to confirm proper tube placement. The standard technique is to listen to the lungs to confirm ventilation; this, of course, is an excellent method. Also, you may see misting of the endotracheal tube with each breath, confirming proper endotracheal placement. Another clinical pearl is to listen first over the stomach. You should not hear noise in the stomach when a breath is being given. If you do hear a noise, the tube is in the esophagus. Modern ICUs have a self-contained chemical sensor built in to the respiratory circuit for cardiac arrest; a color change indicates gas exchange and successful intubation. Check with your respiratory therapist to become familiar with the equipment on hand in your own ICU.

In certain cases, the house officer responding to the arrest situation may not yet be proficient at intubation. In such a case, while a call is placed to the always present, in-house anesthesiologist, mask ventilation should suffice. Again, the use of a mask is best learned via a rotation on the anesthesia service. It is essential to maintain a tight seal with the facial tissues and to be certain that the airway is clear. **An old adage holds that any patient can be ventilated indefinitely with a mask,** and there is much, if not universal, truth in this adage. **The house officer should remember to use mask ventilation if he is unable to intubate reliably and promptly.** The respiratory therapist, who will be responding immediately to the arrest situation, is usually an exceptional ally in performing mask ventilation.

Effective external mechanical cardiac compression is learned through experience. Common errors include trying to perform compression on a soft mattress and being under-vigorous. A rigid board must be placed under the chest for compression to be effective. Very vigorous depression of the sternum must be attained; ribs and the sternum may be fractured, but this is a small price to pay for sustenance of circulation. **Contemporary evidence favors not only vigorous compression, but also a rapid rate of compression, 120 per minute being optimal.**[5] The house officer should be aware that CPR is almost never done effectively on TV; the slow, gentle compressions often shown will certainly be ineffective. The house officer should banish that image from his clinical consciousness.

In the ICU, the arterial line will provide a measure of the effectiveness of external compression. An experienced operator can achieve BPs of 80 mm Hg or more with each compression.

In the patient who is within several days of cardiac surgery, the median sternotomy wound can be opened easily and quickly to provide access for internal massage. It is prudent to splash the chest with antiseptic before reopening the incision. Internal massage may be done with one hand or bimanually. Internal massage is tiring (the skeletal muscles of the hand are not built for the sustained performance requirements of the heart); the operator may find it necessary to switch back and forth between one and two hands. Again, the arterial line provides an index of effectiveness. The house officer should bear in mind that the heart is delicate. Indiscrete manipulation may produce a tear of the cardiac chambers. Do not put your thumb over the right ventricle; this is likely to penetrate the thin wall of the distended right ventricle, resulting in a lethal injury. Rather, if using one hand, put your palm over the right ventricle and your apposed fingers around the side and back of the heart. Beware of internal mammary and vein grafts, which are easily disrupted. Whenever possible, internal massage should be performed by an experienced team member. After achieving successful cardiac resuscitation by open massage, copious irrigation with antibiotic solution should be carried out, and a decision as to primary or delayed closure of the sternotomy incision made; this decision depends on the degree of contamination of the wound.

We tend to favor external cardiac compression because of all the above-listed concerns regarding internal massage. External massage will suffice for a bradycardic or tachyarrhythmic arrest. The exception is an arrest from cardiac bleeding and tamponade, where the open approach will permit relief of tamponade as well as manual cardiac compression.

Without adequate mechanical ventilation and circulation, resuscitation cannot be effective. When adequate ventilation and circulation are provided artificially, the patient's own rhythm, rate, and contractility are, for the moment, not relevant. In this way, critical time is gained to normalize rhythm and contractility, so that the patient's own system may safely and adequately resume circulation.

It has recently been shown that monitoring the end-tidal CO_2 in the endotracheal tube allows on-line assessment of the adequacy of mechanical resuscitation and early recognition of resumption of adequate native hemodynamics. The principle behind this monitoring is that, in the absence of effective circulation, no CO_2 is delivered to the lungs by the bloodstream, and end-tidal CO_2 is low. With effective resuscitation, and especially with resumption of native hemodynamics, increase in end-tidal CO_2 is seen.[6] Noting end-tidal CO_2 also usefully confirms successful intubation.

✚ ARRHYTHMIAS DURING ARREST

The rhythms seen most commonly during arrest are (1) a very slow rhythm (a profound bradycardia or even asystole) and (2) a serious ventricular arrhythmia (rapid ventricular tachycardia or ventricular fibrillation).

The approach for bradycardia is clearly outlined in Chapter 2. Atropine 0.5 mg IV is tried twice. If there is no response, then isoproterenol is given by infusion. If the patient still does not respond, external pacing is instituted.

Chapter 2 also covers the treatment of ventricular tachycardia and ventricular fibrillation. Ventricular tachycardia is treated by cardioversion if vital signs are not maintained. Ventricular fibrillation is always treated by defibrillation. A very fine fibrillation can be coarsened by administration of epinephrine to increase the likelihood of successful defibrillation. A very fine fibrillation may also masquerade as asystole, especially on cursory examination; check carefully for fibrillatory waves, or even defibrillate, on the off-chance of a fine fibrillation.

In the case of ventricular fibrillation, an immediate defibrillation is essential; you may even defibrillate before beginning CPR. **If you defibrillate immediately and without hesitation, you will likely be successful, and native vital signs will be restored.** With each passing second of delay, the chance of defibrillation—and of a successful overall resuscitation—diminishes dramatically.

It is not uncommon to be at the nursing or monitoring station, to hear the alarms sound, and to see an EKG pattern of ventricular fibrillation. Some, if not most, of these occurrences may represent false alarms; a lead may have been disconnected from the patient, or the patient may be causing electrical interference, by brushing his teeth or shivering, for example. But some of these instances will be real and require immediate defibrillation—without delay or hesitation. The house officer may be timid regarding a procedure such as defibrillation. He must not be. Simply follow this sequence: (1) See if the patient is conscious. If he is conscious, then the EKG tracing is spurious. (2) Feel for a femoral or carotid pulse. **If you feel no pulse in an unconscious patient, with the EKG strip showing ventricular fibrillation, DEFIBRILLATE. Do not hesitate.** You cannot reasonably be criticized if you follow these simple guidelines. Rather, you may well save a life; hesitation will ensure a mortal outcome.

✚ PHARMACOLOGY OF RESUSCITATION

Aside from oxygen, only a handful of drugs are essential for resuscitation:[2]

- Sodium bicarbonate
- Atropine
- Lidocaine (or Amiodarone)
- Calcium chloride
- Epinephrine
- Norepinephrine (or Vasopressin)

These drugs are available on "code carts" in prepackaged syringes designed for rapid intravenous bolus administration. Table 11.1 lists the drugs, their prepackaged available forms, commonly used doses, useful actions, and unwanted side effects.

Sodium Bicarbonate

Sodium bicarbonate comes in 50-mL vials with 44 mEq per vial (almost 1 mEq/mL). The dose is 1 mL/kg body weight. This drug is used to correct the metabolic acidosis of cardiac arrest. Acidosis, of course, causes arrhythmias and impairs contractility. We commonly administer 2 ampules of sodium bicarbonate when arrest has been sustained more than a few minutes. Subsequent dosage is guided by arterial blood gas determination.

The house officer should note that acidosis in arrest usually results from a combination of metabolic (from anaerobic metabolism and lactic acid production) and respiratory factors. Vigorous ventilation will correct the respiratory component. It may also be advantageous

TABLE 11.1   Essential Drugs in Cardiac Arrest

Drug	Available Forms	Dose	Use(s)	Disadvantage(s)
Sodium bicarbonate (NaHCO₃)	50 mL ampule (44 mEq/ ampule)	1 mL/kg	Corrects acidosis	Considerable salt load
Atropine	0.4-0.5 mg/ mL (vial) or 1 mg/10 mL (ampule)	0.4-0.5 mg; repeat × 1 prn	Corrects bradycardia	
Lidocaine	100 mg/10 mL (ampule)	1 mg/kg	Corrects ventricular ectopy	Seizures, myocardial depression
Amiodarone		150 mg load 1 mg/min to follow	Corrects ventricular ectopy	Potent vasodilator, negative inotrope
Calcium chloride (CaCl)	1 g/10 mL (ampule)	2.5-10 mL	Augments contractility	Ventricular irritability
Epinephrine	1:10,000 solution (ampule)	1-10 mL	Augments contractility; restores electrical activity in asystole; enhances defibrillation	Ventricular irritability
Norepinephrine	4 mg/4 mL (ampule)	Give by continuous infusion at 0.02-0.2 μug/kg/min	Augments contractility; restores arteriolar tone and increases BP to improve coronary perfusion following restoration of cardiac rhythm	Generalized vasoconstriction, increased afterload
Vasopressin		1-2 units bolus	Increases blood pressure	Can overshoot and cause hypertension

to overventilate down to a low pCO_2 (25 to 30 mm Hg) to compensate for metabolic acidosis.

The main disadvantage of sodium bicarbonate is that it represents a major sodium load (1 ampule contains about as much sodium as a liter of D51/2NS). Also, overadministration of sodium bicarbonate may lead to alkalosis, with resultant hypokalemia and an unfavorable shift of the oxyhemoglobin dissociation curve. Furthermore, acidosis usually corrects quickly once effective circulation is restored. Routine administration of sodium bicarbonate in arrest situations has been questioned, but we favor use of this drug except in very brief circulatory interruptions. It is well known that inotropic medications (and even endogenous catecholamines) are ineffective in an acidotic milieu, and this is a major reason for our favoring bicarbonate use. Many centers continue frequent use of bicarbonate; however, we recommend that you guide therapy by blood gas determination rather than continuing routine administration at intervals, as was previously practiced.

Atropine

Atropine has been discussed in Chapter 2. It comes as 0.4 or 0.5 mg/mL in vials and as 1 mg/10 mL in prefilled syringes. The dose is 0.4 or 0.5 mg, repeated in several minutes if necessary. As discussed in Chapter 2, atropine is the first-line agent in the treatment of bradycardia.

Parasympatholytic side effects are not of priority in the desperate setting of cardiac arrest.

Lidocaine (or Amiodarone)

As discussed in Chapter 2, lidocaine has long been the mainstay of the treatment of ventricular ectopic beats. The dose is 1 mg/kg body weight, followed by a continuous infusion of 1 to 4 mg/min. In actual practice, we often give 100 mg in a single dose to an adult with a serious ventricular arrhythmia. This drug may be used in the setting of cardiac arrest to help prevent reversion to ventricular fibrillation after successful defibrillation. It may also be used to treat and prevent recurrence of ventricular tachycardia or to treat premature ventricular contractions following cardiac arrest.

Lidocaine will cause seizures in high doses. It can also suppress myocardial contractility.

Many authorities now favor amiodarone over lidocaine. In urgent situations, amiodarone is given IV in a 150 mg bolus (may repeat ×1), followed by a drip at 1 mg/min. β-blocking medications are also currently favored for their ability to discourage or suppress the tendency toward ventricular ectopic beats.

Calcium Chloride

Calcium chloride is used as described earlier for near arrest. Overuse will result in excessive ventricular irritability.

The appropriateness of calcium administration has recently been questioned. There has been ongoing concern about detrimental effects by calcium on injured cells. These recent investigations have led to removal of calcium from the American Heart Association's list of drugs recommended for resuscitation.[7-8] Nonetheless, many institutions, our own included, continue judicious use of this powerful inotrope.

Epinephrine

Epinephrine is discussed as a continuous infusion agent in Chapter 7. In cardiac arrest, it can be used as a bolus agent to augment myocardial contractility and to raise BP. It is effective also in restoring rhythm in asystole and in coarsening ventricular fibrillation to enhance defibrillation. On the code cart, epinephrine comes as a 1:10,000 solution in 10-cc automatic syringes. The dose is titrated to effect. From 1 to 10 mL can be given. Giving too much epinephrine will cause ventricular irritability and may precipitate ventricular fibrillation. **If we give you a full 1 mg of epinephrine (10 cc) in a single rapid bolus, there is a good chance you will fibrillate;** use discretion with this powerful inotrope, which has strong pro-arrhythmic tendencies.

Norepinephrine (or Vasopressin)

Norepinephrine can be very effective for adjunctive treatment in cardiac arrest. It is usually administered by continuous infusion during resuscitation to restore and maintain blood pressure after an effective heartbeat and ventilation have been established. Alternatively, a bolus of 1 to 2 units of vasopressin can be used to restore blood pressure immediately. Some evidence supports the administration of a massive dose of vasopressin (40 units) in an arrest setting. A continuous infusion of vasopressin may then follow, if necessary.

Other Drugs

A number of other drugs may be useful in cardiac arrest. Morphine may be given intravenously in 2-mg increments. This drug is useful, of course, in pulmonary edema. Morphine may help to alleviate the pain of an acute myocardial infarction. Morphine may be necessary as well for sedation in case of successful resuscitation.

Isoproterenol is useful for bradycardias. All the inotropic agents discussed in Chapter 7 may at times be useful.

Our recommendations in this chapter take into account standard guidelines but deviate in certain respects, reflecting our own experience and the particular setting of the postoperative cardiac ICU.

✚ CARDIAC ARREST IN SPECIFIC SETTINGS

Arrest Following Cardiac Surgery

Arrhythmia is a common cause of arrest following cardiac surgery. More often than not, the automatic EKG monitor or the nurse will be able to provide the information that an arrhythmia was the primary event.

Overdistention of the heart by injudicious fluid administration may lead to a vicious cycle of increased wall tension, increased oxygen requirement, decreased cardiac output, and decreased oxygen supply. Arrest may result. Fortunately, invasive hemodynamic monitoring helps to prevent this scenario.

Primary myocardial pump failure may lead to arrest. In some cases, the intra-aortic balloon pump may be needed as part of the resuscitative efforts.

Sudden onset of bleeding with cardiac tamponade is always a possibility in cardiac arrest following open heart surgery. In fact, in the first few hours following surgery, if an arrest is unexplained and ordinary measures are nonproductive, opening the chest for internal massage may be indicated to rule out or relieve tamponade. **After the first postoperative night has passed, bleeding is very unlikely, and resuscitation may be best performed externally.** When days have passed, bleeding is very unlikely; furthermore, the sternum may not open easily after several days. There are some exceptions, however, to the rule that bleeding occurs early; specifically, if the patient is being anticoagulated, especially with heparin, bleeding can occur at any point in the hospitalization, especially if an aortic graft is in place. This possibility may argue, in these special circumstances, in favor of an open approach to resuscitation.

A few more points regarding resuscitation in tamponade deserve emphasis. Even a slight decompression, say, improving stroke volume by even 10 cc, can improve cardiac output by nearly a liter (presuming a tachycardia of 100 bpm). A house officer without the experience (or perhaps the early confidence) to re-open the entire sternotomy can produce significant amelioration by simply opening the lowest stitches of the sternotomy closure. By opening the skin and linea alba, fluid under pressure will be released from the pericardial space; this may be just enough to restore hemodynamics until experienced help arrives. Remember, as well, that **imaging, even echocardiography, is unreliable for the diagnosis of tamponade in the postoperative setting, in which localized clots (as over the right atrium or the SVC or IVC) can produce localized, hemodynamically devastating tamponade.**

Arrest Following Thoracic Surgery

A number of problems may lead to cardiac arrest following noncardiac thoracic surgery. These include post-pneumonectomy space problems, intra-thoracic bleeding, tension pneumothorax, cardiac herniation, and lobar torsion. A detailed discussion of these problems is found in Chapter 19, Problems Following Noncardiac Thoracic Surgery.

Extraordinary salvage may be attained by properly administered resuscitative efforts. In our unit, we have had a number of patients survive following resuscitations as long as 2.5 hours. This is an entirely different setting than that of patients found irretrievable after unknown duration of arrest on the medical floors. The house officer may not understand the cardiac surgeon's persistence in some cases. It is the surgeon's prior experience that makes clear that survival is possible following apparently desperate circumstances and provides the impetus for vigorous continuation of efforts.

✚ RESUSCITATION BY CARDIOPULMONARY BYPASS (RESUSCITATION BY ECMO)

With the refinement of Seldinger over-the-wire techniques for cannulation, it has proved possible to cannulate both the femoral artery and vein percutaneously and use bedside cardiopulmonary bypass for cardiopulmonary resuscitation. Initial clinical success has been reported.[9] The circuit is that of a standard ECMO set-up (extracorporial membrane oxygenation), which is available in many ICUs.

If percutaneous institution of cardiopulmonary bypass continues to prove effective, this method may come to represent the ultimate form of resuscitation: oxygenation and circulation are maintained by the heart-lung machine while the native circulatory system is diagnosed and restored.

REFERENCES

1. Nuemar RW, Nolan JP, Adrie C, et al. Post cardiac arrest syndrome. *Circulation.* 2008;118:2452-2483.

2. Gunaydin B. Pharmacotherapy in cardiopulmonary resuscitation (CPR). *Turk J Med Sci.* 2005;35:357-364.

3. Mclntyre KM, Lewis AJ. *Textbook of Advanced Cardiac Life Support.* Dallas, TX: American Heart Association; 1981.

4. Elefteriades JA. Cardiopulmonary resuscitation. In: Baue AE, Geha AS, Hammond GL, Laks H, Naunheim KS, eds. *Glenn's Thoracic and Cardiovascular Surgery.* 5th ed. Norwalk, CT: Appleton & Lange; 1991.

5. Maier GW, Newton JR, Wolfe A, et al. The influence of manual chest compression rate on hemodynamic support during cardiac arrest: high-impulse cardiopulmonary resuscitation. *Circulation.* 1986;75 (Suppl IV):IV-51-59.

6. Garnett AR, Ornato JP, Gonzales ER, Johnson B. End-tidal carbon dioxide monitoring during cardiopulmonary resuscitation. *JAMA.* 1987;257:512-515.

7. Steuven HA, Thompson B, Aprahamian C, Darin JC. Use of calcium in prehospital cardiac arrest. *Ann Emerg Med.* 1983;12:136-139.

8. White BC, Winegar CD, Wilson RF, et al. Possible role of calcium blockers in cerebral resuscitation: a review of the literature and synthesis for future studies. *Crit Care Med.* 1983;11:202-207.

9. Phillips SJ, Ballentine B, Slonine D, et al. Percutaneous initiation of cardiopulmonary bypass. *Ann Thorac Surg.* 1983;36:223-225.

SUGGESTED FURTHER READING

Nuemar RW, Nolan JP, Adrie C, et al. Post cardiac arrest syndrome. *Circulation.* 2008;118:2452-2483.

This is highly recommended for the house officer with interest in and responsibility for ICU care.

Gunaydin B. Pharmacotherapy in cardiopulmonary resuscitation (CPR). *Turk J Med Sci.* 2005;35:357-364.

A good, up-to-date review. Well described and illustrated.

Masterson T, Rothenhaus T. *Emergency Medicine Pocket Survival Guides: CPR/ED for the Professional Rescuer: Participants Manual.* Red Cross. 2006.

Elefteriades JA. Cardiopulmonary resuscitation. In: Baue AE, Geha AS, Hammond GL, Laks H, Naunheim KS, eds. *Glenn's Thoracic and Cardiovascular Surgery.* 5th ed. Norwalk, CT: Appleton & Lange; 1991.
Traditional, fundamental recommendations.

McIntyre KM, Lewis AJ. *Textbook of Advanced Cardiac Life Support.* Dallas, TX: American Heart Association; 1981.
This is highly recommended for the house officer with interest in and responsibility for ICU care.

12

THORACIC IMAGING IN ACUTE DISEASE

D iagnostic imaging of thoracic organs has virtually exploded with powerful techniques in the last several decades. The present chapter will provide an overview of available techniques and their application in patients with acute cardiopulmonary disease. Specific references to diagnostic techniques are included as well in the chapters on particular disease entities.

✚ CXR

Having "grown up" in the age of advanced diagnostic imaging techniques, many of today's house officers underestimate the importance and power of the chest x-ray (CXR). The chest x-ray remains the gold standard for initial evaluation in the acute-care setting of the lungs (pneumothorax, hemothorax, pleural effusion, infiltrate, mass lesion, cavity, edema), the heart (cardiomegaly, pericardial fullness, congestive heart failure, herniation), the mediastinum (widening, pneumomediastinum), and the aorta (ascending aortic shadow, aortic knob, descending aortic shadow, widening, tortuosity). In addition, the chest x-ray confirms the position of lines,

The House Officer's Guide to ICU Care: Fundamentals of Management of the Heart and Lungs, 3rd ed. © 2013 John A. Elefteriades, Curtis Tribble, Alexander S. Geha, Mark D. Siegel, and Lawrence S. Cohen, eds. Cardiotext Publishing, ISBN: 978-1-935395-68-3.

drains, and tubes in the heart, great vessels, and pleural spaces. The cardiologist, the cardiac surgeon, and the pulmonologist rely heavily on the chest x-ray, from which, based on training and experience, they extract a tremendous amount of information. Respect the CXR and learn to glean the tremendous amount of information contained in it.

✚ ECHOCARDIOGRAPHY

Echocardiography offers a wealth of information, is available on an emergency basis, can be performed at the bedside, and is essentially risk-free. Vital information is provided about the pericardial space (effusion, clot, tamponade), the cardiac chambers (size, volume status, contractility of left and right ventricles, thrombus, masses), the cardiac valves (stenosis, regurgitation, masses, vegetations), and the aorta (atheroma, dilatation, dissection). With the advent of transesophageal echocardiography, which can also be performed portably at the bedside in critically ill ICU patients, even more complete, high-quality, and precise images can be obtained than with the surface echo (Figure 12.1). The aorta is especially well visualized. Biplane and omniplane probes are now available that improve even more the accuracy and scope of the transesophageal images.

It is important to keep in mind certain specific limitations of echocardiography as regards acute ICU care:

- Windows for transthoracic echocardiography can be difficult early after cardiac surgery.
- Tamponade can be very localized, without standard echocardiographic manifestations, early after cardiac surgery.
- Gaining access for transesophageal echocardiography can be difficult in the early postoperative phase due to edema of the mouth, tongue, and pharynx.

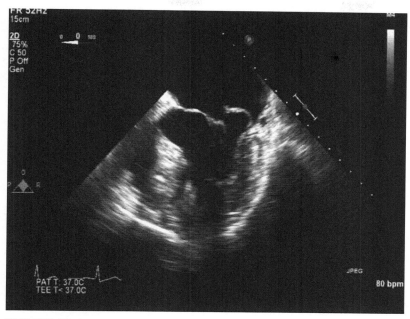

FIGURE 12.1

Transesophageal echo demonstrating flail mitral leaflet (indicated).

✚ CT SCAN

In the cardiothoracic acute-care setting, computerized axial tomography (CT scan) is most useful for the evaluation of the pleural space (effusion, hemorrhage) and of the aorta (Figure 12.2). The CT scan, of course, is not a bedside test. Intravenous radiographic contrast, with its attendant risks (hypersensitivity reaction, volume overload from osmotic expansion of the intravascular space, acute tubular necrosis), is usually required. Exciting multiplane reconstructions are being applied to CT scans, and dramatically detailed aortic images can be obtained; CT coronary angiography is now entering its own as a potential alternative to standard catheterization laboratory coronary angiography.

The house officer should also not underestimate the risks of a "road trip" to the x-ray department in a critically ill patient. Tubes

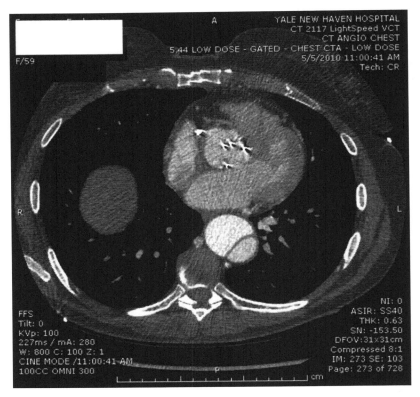

FIGURE 12.2

CT scan demonstrating descending aortic dissection. Note two lumens separated by intimal flap.

and wires can get hooked on doorknobs, and monitoring and treating the patient can be difficult and suboptimal; the house officer must evaluate carefully the risks and benefits of an imaging study before setting sail for the dark corridors of the radiology department.

✚ MRI

Magnetic resonance imaging (MRI) has in recent years been applied to cardiac and aortic imaging and has proved to be a very powerful technique. The cardiac anatomy is visualized with a detail and clarity rivaled only by direct operative exposure (see Figure 12.3). Chamber size and wall thickness, especially of the left ventricle, are beautifully displayed. Ventricular function can be assessed. The aorta is precisely displayed throughout its extent. No radiopaque contrast is required. Images can be obtained in multiple planes (coronal, sagittal, axial, and various obliques). Exciting three-dimensional reconstructions can be performed. Dynamic images, in which heart function can be observed "in motion" and "beat by beat," can be viewed on a computer. MRI, of course, cannot be performed portably, but requires transport of the patient to the protected MRI suite. Metallic foreign bodies in the chest may contraindicate MRI scanning because of the danger of displacement by the magnetic field or induction of internal electric currents. Metallic vessel clips used during surgery and sternal wires generally do not interfere with MRI, but pacemaker or defibrillator hardware and bullet fragments may do so.

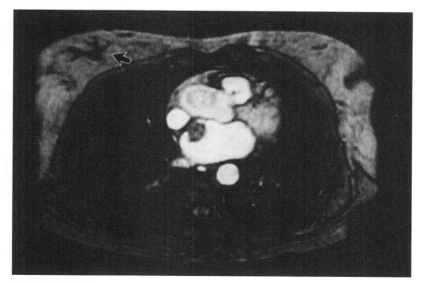

FIGURE 12.3

MRI image of intracardiac tumor (myxoma in left atrium; indicated).

These are the diagnostic imaging techniques available to the house officer to complement his or her assessment of the critically ill cardiopulmonary ICU patient.

Special Note: Aortic Imaging in the Present Era

The cardiologist and the cardiac surgeon have long considered angiography the optimal tool for evaluation of the aorta for aneurysm or dissection, especially in the critically ill patient. Aortic imaging has passed through a transition phase in which aortography has been superseded by other powerful modern imaging techniques.

CT scan has been used clinically for decades for aortic imaging. With the use of contrast, the aorta is well demonstrated, but traditionally only in the axial plane. CT imaging in coronal and sagittal planes is now feasible, although image quality often is suboptimal outside of the standard axial planes. In the case of aneurysm, aortic dimension, wall thickness, and thrombus are well visualized. Size estimation is hampered at the level of the aortic arch, where the axial plane of the CT scan cuts the aorta obliquely, exaggerating the dimensions.[1-2] In the case of dissection, CT scan clearly demonstrates the dissection planes—in fact, with considerably greater sensitivity than angiography.[3-5] CT scan also excels at diagnosing traumatic aortic injury and has replaced angiopraphy as the technique of choice.

MRI provides unparalleled imaging of the thoracic aorta, without radiopaque contrast medium. In aneurysm disease, dimensions of the aorta are clearly seen, without the axial limitations of CT scanning. In dissection, the true and false lumens and the intervening flap are visualized and their respective flow patterns are demonstrated.

MRI is becoming a preferred modality for aortic imaging, challenging CT scanning. MRI offers a clarity of image that rivals angiography. The images of MRI can be taken in any plane preferred by the radiologist or clinician. The whole aorta can be displayed at one

time in one image in the sagittal or coronal perspective, in contradistinction to aortography, in which only a short portion of the
aorta is opacified by a specific bolus of dye. Figures 12.4 to 12.6
demonstrate the imaging power of the MRI technique.

We tend to prefer CT scan in the critically ill patient, because it
is usually more easily and promptly available, and because the patient care staff has better access to the patient in the CT scanner
than in the metal-protected MRI suite.

Transesophageal echocardiography, especially with multiplane
probes, provides immediate and sensitive information regarding
aortic emergencies at very little risk. Experience with ruling out
traumatic aortic injury is growing; a good view of the luminal surface of the aorta at the aortic isthmus is routinely obtained. Transesophageal echo is proving sensitive and specific for aortic dissection.

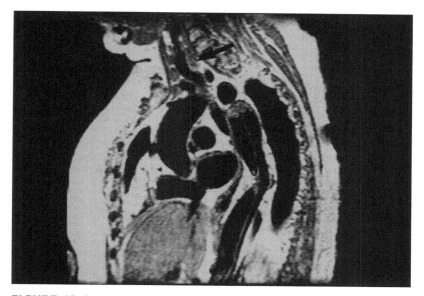

FIGURE 12.4

MRI image of descending aortic dissection (indicated). Note how nearly
the entire thoracic aorta can be displayed on one image.

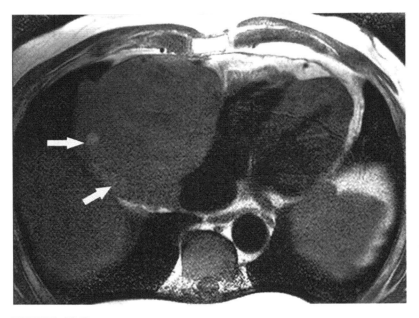

FIGURE 12.5

MRI 3-dimensional image of massive cardiac tumor (teratoma).

Source: Reprinted with permission from Sparrow PJ, Kurian JB, Jones TR, Sivananthan M. MR imaging of cardiac tumors. *Radiographics.* 2005;25: 1255-1276.

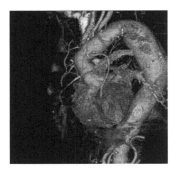

FIGURE 12.6

MRI 3-dimensional reconstruction of aneurysmal descending aorta.

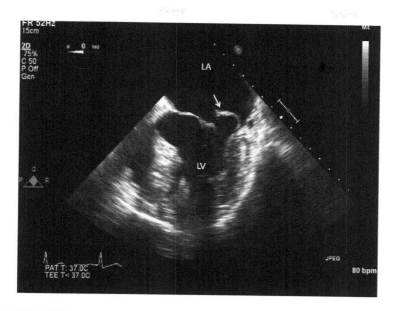

FIGURE 12.7

Transesophageal echo demonstrating ascending aortic dissection. Note two lumens separated by flap.

In acute aortic dissection, we commonly perform echocardiography at the bedside in the ICU and move directly to the operating room without any further tests when the diagnosis is confirmed (Figure 12.7).

Multiple studies have defined the relative roles of these powerful tests in aortic imaging for trauma, aneurysm, and dissection.[3-5] In cases of aortic dissection, a common issue for house officers, all three of these techniques have sensitivities and specificities in the 98% or higher range.

Figures 12.8 to 12.11 present some valuable specifics regarding aortic imaging that will be of use to the house officer.

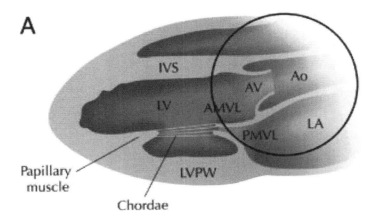

Parasternal long-axis view

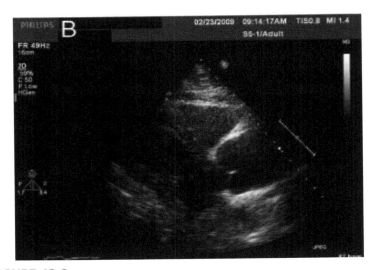

FIGURE 12.8

Limitations of transthoracic echocardiography. Limited distance above the aortic valve (AV) for which the ascending aorta (Ao) can be seen on transthoracic echocardiography. Schematic (**A**) and actual echocardiographic (**B**) image. AMVL = anterior mitral valve leaflet; IVS = interventricular septum; LA = left atrium; LV = left ventricle; LVPW = left ventricular posterior wall.

Source: Panel A illustration by Rob Flewell. Elefteriades JA, Farkas EA. Thoracic aortic aneurysm: clinically pertinent controversies and uncertainties. *J Am Coll Cardiol.* 2010;55:841-857. With permission from Elsevier.

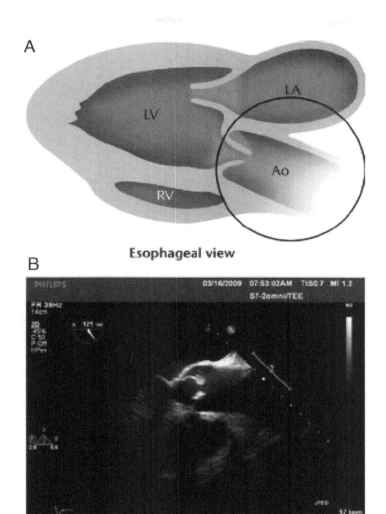

FIGURE 12.9

Limitations of transesophageal echocardiography. Limited distance above the aortic valve for which the ascending aorta can be seen on transesophageal echocardiography. The tracheal air column interferes with visualization of the upper ascending aorta. Schematic (**A**) and actual echocardiographic image (**B**). RV = right ventricle; other abbreviations as in Figure 12.8.

Source: Panel A illustration by Rob Flewell. Elefteriades JA, Farkas EA. Thoracic aortic aneurysm: clinically pertinent controversies and uncertainties. *J Am Coll Cardiol.* 2010;55:841-857. With permission from Elsevier.

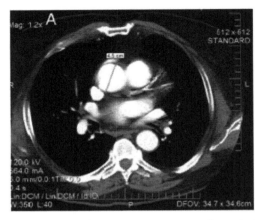

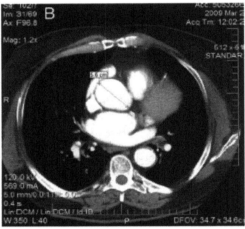

FIGURE 12.10

Limitations of axial imaging. Difficulty in determining whether a given axial computed tomography (CT) image is still in the aorta or passing partially through the aorta and the left ventricular (LV) outflow track. This factor can lead to gross misinterpretations of aortic diameter. (**A**) and (**B**) differ by only 1 CT level, yet yield markedly different diameters. Is **Panel B** still in the aorta? Does it represent the dimension at the sinuses, or does it run obliquely through both aorta and LV outflow tract? It can be difficult or impossible to ascertain these answers when a purely axial technique is used.

Source: Reproduced with permission from Elefteriades JA, Farkas EA. Thoracic aortic aneurysm: clinically pertinent controversies and uncertainties. *J Am Coll Cardiol.* 2010;55:841-857. With permission from Elsevier.

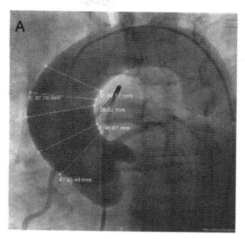

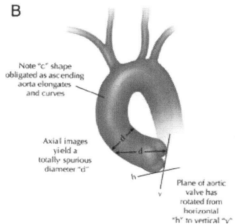

FIGURE 12.11

Confounding of ascending aortic measurements due to elongation and C shape of ascending aorta. Aortogram (**A**) and schematic (**B**) showing gross elongation of the ascending aorta, forcing the aorta into a C shape and obligating the aortic valve to take a nearly vertical plane of orientation. On an axial CT image, this common anatomy would markedly confound measurement of proximal aortic diameter. Note the difference between a horizontal diameter (as in an axial image) and a diameter perpendicular to the long axis of the aorta.

Source: Figure illustration by Rob Flewell. Elefteriades JA, Farkas EA. Thoracic aortic aneurysm: clinically pertinent controversies and uncertainties. *J Am Coll Cardiol.* 2010;55:841-857. With permission from Elsevier.

REFERENCES

1. Elefteriades JA, Hartleroad J, Gusberg RT, et al. Long-term experience with descending aortic dissection: the complication-specific approach. *Ann Thorac Surg.* 1992;53:11-21.
2. Elefteriades JA, Farkas EA. Thoracic aortic aneurysm: clinically pertinent controversies and uncertainties. *J Am Coll Cardiol.* 2010;55: 841-857.
3. Shiga T, Wajima Z, Apfel CC, Inoue T, Ohe T. Diagnostic accuracy of transesophageal echocardiography, helical computed tomography, and magnetic resonance imaging for suspected thoracic aortic dissection: systematic review and meta-analysis. *Arch Intern Med.* 2006;166:1350-1356.
4. Nienaber CA, von Kodolitsh Y, Nicolas V, et al. The diagnosis of thoracic aortic dissection by noninvasive imaging procedures. *N Engl J Med.* 1993;328:1-9.
5. Cigarroa JE, Isselbacher EM, De Sanctis RW, Eagle KA. Diagnostic imaging in the evaluation of suspected aortic dissection: old standards and new directions. *N Engl J Med.* 1993;328:35-43.

SUGGESTED FURTHER READING

Elefteriades JA, Farkas EA. Thoracic aortic aneurysm: clinically pertinent controversies and uncertainties. *J Am Coll Cardiol.* 2010;55:841-857. A full review of the strengths and limitations of various imaging techniques for aortic aneurysms and dissections.

MANAGEMENT OF ACUTE CORONARY ISCHEMIA

written with **John K. Forrest, MD**
Section of Cardiovascular Medicine,
Yale University School of Medicine

The acute coronary ischemic syndromes are comprised of unstable angina, acute non-ST-segment elevation myocardial infarction, and ST-segment elevation myocardial infarction (see Table 13.1). Each of these syndromes requires acute hospital care. Furthermore, rapid diagnosis and treatment are essential to saving cardiac muscle—and saving lives. As they say, "time is muscle" with these syndromes. This chapter will describe the etiology and management of each of these cardiac emergencies. The emphasis is on basic understanding of the ischemic syndromes and on the general patterns of care with which the house officer must be familiar in order to initiate appropriate and prompt treatment.

TABLE 13.1   Acute Ischemic Syndromes

- Unstable angina
- Acute non-ST-segment elevation myocardial infarction (NSTEMI)
- Acute ST-segment elevation myocardial infarction (STEMI)

The House Officer's Guide to ICU Care: Fundamentals of Management of the Heart and Lungs, 3rd ed. © 2013 John A. Elefteriades, Curtis Tribble, Alexander S. Geha, Mark D. Siegel, and Lawrence S. Cohen, eds. Cardiotext Publishing, ISBN: 978-1-935395-68-3.

✚ UNSTABLE ANGINA AND ACUTE NON-ST-SEGMENT ELEVATION MYOCARDIAL INFARCTION

The diagnosis of unstable angina rests on several clinical features: (1) new-onset angina, which is often brought on by minimal exertion and significantly limits activity; (2) the transition from a stable exertion-related anginal pattern to angina that is more frequent, lasts longer, and occurs with less exertion; or (3) angina at rest that frequently lasts more than 20 minutes in duration. These categories reflect new onset of angina or worsening of an established anginal pattern. Angina at rest presents a worrisome situation, as coronary blood supply is inadequate even in the baseline state without the increased demands of physical exertion.

The spectrum of patients represented by the preceding criteria is of course quite broad. Many patients have stable angina for years with little or no change in their anginal pattern. Without apparent reason, the stable pattern may become unstable.

The diagnosis of an acute non-ST-segment elevation myocardial infarction (NSTEMI) differs from that of unstable angina in that it is accompanied by a rise in cardiac enzymes (troponin) due to myocardial cell injury. **Because troponins may not be elevated for up to 6 hours after presentation, unstable angina and acute NSTEMI frequently cannot be distinguished on initial presentation, and thus their initial management is similar.**

Serial coronary angiograms before and after the onset of accelerating angina often show a significant progression in a stenotic lesion, which may be due to plaque fissuring or rupture. These findings suggest that plaque rupture can change the geometric shape of the plaque, thereby increasing the degree of stenosis. The development of rest angina suggests the presence of a partially occlusive thrombus at the site of plaque fissure. The presence of a thrombus explains the phenomenon that angina can wax and wane, as the clot may undergo spontaneous thrombolysis. It also explains the progression of unstable angina to myocardial infarction if the clot becomes totally occlusive. In addition to plaque fissuring and thrombosis, vasoconstriction plays a role in the clinical presentation of patients with unstable angina. Quantitative angiography has demonstrated abnormalities in coronary artery tone in patients with unstable angina. Alterations in coronary tone at the site of plaques may initiate thrombosis and in turn lead to more spasm secondary to the release of thromboxane A_2, serotonin, prostanoids, and platelet-derived growth factor. **Whereas patients with stable angina develop symptoms due to an increase in myocardial oxygen demand, patients with unstable angina develop symptoms due to a dynamic decrease in myocardial oxygen delivery.** Symptoms are therefore unpredictable and may occur at rest. The triad of plaque fissuring, thrombosis, and coronary vasospasm interact to make unstable angina a most serious and compelling syndrome.

The chest discomfort associated with unstable angina may be similar to that of patients with stable angina but is often more severe and more prolonged, and may come on at rest. At times it will wake patients from their sleep. Rest and the administration of sublingual nitroglycerin will often afford only temporary relief. There is no necessary relationship to exertion. **In unstable angina and in acute NSTEMI, the electrocardiogram will frequently display transient ST-segment depression or prominent T-wave inversions.** These changes may revert to normal after the relief of pain.

Through the Thrombolysis in Myocardial Infarction (TIMI) 11B and ESSENCE[1-2] studies, 7 independent factors were identified that predict outcome in patients with unstable angina or an acute NSTEMI. Each risk factor is given a score of 1 if present or 0 if absent. A score of 0 to 1 is considered low risk, 2 to 3 intermediate risk, and 4 to 7 high risk (Table 13.2). A higher TIMI risk score is associated with increased events at 2 weeks, including all-cause mortality, new or recurrent myocardial infarction (MI), or severe recurrent ischemia requiring revascularization. Patients with TIMI risk score of 0 or 1 have a 4.7% risk of having an event within 2

TABLE 13.2 TIMI Risk Score

- Age > 65
- Presence of at least three risk factors for coronary artery disease (hypertension, diabetes, hyperlipidemia, current smoker, or positive family history of an early MI)
- Prior coronary stenosis of > 50%
- Presence of ST-segment deviation > 0.5 mm on admission EKG
- At least 2 anginal episodes in prior 24 hours
- Elevated serum cardiac markers
- Use of aspirin in prior 7 days

weeks; score of 2, 8.3%; score of 3, 13%; score of 4, 20%; score of 5, 26%; and score of 6 or greater 41%.[3]

The pathophysiology of patients with unstable angina and acute NSTEMI includes changes related to the underlying coronary atherosclerosis, platelet aggregation, thrombosis, coronary spasm, and often plaque rupture.[4-7] Appropriate management of these syndromes therefore must be directed toward a multifactorial approach that addresses these pathophysiologic mechanisms.

Unstable angina and acute NSTEMI are serious conditions, and patients with these diagnoses should be admitted to the hospital. Certain general supportive measures are important. Assessment of the patient's hemodynamic status, initiation of antithrombotic therapy, relief of ischemic pain, choice of management strategy (invasive versus medical), and the display to the patient of a competent hospital staff are all beneficial. An intravenous line should be placed and the patient should have continuous electrocardiographic monitoring.

Anticoagulants and antiplatelet agents are cornerstones of effective therapy (see Table 13.3). In the absence of an absolute contraindication, antiplatelet therapy is indicated in all patients with a

TABLE 13.3. Management of Unstable Angina

- Anticoagulants and antiplatelet drugs (heparin, aspirin, and clopidogrel)
- Nitrates
- β-blockers
- Decision regarding early interventional vs non-interventional approach
- No role for thrombolytic therapy

unstable angina and non-ST-segment elevation myocardial infarction.[8] If the patient is not taking aspirin when first seen in the emergency department, 325 mg of aspirin should be either chewed or swallowed. In addition to aspirin, patients presenting with unstable angina or acute NSTEMI should be started on intravenous unfractionated heparin. A bolus of 70 to 100 U/kg will saturate heparin receptors in the liver and elsewhere. This should be followed by a dose ranging from approximately 1000 U/h to 1300 U/h, depending on patient size and aimed at keeping the activated partial thromboplastin time (aPTT) at 2.0 to 2.5 times control. An as alternative to unfractionated heparin, low-molecular weight heparins (eg, enoxaparin) have been shown to have similar effectiveness. Thienopyridines (eg, clopidogrel) have also been shown in multiple studies to have additive benefits in combination with aspirin therapy. In the CURE trial,[9] which randomly assigned patients presenting within 24 hours after the onset of an acute NSTEMI, it was found that the combination of aspirin and clopidogrel (300 mg loading dose followed by 75 mg daily) led to fewer myocardial infarctions (5.2% vs 6.7%), although there was a slight increase in major bleeding (3.7% vs 2.7%). The patients who derived the greatest risk from clopidogrel were those with higher TIMI risk scores. Patients presenting with unstable angina and acute NSTEMI should thus be loaded with 300 to 600 mg of clopidogrel and thereafter started on 75 mg of clopidogrel daily. Clopidogrel should be continued for at least 1 month and ideally for up to 1 year after myocardial infarction. Given the increased risk of surgical bleeding on clopidogrel, clopidogrel should be withheld for 5 to 7 days prior to planned coronary artery bypass graft surgery (CABG) if possible (although this is controversial).

Nitrate therapy is also indicated in the treatment of a patient with unstable angina or acute NSTEMI. Sublingual, oral, topical, or intravenous administration is helpful in relieving the vasospastic component and in reducing left ventricular preload and afterload. If sublingual, oral, or transdermal nitroglycerin, individually or in concert, do not provide pain relief, then intravenous nitroglycerin should be started. A starting dose is usually 0.5 µg/kg/min, but this dose may be increased sequentially to as much as 5 µg/kg/min. Hypotension is usually the limiting factor. It is remarkable how much intravenous nitroglycerin may be tolerated by a patient. The dose of 5 µg is equal to a sublingual nitroglycerin tablet. Therefore patients being administered this dose of intravenous nitroglycerin are taking the equivalent of a sublingual nitroglycerin tablet each minute. Pharmacologic tolerance to intravenous nitroglycerin therapy may start to develop after 24 hours.

β-blockers have a valuable role in the treatment of patients with unstable angina and acute non-ST-segment elevation myocardial infarction. This is particularly true if the resting heart rate is 75 or above. Metoprolol (Lopressor) 15 mg IV divided into 3 equal doses or intravenous propranolol (1 mg boluses) to a total of 10 to 12 mg will begin to achieve a bradycardic response. Sufficient follow-up oral therapy should be delivered with the goal of keeping the resting heart rate between 55 and 65 beats per minute. The only limitation of the preceding program is the patient with hypotension or congestive heart failure. In the former case, sufficient fluids should be administered to ensure that the patient is not hypovolemic; in the latter instance, diuretics and afterload reduction should be administered to help control the congestive heart failure.

There has been considerable debate concerning whether there is a role for early thrombolytic therapy in patients with unstable angina or NSTEMI. The TIMI IIIA trial addressed this question by randomizing patients with the preceding syndromes into either a tissue plasminogen activator (t-PA) or a placebo arm.[10] The results showed no difference in the major outcomes (death or myocardial infarction) or in the secondary outcomes (evidence of residual ischemia by Holter or exercise tests). There is an increased risk of significant bleeding with t-PA, and therefore the current recommendation for patients with unstable angina or acute NSTEMI does not include the use of thrombolytics.

The role of early cardiac catheterization in the setting of unstable angina or acute NSTEMI compared with a course of medical management and watchful waiting has been evaluated in several studies. The results demonstrated that for the 2 primary end points—death and myocardial infarction—there was no difference between the 2 strategies. However, patients subjected to early cardiac catheterization were found to have less residual ischemia during stress tests obtained 6 weeks after the initial event.[11-12] Given these findings, it is recommended that **patients who present with unstable angina or acute non-ST-segment elevation myocardial infarction (NSTEMI) who have ongoing pain, persistent ST-segment or T-wave changes, or hemodynamic abnormalities be referred for urgent catheterization if available.**

In the preceding discussion, patients with unstable angina or acute non-ST-segment elevation myocardial infarction have been considered together, as it is often impossible to distinguish between them until the troponin assay returns. Because the troponin assay may be initially negative and not turn positive for up to 6 to 8 hours after presentation, initial clinical management of the 2 conditions is very similar.

✚ ACUTE ST-SEGMENT ELEVATION MYOCARDIAL INFARCTION

The diagnosis of acute ST-segment elevation myocardial infarction (STEMI) is made by the triad of clinical history, the presence of ST-segment elevation on the EKG (Figure 13.1), and a rise in serum cardiac enzymes.

Despite advances in diagnostic examinations to detect acute myocardial infarction, the history remains a pivotal diagnostic tool. Although a small number of patients with acute myocardial infarction may feel no pain, the vast majority of patients do have clear-cut symptomatic evidence that there is a major calamity. The pain is generally substernal, although it may begin in the epigastrium. It builds to a climax and does not recede. It may radiate to the

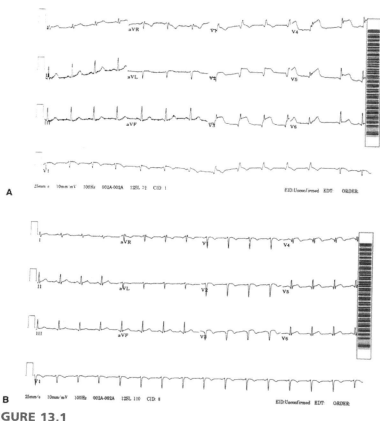

FIGURE 13.1

Panel A: EKG of a 48-year-old woman with acute anterior-wall myocardial infarction. **Panel B:** EKG of the same patient 1 day later with evolution of anterior-wall myocardial infarction.

shoulders, jaw, or arms. The patient is likely to remain still, for even small movement seems to exacerbate the discomfort. Nausea and vomiting occur in half of all patients with acute myocardial infarction. Other symptoms include weakness, dizziness, exhaustion, and at times hiccups. Syncope may at times be the presenting symptom, possibly reflecting ventricular arrhythmias.

The physical examination of the patient experiencing an acute myocardial infarction is important (see Table 13.4). Patients are

TABLE 13.4 Common Findings on Physical Examination in Acute Myocardial Infarction

These items should direct the house officer's examination.
- General: state of distress
- Respiratory: dyspnea, orthopnea, cyanosis
- Pulse: tachycardia (unless on prior β-blocker Rx)
- BP: mild hypotension
- Carotid pulse: small volume
- Jugular venous pulse: distended veins, prominent a wave, prominent v wave (tricuspid regurgitation)
- Cardiac auscultation and palpation: systolic murmur (mitral regurgitation), extra third or fourth heart sound or impulse (left ventricular failure), friction rub (transmural infarction [early] or pericarditis [later])

uniformly distressed and uncomfortable. They may be restless or remain perfectly still. Patients with acute left ventricular failure will sit up, gasp for breath, and have a dusky hue. There is generally a tachycardia, except in patients who have been taking a β-blocker or in those who are having an inferior-wall myocardial infarction, in which case there may be vagally induced bradycardia. There may be a range of blood pressure responses. In general, the blood pressure will be lower than is normal for the patient prior to the onset of myocardial infarction. In some patients, however, because of a profound adrenergic response, systolic hypertension will be present. The carotid pulse will often be small in volume but sharp in its upstroke. The small volume reflects a diminished stroke volume. The jugular venous pulse may be normal, but certain circumstances may lead to abnormalities. In the presence of left ventricular failure, the jugular venous pressure may be elevated, with particular accentuation of the a wave due to atrial contraction against a noncompliant right ventricle. In the presence of functional or anatomic tricuspid regurgitation, there may be large v waves. In right ventricular infarction, the jugular venous pressure will be elevated, as it will be in cardiogenic shock. Palpation of the heart may reveal a presystolic impulse coincident with a fourth heart sound. If there is cardiac decompensation, an outward movement of the left ventricle may be palpated in early diastole coincident with a third heart sound. The first heart sound is often muffled because of a decrease in left ventricular contractility. Also, if there is prolongation of the PR interval, the first heart sound will be soft. The second heart sound may be paradoxically split if there is isolated left ventricular dysfunction. The presence of a third or fourth heart sound denotes left ventricular dysfunction. A murmur of mitral regurgitation may be heard if there is papillary muscle dysfunction. A pericardial friction rub may be present, especially if there is a transmural myocardial infarction. Friction rubs may be evanescent and may require frequent auscultation in order to be heard. A friction rub may be heard on the first day, but more commonly it is heard on day 2 or 3. A friction rub heard for the first time several weeks after myocardial infarction is more likely a feature of the postmyocardial infarction syndrome.

The pathologic sequence of myocardial infarction involves ischemia, injury, and necrosis; the electrocardiographic representations of these (respectively) are T wave changes, ST-segment elevation, and the development of Q waves (see Table 13.5). Although there is usually little problem in diagnosing an acute transmural anterior- or inferior-wall infarction, there is less certainty when an infarction involves the lateral wall or posterior wall or is subendocardial (or nontransmural) in location. In the past, the development of a Q wave was the criterion for calling a myocardial infarction transmural, and the lack of development of a Q wave denoted a nontransmural or subendocardial infarction. Pathologic studies have demonstrated that patients with transmural myocardial infarction may not develop Q waves and that a patient developing only ST- and T-wave changes may have transmural necrosis pathologically. Nevertheless, in terms of prognosis, the development or lack of development of Q waves does serve a useful purpose. In patients who ultimately are diagnosed as having sustained a myocardial infarction, the initial electrocardiogram is diagnostic in approximately 50% of patients, abnormal but not diagnostic in approximately

TABLE 13.5 General Significance of Basic EKG Findings in Ischemia and Myocardial Infarction

EKG Finding	Pathological Implication
T-wave inversion	Ischemia
ST-segment elevation	Injury
Q waves	Infarction

35%, and normal in about 15%. The obtainment of serial electrocardiograms increases the diagnostic sensitivity to about 95%.

The earliest change in a classical electrocardiogram of myocardial infarction is an abnormal T wave. The T wave may be prolonged, increased in magnitude, or inverted. This is followed by ST-segment elevation in leads facing the area of injury and ST-segment depression in the reciprocal leads (Figure 13.1A). A Q wave may be present on the initial electrocardiogram or may develop on subsequent tracings (Figures 13.1B, 13.2). In patients who have had previous cardiac events, the diagnostic accuracy of the electrocardiogram poses problems. If there has been a previous transmural myocardial infarction, recognition of new injury in the same region is sometimes difficult. The presence of a left bundle branch block virtually precludes the diagnosis of a new anterior-wall infarction. The presence of conduction abnormalities, left ventricular hypertrophy, or electrolyte abnormalities may make recognition of an acute infarction difficult. The diagnosis of a nontransmural myocardial infarction may be even more difficult, for changes in the ST- and T-wave segments are nonspecific. They may occur in a variety of conditions, including stable and unstable angina pectoris, ventricular hypertrophy, pericarditis, early repolarization, electrolyte abnormalities, and treatment with digitalis. In unstable angina, the deeper the ST-segment depression and the longer it lasts, the more likely is the diagnosis of myocardial infarction. For all the preceding reasons, the diagnosis of myocardial infarction sometimes rests on the pattern of serum cardiac enzymes.

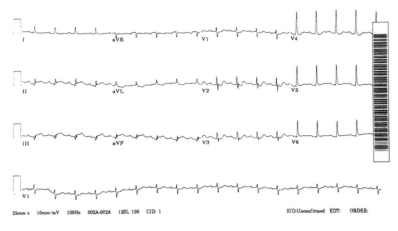

FIGURE 13.2

EKG of a 68-year-old man with acute inferior-wall myocardial infarction.

Note the ST-segment elevation in leads II, III, and a VF. Irreversibly damaged myocardial cells release a variety of enzymes into the circulation. These enzymes act as markers of myocardial necrosis and, in concert with the history and electrocardiogram, confirm the diagnosis. They are rarely of immediate value when the patient first presents, because it takes some time for the markers to reach elevated values in the bloodstream. The most specific of the cardiac biomarkers is troponin. Cardiac troponin I and troponin T are proteins that control the interaction of actin and myosin. **During myocardial ischemia and cell death, troponin is released and can be measured.** Unlike other biomarkers, troponin I appears to be expressed only in the heart and thus a significant rise in cardiac troponin is diagnostic of myocardial injury. While troponin T is also expressed in skeletal muscle, the current assay used to measure troponin T does not detect skeletal muscle forms of the protein and thus is also very specific. Troponins can be detected within 3 to 12 hours of myocardial infarction and peak at 18 to 24 hours (Table 13.6). Compared to the other biomarkers discussed below, troponins also remain present for the longest period of time and can be detected for up to 10 days. (Remember that cardiac biomarkers are released normally during open heart surgery from manipulation and instrumentation of the heart, and their detection after surgery does not carry the same significance as in an ambulatory patient being seen in the emergency department.)

Serum creatine kinase, particularly the myocardial-specific CK-MB isoenzyme, is also useful in establishing the diagnosis of myocardial infarction. Serum CK activity exceeds the normal range within 4 to 8 hours following the onset of acute myocardial infarction. The time to peak CK activity varies somewhat. In patients with neither spontaneous reperfusion nor reperfusion in response to thrombolytic therapy, the peak is at 14 to 24 hours. If there has been reperfusion, CK and CK-MB peak within the first 8 to 10 hours. The timing of the CK collection is quite important. If the patient delays coming to the hospital, the CK level may have already peaked and returned to normal levels. If there is a delay in obtaining CK levels after the patient arrives at the hospital, the abnormal levels may have already abated. It must be recognized that CK elevations may occur in patients with muscle disease, alcohol intoxication, diabetes mellitus, skeletal muscle trauma, vigorous exercise, convulsions, and intramuscular injections. (The same caveats in interpretation after cardiac surgery apply for CK as for troponin.)

For many years, the activity of serum glutamic oxaloacetic acid transaminase (SGOT) was measured. This enzyme is now called aspartate aminotransferase (AST). Levels rise above normal 8 to 12 hours after the onset of chest pain, peak at 18 to 36 hours, and generally fall to normal in 3 to 4 days. This enzyme has not proved to be of great use, as it is elevated in the face of hepatic or skeletal muscle disease, following intramuscular injections, and with shock. Lactic dehydrogenase (LDH), which exceeds the normal range by 24 to 48 hours after the onset of acute myocardial infarction and reaches a peak 3 to 6 days after the onset of this infarct, has in the past also been used to help in diagnosis of myocardial infarction; however, in the setting of newer troponin assays, its use is not of added benefit.

TABLE 13.6 Serum Biomarkers of Myocardial Infarction

	Time Detectable	Time of Peak Elevation	Comments
Troponin I and T	3-12 hours	18-24 hours	Current standard for diagnosis, because of specificity and early onset Remain elevated the longest (up to 10 days)
CK-MB	4-8 hours	14-24 hours	The standard in the pre-troponin era
LDH	24-48 hours	3-6 days	Historical interest
AST (formerly SGOT)	8-12 hours	18-36 hours	Historical interest

The initial diagnosis of a myocardial infarction must be made based on the history and the presenting electrocardiogram. The physician must then make critical judgments concerning early therapy. Because treatment (either thrombolytic therapy or coronary angioplasty) is most useful when performed early, and because efficacy diminishes when administration is delayed, **correct early diagnosis is essential. Again, "time is muscle."** Conversely, a number of conditions that may simulate myocardial infarction—such as acute aortic dissection, acute pericarditis, perforated ulcer, or cholecystitis—may be converted into lethal problems by the inappropriate administration of thrombolytics.

The treatment of patients with acute ST-segment elevation myocardial infarction should focus on (1) relieving ischemic pain, (2) assessment of the hemodynamic state and correction of abnormalities that are present, (3) antithrombotic therapy, (4) β-blocker administration, and (5) initiation of reperfusion therapy with primary percutaneous coronary intervention (PCI) or thrombolysis. This paradigm is similar to that for NSTEMI with the exception that **reperfusion therapy is added for STEMI.** The usage of aspirin and heparin in STEMI is also critically important, and these drugs should be administered immediately, as reviewed previously in the discussion of acute NSTEMI. It has also been demonstrated that the administration of clopidogrel in addition to aspirin in the setting of acute myocardial infarction has added benefit. The PCI-CLARITY study randomized patients presenting with acute myocardial infarction to receive clopidogrel pretreatment versus no clopidogrel pretreatment.[13] At 30-day follow-up, there was found to be a significant reduction in the primary end point of cardiovascular death, MI, or stroke (6.2% in the no pretreatment group versus 3.6% in the clopidogrel group). As a result, it is recommended that patients presenting with a STEMI be given a 300- or 600-mg loading dose of clopidogrel. In addition to antithrombotic medications (aspirin, heparin, and clopidogrel), the use of nitrates and β-blockers is similar for STEMI and acute NSTEMI and has been reviewed earlier in this chapter. **A primary difference in the treatment of STEMI as compared to NSTEMI or unstable angina is that patients with a STEMI require emergent definitive therapy (PCI or thrombolytics) unless there is an absolute contraindication.** For patients undergoing urgent PCI who have been treated with heparin, the administration of glycoprotein IIb/IIIa inhibitors just before PCI has been shown to reduce mortality and reinfarction without an increase in bleeding, and as such, it is recommended.[14-15] These drugs include abciximab (ReoPro), eptifibatide (Integrilin), and tirofiban (Aggrastat).

The primary cause of myocardial ischemic and cell death in STEMI is acute occlusion of the coronary artery due to thrombus formation. As such, removal of the thrombus has been the primary treatment for STEMI for the past 20+ years. Fibrinolytic therapy was the first well-established mechanism by which acute coronary thrombus could be intervened upon.

While fibrinolytic therapy has clear benefit in STEMI, its effectiveness correlates with both restoration of flow and the achievement of complete normalization of blood flow (TIMI 3 flow) in the culprit vessel. (See Table 13.7 for TIMI flow grade definitions.) Thrombolytics are successful in restoring some flow in up to 87% of

TABLE 13.7 TIMI Grading System for Coronary Artery Flow Beyond a Lesion

---

TIMI 0 flow (no perfusion): no antegrade flow beyond a lesion
TIMI 1 flow (penetration without perfusion): faint antegrade flow beyond a lesion, with only partial opacification of the lesion
TIMI 2 flow (partial reperfusion): delayed or sluggish antegrade flow, but with complete filling of the distal territory
TIMI 3 flow (complete perfusion): normal flow, filling the vessel fully

---

patients; however, TIMI 3 flow is achieved in only 50% to 60% of patients treated with thrombolytics. Over the past 17 years, multiple randomized trials have compared thrombolytic therapy to primary percutaneous intervention (first with balloon angioplasty alone and subsequently with stenting). The largest of the thrombolytic versus PCI studies were the DANAMI-2 and PRAGUE-2 trials.[16-17] In DANAMI-2, patients were randomized to receive front-loaded alteplase or to receive primary PCI with stenting. The study was stopped early due to a significant reduction in the primary end point of mortality, reinfarction, or stroke at 30 days (8.0% in PCI group vs 13.7% in thrombolytic group). This reduction can be partially attributed to the fact that TIMI 3 flow is able to be achieved in > 90% of patients undergoing primary PCI as demonstrated in the PAMI and CADILLAC trials.[18-19] In all, there have been more than 20 randomized trials comparing thrombolytics to PCI. These trials have demonstrated a significantly lower incidence of death, reinfarction, and hemorrhagic stroke with PCI versus thrombolytics.[20]

It is important to recognize that the benefit of PCI versus thrombolytics is directly related to timing of the intervention. The mortality benefits of PCI over thrombolytics are directly correlated to timing of reperfusion—in fact, **if it is not feasible for PCI to be performed within 90 minutes of presentation, then thrombolytic therapy should be given, and no PCI performed.** As a result, the current ACC/AHA guidelines recommend primary PCI with stenting for any patient presenting with a STEMI in whom

PCI can be performed within **90 minutes** of initial presentation. If primary PCI is not available on-site at the presenting institution, then transport of the patient to a center with primary PCI capabilities remains **beneficial as long as the door-to-balloon time, including time for transport, can be accomplished within 90 minutes.** If this is not possible, then treatment with thrombolytic therapy and subsequent transfer to a center where rescue PCI can be done if indicated are recommended. Indications for emergent angiography and PCI after thrombolytic therapy include failed fibrinolysis or threatened reocclusion. In patients who have received successful fibrinolysis, routine PCI following fibrinolysis should be considered prior to hospital discharge.

Both drug-eluting stents (DES) and bare-metal stents (BMS) have been used in the setting of STEMI. Meta-analyses comparing DES to BMS have demonstrated a decrease in the need for subsequent target lesion revascularization in patients who receive DES.[21] The most recent study to compare DES to BMS was the HORIZONS-AMI study, which enrolled patients presenting with STEMI and randomized them to either Taxus DES or Express BMS.[22] In patients with STEMI undergoing primary PCI, the use of Taxus DES rather than Express BMS resulted in comparable rates of stent thrombosis, reinfarction, and death at 2 years, with a significant reduction in restenosis and need for additional target vessel revascularization in all lesions except those at low risk for restenosis. Although these early data are favorable, further long-term data and randomized trials are needed to determine conclusively if new DES are safer or more effective than BMS in STEMI.

Post acute myocardial infarction, there are a number of drugs that should be started and continued upon discharge. In addition to the aforementioned aspirin, clopidogrel, and β-blocker, patients should also be started on statin therapy and angiotensin converting enzyme (ACE) inhibitor therapy unless contraindicated due to allergies or renal insufficiency. The statins attack the fundamental arteriosclerotic process that resulted in coronary artery disease in the first place. The ACE inhibitors unload the left ventricle and prevent its adverse dilatation after injury. The use of an ACE inhibitor is of particular importance in patients with depressed left ventricular function or in patients with an anterior-wall myocardial infarction to prevent adverse remodeling of the left ventricle.

The early treatment of acute ischemic syndromes can be imposing to the house officer. Senior staff often talk about details of catheterization or endovascular therapy, taking the fundamentals for granted, so that basic tenets remain obscure. The approaches detailed above represent current accepted therapeutic patterns. The house officer can follow the therapeutic paradigms outlined with assurance that his or her therapies are appropriate.

REFERENCES

1. Goodman SG, Cohen M, Bigonzi F, et al. Randomized trial of low molecular weight heparin (enoxaparin) versus unfractionated heparin for unstable coronary artery disease: one-year results of the ESSENCE study. Efficacy and safety of subcutaneous enoxaparin in non-Q-wave coronary events. *J Am Coll Cardiol.* 2000;35:693-698.
2. Antman EM, McCabe CH, Gurfinkel EP, et al. Enoxaparin prevents death and cardiac ischemic events in unstable angina/non-Q-wave myocardial infarction: results of the Thrombolysis in Myocardial Infarction (TIMI) 11B trial. *Circulation.* 1999;100:1593-1601.
3. Antman EM, Cohen M, Bernink PJ, et al. The TIMI risk score for unstable angina and non-ST elevation MI: a method for prognostication and therapeutic decision making. *JAMA.* 284:835-842.
4. Davies MJ, Thomas AC. Plaque assuring: the cause of acute myocardial infarction, sudden ischemic death, and crescendo angina. *Br Heart J.* 1985;53:363-373.
5. Falk E. Morphologic features of unstable atherothrombotic plaques underlying acute coronary syndromes. *Am J Cardiol.* 1989;63:114E-120E.
6. Holmes DR Jr, Hartzler GO, Smith HC, Fuster V. Coronary artery thrombosis in patients with unstable angina. *Br Heart J.* 1981;45:411-416.

7. Lam JYT, Chesebro JH, Steele PM, Badimon L, Fuster V. Is vasospasm related to platelet deposition? Relationship in porcine preparation of arterial injury in vivo. *Circulation.* 1987;75:243-248.

8. Theroux P, Ouimet H, McCans J, et al. Aspirin, heparin, or both to treat unstable angina. *N Engl J Med.* 1988;319:1105-1111.

9. Yusuf S, Zhao S, Mehta SR, et al. Effects of clopidogrel in addition to aspirin in patients with acute coronary syndromes without ST-segment elevation. *N Engl J Med.* 2001;345:494-502.

10. The TIMI Study Group: Early effects of tissue-type plasminogen activator added to conventional therapy on the culprit lesion in patients presenting with ischemic cardiac pain at rest. Results of the thrombolysis in myocardial ischemia (TIMI IIIA) trial. *Circulation.* 1993;87:38-52.

11. Grines CL, Browne KF, Marco J, et al. A comparison of immediate angioplasty with thrombolytic therapy for acute myocardial infarction. *N Engl J Med.* 1993;328:673-679.

12. The TIMI Study Group. Comparison of invasive and conservative strategies after treatment with intravenous tissue plasminogen activator in acute myocardial infarction: results of the Thrombolysis in Myocardial Infarction (TIMI) phase II trial. *N Engl J Med.* 1989;320:618-627.

13. Sabatin MS, Cannon CP, Gibson CM, et al. Effect of clopidogrel pretreatment before percutaneous coronary intervention in patients with ST-elevation myocardial infarction treated with fibrinolytics: the PCI-CLARITY study. *JAMA.* 2005;291:1224-1232.

14. Boersma E, Harrington RA, Moliterno DJ, et al. Platelet glycoprotein IIb/IIIa inhibitors in acute coronary syndromes: a meta-analysis of all major randomized clinical trials. *Lancet.* 2002;359;189-198.

15. De Luca G, Suryapranata H, Stone GW, et al. Abciximab as adjunctive therapy to reperfusion in acute ST-segment elevation myocardial infarction: a meta-analysis of randomized trials. *JAMA.* 2005;293;1759-1765.

16. Busk M, Maeng M, Rasmussen K, et al. The Danish multicentre randomized study of fibrinolytic therapy vs primary angioplasty in acute myocardial infarction (the DANAMI-2 trial): outcome after 3 years follow-up. *Eur Heart J.* 2008;29:1259-1266.

17. Widimsky P, Budesinsky T, Vorac D, et al. Long distance transport for primary angioplasty vs. immediate thrombolysis in acute myocardial infarction. Final results of the randomized national multicentre trial PRAGUE-2. *Eur Heart J.* 2003;24:94-104.

18. Mehta RH, Harjai KJ, Cox D, et al. Clinical and angiographic correlates and outcomes of suboptimal coronary flow in patients with acute myocardial infarction undergoing primary percutaneous coronary intervention. *J Am Coll Cardiol.* 2003:42:1739-1746.

19. Stone GW, Grines CL, Cox DA, et al. Comparison of angioplasty with stenting, with or without abciximab in acute myocardial infarction. *NEJM.* 2002;346:957-966.

20. Keeley EC, Boura JA, Grines CL. Primary angioplasty versus thrombolytic therapy for acute myocardial infarction: a quantitative review of 23 randomized trials. *Lancet.* 2003;361:13-20.

21. Babapulle MN, Joseph L, Belisle P, Brophy JM, Eisengerg MJ. A hierarchical Bayesian meta-analysis of randomized clinical trials of drug-eluting stents. *Lancet.* 2004;364:583-591.

22. Mehran R, Brodie B, Cox C, et al. The Harmonizing Outcomes with Revascularization and Stents in Acute Myocardial Infarctions (HORIZONS-AMI) trial: study design and rationale. *Am Heart J.* 2008;156;44-56.

14

ACUTE MANAGEMENT OF VALVULAR HEART DISEASE

authored in Second Edition with **John F. Setaro, MD**
Section of Cardiovascular Medicine,
Yale University School of Medicine

To maintain cellular viability throughout the body, cardiac output must be maintained. The integrity of forward cardiac output is safeguarded by the presence of four unidirectional heart valves. Regurgitant, stenotic, or mixed lesions of one or more valves may exist in a subclinical fashion for many years. Superimposition of an additional burden—via disease progression or cardiac ischemia, volume overload, or infection—may lead to an emergent presentation of the valvular heart disease. In other cases, a new catastrophic mechanical valvular event may precipitate a sudden critical illness in a patient who previously had normal valve structure and function. The present chapter provides background information on valvular physiology and practical information on management to allow the house officer to treat valvular disease in the acutely ill patient accurately and effectively.

The House Officer's Guide to ICU Care: Fundamentals of Management of the Heart and Lungs, 3rd ed. © 2013 John A. Elefteriades, Curtis Tribble, Alexander S. Geha, Mark D. Siegel, and Lawrence S. Cohen, eds. Cardiotext Publishing, ISBN: 978-1-935395-68-3.

✚ BASIC PHYSIOLOGY OF REGURGITANT AND STENOTIC LESIONS

Valvular regurgitation (*incompetence* or *insufficiency* are synonyms found in the medical literature) implies leaking, or retrograde flow of blood, due to a diseased valve. To cope with the regurgitation (either aortic or mitral), the left ventricle enlarges in order to maintain adequate forward flow;[1] this represents a state of dilation, or **volume overload**. Since some portion of the blood, with each heartbeat, goes backward through the leaky valve, the only way for the heart to maintain a normal net forward flow is to enlarge and eject more blood with each beat. Then, even though some of the ejected blood goes backward, there is still enough going forward to meet the body's needs.

Valvular stenosis, or obstruction to the forward flow of blood, imposes a **pressure overload** on the cardiac chamber proximal to the affected valve. In mitral stenosis, this overload is exerted on the left atrium and, consequently, on the lungs. In aortic stenosis, the pressure overload is exerted on the left ventricle. To cope with the increased afterload and to reduce wall stress by the law of Laplace, the left ventricle hypertrophies.[2]

When valvular lesions are acute, no immediate cardiac adaptation is feasible, and swift clinical decompensation may be witnessed. Even in the chronic state, dilation and/or hypertrophy exact a toll of increased myocardial oxygen demand, predisposing to ischemia in addition to heart failure.

In the critical setting where significant cardiopulmonary compromise exists on the basis of a valvular disorder, regulation of circulating volume and manipulation of hemodynamics are essential. **A Swan-Ganz catheter is nearly always necessary in the critically ill patient with acutely presenting valvular heart disease.** Central venous pressure measurements do not suffice, especially in patients with concomitant lung disease and elevated right heart pressures on a pulmonary basis. The Swan-Ganz catheter permits assessment of right atrial, right ventricular, pulmonary artery, and pulmonary capillary wedge pressure (functionally equivalent to left atrial or left ventricular end-diastolic pressure). (See also Chapter 5, Hemodynamic Monitoring and the Swan-Ganz Catheter.) The pulmonary artery catheter also allows the measurement of oxygen saturation in several chambers as well as determination of cardiac output by thermodilution. Pulmonary and systemic vascular resistance can be calculated from the pressures measured and the cardiac output. On the basis of this information, volume status can be optimized and appropriate pharmacologic manipulations can be carried out. (See also Chapter 6, Hemodynamic Management.)

✚ ENDOCARDITIS, ARRHYTHMIAS, AND THROMBUS FORMATION AND EMBOLIZATION

Before considering each valve lesion individually, certain critical general points regarding endocarditis, arrhythmias, and thrombus formation and embolization will be made.

Endocarditis

Whenever a patient presents with a new valvular disorder or an exacerbation of a chronic valvular disorder, the possibility of infectious endocarditis should be entertained. Rheumatic or prosthetic valves are particularly susceptible to infection (Figure 14.1). Endocarditis may follow the placement of intravascular cannulae, for instance, in patients receiving dialysis, chemotherapy, or parenteral nutrition. Endocarditis is always a possibility in intravenous drug users. Endocarditis can also complicate dental, gastrointestinal, or genitourinary instrumentation.[3] Multiple blood cultures should precede the institution of antibiotic therapy if suspicion for endocarditis is high. Evidence for fungal as well as bacterial involvement must be sought. When endocarditis is suspected clinically in a patient with decompensated valvular heart disease, presumptive antimicrobial treatment should be started prior to confirmation by culture.

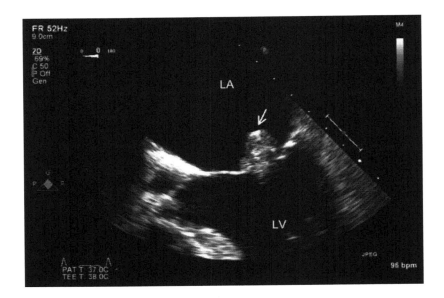

FIGURE 14.1

Infectious endocarditis visualized by transesophageal echocardiography shows an echogenic mass on the anterior mitral leaflet indicated by the arrow. LV = left ventricle, LA = left atrium.

Arrhythmias

Disturbances of heart rhythm, rate, and electrical conduction often accompany acute valvular disease. Such phenomena can represent markers of the severity of the pathologic process and tend to complicate management because of their interference with hemodynamic stability, physiologic atrioventricular transport, and appropriate diastolic filling. Control of ventricular rate in atrial arrhythmias (see Chapter 2, Arrhythmias) is extremely important in the face of acute valvular decompensation.

Thrombus/Embolization

Abnormal valve structure, combined with arrhythmias and blood pooling proximal to stenotic valves, tends to foster thrombus formation, with possible distant embolization. The classic scenario involves mitral stenosis with atrial fibrillation and left atrial enlargement.

Anticoagulation is usually indicated in mitral valvular stenosis with atrial fibrillation, and in the acute setting, an intravenous heparin infusion to maintain a PTT of 60 to 90 seconds is desirable.

Specific Valvular Lesions

There are only four cardinally important valvular heart lesions with which the house officer needs to be concerned. These are

- Aortic regurgitation
- Mitral regurgitation
- Aortic stenosis
- Mitral stenosis

These will be covered individually immediately below. Tricuspid regurgitation, although not usually the cause of acute hemodynamic collapse, will also be addressed.

✚ AORTIC REGURGITATION
Etiology

Acute aortic valvular regurgitation is typically caused, in descending frequency, by infectious endocarditis, aortic dissection, and chest trauma.[4] Congenital (bicuspid) or rheumatic abnormalities and the presence of a valvular prosthesis or connective tissue disease can predispose to infection, with consequent valve destruction. Hypertension and Marfan's syndrome (and Ehler-Danlos or Loeys-Dietz syndrome) are risk factors for aortic dissection, which may extend retrograde to distort aortic valve geometry. (See Chapter 20, Aortic Emergencies.)

Blunt or penetrating trauma may cause aortic valvular insufficiency, as can a variety of intracardiac catheterization and invasive therapeutic procedures.

Clinical Presentation

Acute congestive heart failure with a new or intensified blowing diastolic murmur at the left sternal border should raise the suspicion of acute aortic insufficiency.

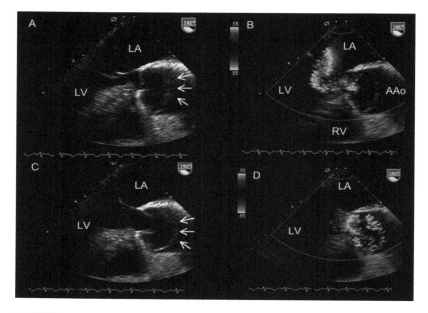

FIGURE 14.2A

Transesophageal echocardiogram in a patient with an ascending aortic dissection (**arrows**) seen in systole (**Panel A**) and diastole (**Panel C**). There is severe aortic regurgitation seen in **Panel B** and systolic filling of the true lumen in **Panel D**. LV = left ventricle, LA = left atrium, AAo = Ascending aorta, RV = right ventricle.

On cardiac auscultation, a softening of S_1 may be heard, ascribable to preclosure of the mitral valve by the regurgitant blood. An apical diastolic murmur (Austin Flint) may be heard, at times leading to confusion with mitral stenosis. The cause of the Austin Flint murmur in aortic insufficiency has not been determined with certainty; it is speculated that apical vibrations from the regurgitant flow or functional mitral inflow abnormalities related to preclosure of the mitral valve may obtain a valuable resource. The lung exam may reflect acute left ventricular failure. The bounding, collapsing ("water-hammer") pulses observed throughout the body in chronic aortic regurgitation are less prominent in acute regurgitation.

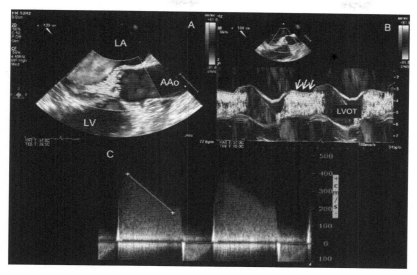

FIGURE 14.2B

Transesophageal echocardiogram in a patient with severe aortic regurgitation in **Panel A**. On M-mode echo, the regurgitant jet fills the entire left ventricular outflow tract (**Panel B**) and there is a steep deceleration slope of the continuous wave Doppler flow (indicated by the white line, **Panel C**) supporting the diagnosis of severe aortic regurgitation.

Diagnostic Methods

The EKG may show sinus tachycardia and voltage or strain signs of hypertrophy, depending on the chronicity of the aortic regurgitation. Conduction disturbances (heart block) point to aortic ring abscess in cases of endocarditis. The chest x-ray will show pulmonary congestion, though acute cardiomegaly may not yet be manifested. A widened mediastinum or pleural effusion may raise concerns regarding associated aortic dissection. Transthoracic or transesophageal echocardiography is useful in defining the presence and severity of aortic regurgitation, as well as the presence or absence of valvular vegetation or aortic dissection (Figure 14.2A, 14.2B). (See Chapter 12, Thoracic Imaging in Acute Disease.)

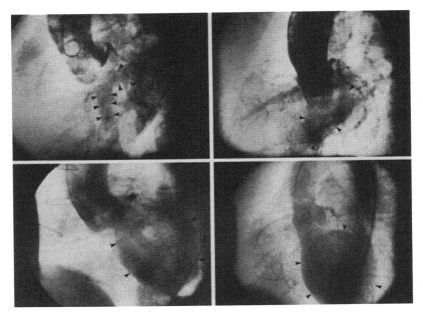

FIGURE 14.3

Angiographic view of grading of aortic regurgitation, 1+ to 4+, starting at upper left. Arrows delineate the opacification of the left ventricle.

Source: Reproduced with permission from Yang SS, Bentivoglio LG, Maranhao V, Goldberg H. *From Cardiac Catheterization Data to Hemodynamic Parameters.* 3rd ed. Philadelphia: FA Davis; 1988:154.

Contrast-enhanced computerized tomography and magnetic resonance imaging are excellent methods for assessing the thoracic aorta. In terms of assessing the severity of aortic insufficiency, aortography has traditionally been the gold standard. Insufficiency is graded angiographically, in terms of severity, on a scale of 0 to 4+ according to the rapidity and completeness of opacification of the left ventricle following aortic injection of dye (Figure 14.3). In the current era, echocardiography, which can assess aortic valve function very precisely, has challenged aortography as the gold standard for assessment of the severity of aortic regurgitation.

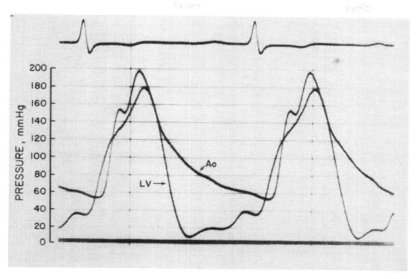

FIGURE 14.4

Left ventricular (LV) and aortic (Ao) pressures nearly equalize at end-diastole in a case of severe aortic insufficiency.

Source: Reprinted with permission from Grossman W, Baim DS. *Cardiac Catheterization, Angiography, and Intervention.* 5th ed. Philadelphia: Lea & Febiger; 1995.

Hemodynamic Profile

Pulmonary capillary wedge and left ventricular end-diastolic pressures may be considerably elevated in acute aortic insufficiency, for instance, at or above the range of 25 to 30 mm Hg. **Aortic and left ventricular diastolic pressures may nearly equalize,** reflecting the loss of a competent valve to maintain the aortic diastolic pressure (Figure 14.4).

Pharmacologic Management

Afterload reduction with a potent vasodilator (such as nitroprusside) is the mainstay of treatment of acute aortic insufficiency. Arterial dilatation lessens impedance to aortic outflow and increases forward flow of blood, thereby lowering left ventricular chamber volume, ventricular wall stress, and myocardial oxygen demand. In cases of aortic dissection, intravenous β-blockers (or calcium antagonists) are useful to slow the rate of rise of developed left ventricular and aortic pressure. Intravenous diuretics are used as necessary to maintain euvolemia. Oxygen should be administered. **There is no role for intra-aortic balloon counterpulsation in aortic insufficiency;** in fact, the IABP may aggravate left ventricular volume overload by driving blood backward through the incompetent aortic valve. Antibiotics should be started (after blood cultures have been drawn) if infectious endocarditis is suspected.

Operative Correction

Acute aortic valvular regurgitation is largely a surgical disorder.[4] Refractory heart failure, complications of endocarditis (systemic embolization, uncontrolled sepsis), or presence of ascending aortic dissection mandate urgent operation. Even when urgent intervention is not necessary, early intervention for valve replacement usually becomes necessary because of left ventricular dilation from the acute aortic insufficiency, which is usually very poorly tolerated.

✚ MITRAL REGURGITATION

Etiology

Mitral valvular regurgitation may exist on the basis of rheumatic valvular disease, infectious endocarditis, coronary artery disease with ischemia or infarction, or myxomatous degeneration with prolapse or ruptured chordae tendineae.

Clinical Presentation

The patient with acute mitral regurgitation may present in extremis, with dyspnea and hypotension. The most dramatic presentations are observed with chordal rupture, endocarditis, or ischemically mediated papillary muscle dysfunction, necrosis, or rupture.

Sinus tachycardia is often present. **A loud, blowing, holosystolic murmur is audible at the apex, radiating into the axilla.** Particularly in older patients, the systolic murmur of mitral regurgitation may simulate that of aortic stenosis. The location of the murmur at the axilla helps to distinguish mitral regurgitation. Also, the murmur of mitral regurgitation is holosytolic, whereas that of aortic stenosis has a non-holosystolic, crescendo-decresendo profile. A lack of augmentation after a premature ventricular contraction may assist in identifying the murmur as mitral regurgitation rather than as aortic stenosis. A third heart sound and a hyperdynamic precordium may be discovered.

Diagnostic Methods

The EKG is likely to demonstrate an inferior or posterior infarct if papillary muscle necrosis is culpable. Otherwise, sinus tachycardia or atrial arrhythmias may be observed, often with a left axis deviation and left atrial enlargement. Left atrial and left ventricular enlargement, with pulmonary congestion, will be in evidence on chest x-ray. Echocardiography, especially using the transesophageal approach (Figure 14.5), is an essential tool in assessing the cause and

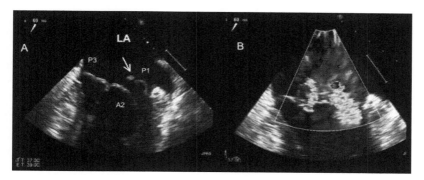

FIGURE 14.5

Transesophageal echo at the mid-esophageal level at 60 degrees showing a P1 flail leaflet, ruptured chord indicated by the arrow, and severe mitral regurgitation.

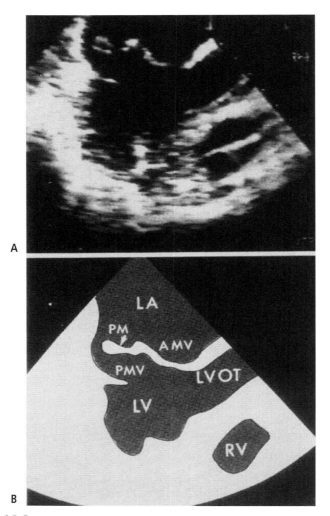

FIGURE 14.6

Transesophageal echocardiographic view of ruptured papillary muscles appearing as a free appendage attached to the mitral valve and observed in the left atrium. LA = left atrium, LV = left ventricle, LVOT = left ventricular outflow tract, RV = right ventricle, PM = posterior papillary muscle, PMV = posterior mitral valve leaflet, AMV = anterior mitral valve leaflet.

Source: Reprinted with permission from Zotz RJ, Dohmen G, Genth S, Erbel R, Meyer J. Diagnosis of papillary muscle rupture after acute myocardial infarction by transthoracic and transesophageal echocardiography. *Clin Cardiol.* 1993;19:665-670.

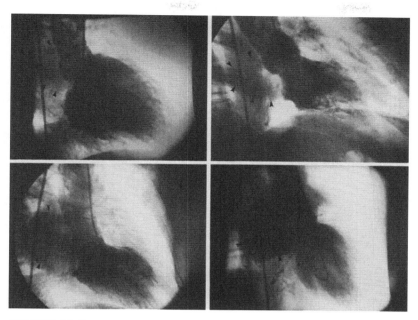

FIGURE 14.7

Angiographic view of grading of mitral regurgitation, 1+ to 4+, starting at upper left. Arrows delineate the opacification of the left atrium.

Source: Reprinted with permission from Yang SS, Bentivoglio LG, Maranhao V, Goldberg H. *From Cardiac Catheterization Data to Hemodynamic Parameters.* 3rd ed. Philadelphia; FA Davis; 1988:155.

degree of mitral valvular regurgitation[5] (Figure 14.6). Left ventriculography will provide information relating to ventricular function and angiographic grading of degree of regurgitation, Grades 1 to 4+ (Figure 14.7). Coronary arteriography is useful in defining anatomic lesions responsible for the ischemic event and guides percutaneous (angioplasty) or surgical coronary revascularization.

Echocardiography (either transthoracic or transesophageal) can very accurately assess the severity of mitral regurgitation and its anatomic basis.

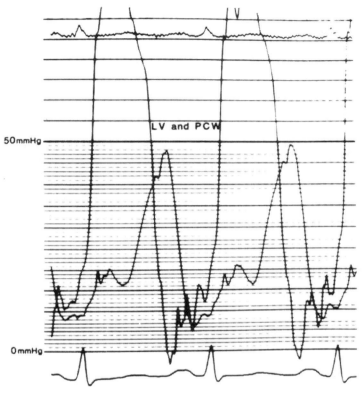

FIGURE 14.8

Acute mitral regurgitation with large v wave to 50 mm Hg.
PCW = pulmonary capillary wedge, LV = left ventricle.

Source: Reprinted with permission from Pepine CJ, Hill JA, Lambert R.
Diagnostic and Therapeutic Cardiac Catheterization. 3rd ed. Baltimore, MD:
Williams & Wilkins; 1998.

Hemodynamic Profile

The ejection of a quantity of the left ventricular stroke volume
into the low-pressure left atrial chamber results in a rise of the
left-sided filling pressures and the appearance of a characteristic
v, or "ventricular," wave in the pulmonary capillary wedge tracing recorded by the Swan-Ganz catheter (Figures 14.8 and 14.9).

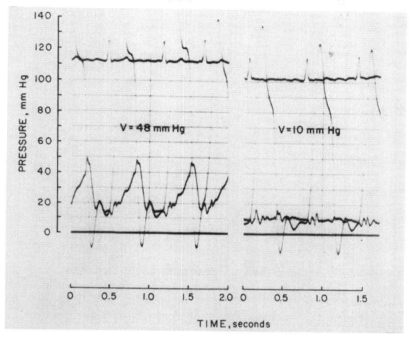

FIGURE 14.9

Severe mitral regurgitation with v wave to 48 mm Hg (**left**) before and after (**right**) infusion of afterload reducing vasodilator nitroprusside with reduction of v wave to 10 mm Hg.

Source: Reprinted with permission from Harshaw CW, et al. *Ann Intern Med.* 1975;83:312.

In acute, severe mitral regurgitation, volume overload may enlarge all chambers until the pericardial limit is reached, causing equalization of chamber pressures in diastole, as would be the case in pericardial constriction (Figure 14.10).

Pharmacologic Management

Vasodilator therapy, typically with nitroprusside (though in ischemic states, nitroglycerin may have a role as well), serves to reduce left ventricular afterload and permits a greater

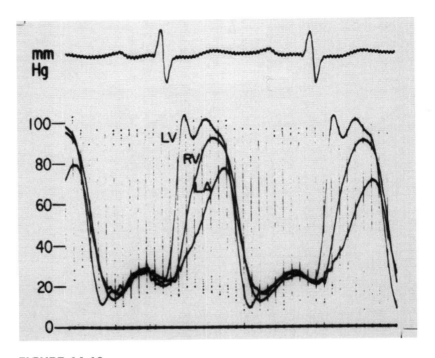

FIGURE 14.10

Acute mitral regurgitation with volume overload and equalization of pressures in diastole, simulating pericardial constriction. LV = left ventricle, RV = right ventricle, LA = left atrium.

Source: Reprinted with permission from Bartle SH, Hermann HJ. *Circulation.* 1967;36:839.

proportion of the stroke volume to flow antegrade into the aorta, rather than retrograde across the incompetent mitral valve into the left atrium (Figure 14.9). Control of volume state through diuresis, although indicated, may be of limited benefit in acute states of pulmonary congestion, and mechanical ventilatory support is often needed. Digitalis may be useful for rate control in atrial fibrillation. **Placement of the IABP may be of great benefit in acute mitral regurgitation. The systolic unloading of the systemic vasculature encourages forward flow from the left ventricle rather than regurgitation into the left atrium.**

Operative Correction

Definitive treatment for hemodynamically intolerable acute mitral regurgitation of whatever etiology is surgical, and medical manipulations should be directed toward that end.[6] Current surgical possibilities include valve repair as well as replacement. Percutaneous angioplasty can help to stabilize patients with ischemic mitral regurgitation on a short-term or occasionally even a definitive basis. In any case, surgical consultation is required for optimal management.

✚ TRICUSPID REGURGITATION
Etiology

Tricuspid regurgitation may exist on an organic or a functional basis. Organic causes include primary valvular diseases such as rheumatic heart disease, infectious endocarditis, myxomatous degeneration, Ebstein anomaly, right ventricular infarction, or carcinoid disease. (When the etiology is rheumatic, there is nearly always concomitant mitral disease.) Functional tricuspid regurgitation occurs on the basis of left heart failure, or primary lung or right ventricular etiologies, which result in right-sided hypertension or volume overload.

Clinical Presentation

Patients may present with markers of right heart failure, including dyspnea, liver enlargement, and edema. If the valve is infected, fever and septic pulmonary emboli are observed. If there is a patent foramen ovale or an atrial septal defect, systemic embolism is a risk.

Severe tricuspid regurgitation may present with tachycardia, atrial fibrillation, borderline blood pressure, dyspnea, orthopnea, elevated pulsatile neck veins and liver, and peripheral edema. A characteristic holosystolic murmur is audible at the lower left

sternal border that increases with inspiration. Stigmata of endocarditis may be visible (such as splinter hemorrhages), and lung findings may point to septic embolism (rounded infarcts, with or without cavitation).

Diagnostic Methods

The EKG can be remarkable for signs of right heart strain, atrial arrhythmias, and right atrial enlargement. The chest x-ray shows an enlarged right atrium and right ventricle in organic tricuspid regurgitation, whereas findings of pulmonary congestion (vessel engorgement) or pulmonary hypertension (enlarged main pulmonary arteries) predominate in cases of functional tricuspid regurgitation. Echocardiography reveals right ventricular enlargement and may demonstrate signs of endocarditis. Doppler techniques can provide an accurate estimate of the severity of tricuspid regurgitation (Figure 14.11).

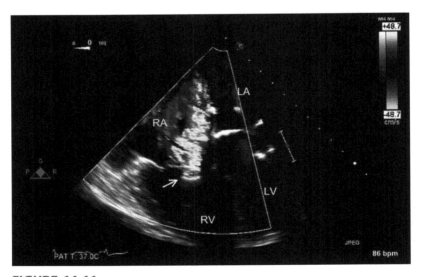

FIGURE 14.11

Transesophageal echo of the right ventricle and tricuspid valve shows severe tricuspid regurgitation by color flow Doppler shown by the arrow. RA = right atrium, RV = right ventricle, LA = left atrium, and LV = left ventricle.

Hemodynamic Profile

Hemodynamically, tricuspid regurgitation is notable for an increase in right atrial pressure with prominent v, or "ventricular," waves in the right atrial trace. Recorded right atrial wave forms may overlap those of the right ventricle to a considerable degree.

Pharmacologic Management

Diuretics to correct volume excess are the key element in treatment of tricuspid insufficiency. Treatment of underlying or coexisting pulmonary disease may be helpful. If functional tricuspid regurgitation has resulted from left heart failure, specific measures, such as diuretics, afterload reducers, or anti-ischemics, should be employed to treat the underlying cardiac disorders. Digitalis may be useful if atrial arrhythmias appear.

Operative Correction

Refractory tricuspid regurgitation, particularly if the valve is the source of uncontrollable septic emboli, may warrant surgical treatment. Valve excision, repair (by annuloplasty), or replacement may be necessary.

(Valve excision, although very helpful in putting an immediate end to septic pulmonary emboli, does, of course, leave wide-open tricuspid insufficiency; this is often very well tolerated. If addicts remain drug-free, they can undergo elective valve replacement at a later date to control peripheral edema symptoms.)

✛ AORTIC STENOSIS

Etiology

Younger and middle-aged patients with severe aortic stenosis have a higher frequency of congenitally abnormal valves (especially bicuspid) in comparison to elderly patients, who are more likely to have senile, degenerative, calcific aortic stenosis[7] (Figure 14.12). It can be said that the bicuspid valve "wears out" 1 to 2 decades

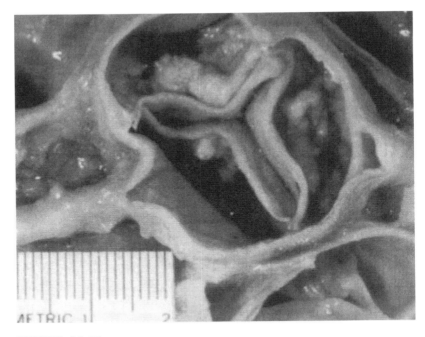

FIGURE 14.12

Severe degenerative aortic stenosis, with quantities of calcium in sinuses of Valsalva. Commissures are not fused.

Source: Reprinted with permission from Waller BF, McKay C, Van Tassel JW, Taliercio C, Howard J, Green F. Catheter balloon valvuloplasty of stenotic aortic valves. Part I. Anatomic basis and mechanisms of balloon dilation. *Clin Cardiol.* 1991;14:836-846.

before its normally tricuspid counterpart. Aortic stenosis may also occur on a rheumatic basis, in which case there is always concomitant mitral disease.

Clinical Presentation

Angina, syncope, and dyspnea (left ventricular failure) represent the three cardinal symptoms of aortic valvular stenosis. Yet patients may remain symptom-free until late in the course of aortic stenosis. Exercise intolerance and fatigue may herald a major deterioration.

As is well known, prognosis without valve replacement is poor once symptoms develop (Figure 14.13). The prognosis is so poor

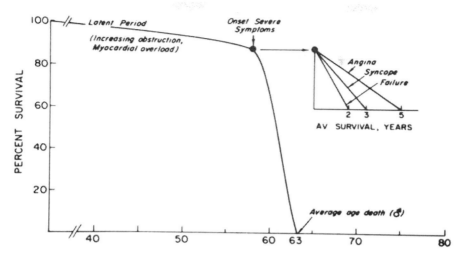

FIGURE 14.13

Natural history of aortic stenosis. Note dismal outlook once symptoms have developed.

Source: Reproduced with permission from Ross J Jr, Braunwald E. Aortic stenosis. *Circulation.* 1968:38suppl(V):V-1:V112.

that most surgeons have had a patient arrest and die the night before elective surgery for valve replacement. The house officer must respond immediately and with fullest attention to any calls regarding the patient with critical aortic stenosis, maintaining a high respect for the severity and precarious nature of the hemodynamic status.

Findings on exam favoring severe or critical aortic valvular stenosis include a harsh, crescendo-decrescendo murmur, heard best at the right upper sternal border, radiating into the carotids, often associated with a single second heart sound. A thrill over the aortic area, a left ventricular lift, and a carotid shudder are findings on palpation, with depressed, late carotid upstrokes. Cardiac gallops may be heard. Typically, the characteristic murmur is easily appreciated. Yet, as with any stenotic murmur, **as the lesion progresses to near-complete valve immobility, the murmur may become quite soft—an ominous sign of low forward flow.**

Diagnostic Methods

The EKG typically shows a pattern of left ventricular hypertrophy with strain, and in older patients, conduction delays may be seen, ascribable to calcific infiltration spreading from the valve to septal myocardium and the bundle of His. **Atrial fibrillation is an especially unfavorable rhythm in aortic stenosis, given the need to distend and fill the stiff left ventricle in diastole in this preload-sensitive state.** The chest x-ray demonstrates valve calcification and a prominent left ventricle. The ascending aorta may be enlarged from "poststenotic dilatation." Echocardiography is excellent for identifying aortic stenosis and, by Doppler methods, for quantifying the valve gradient and estimating the valve cross-sectional area.

Hemodynamic Profile

Left ventricular filling pressures may be elevated, cardiac output may be depressed, and a major gradient will exist when aortic and left ventricular pressures are compared (Figure 14.14). In calculations from catheterization laboratory data, valve area is directly proportional to cardiac output and inversely proportional to the valvular gradient. In fact, a useful rule of thumb for the house officer is that the valve area can be approximated by the cardiac output divided by the square root of the gradient. **In an adult, an absolute valve area of less than 0.7 cm² is diagnostic of critical aortic stenosis.** Operation is essential. Valve areas between 0.7 and 1.0 cm² represent significant, but subcritical, aortic stenosis; surgery may be required.

Pharmacologic Management

The patient with severe or critical aortic stenosis is highly preload, or volume, sensitive. The house officer must be careful not to drop filling pressures acutely, such as by nitrate administration. Low filling pressures will be inadequate to distend the stiff, hypertrophied left ventricle in diastole, leading to a depressed

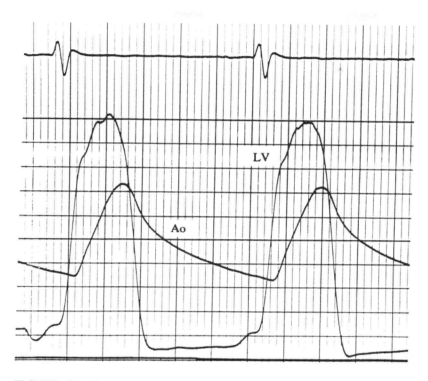

FIGURE 14.14

Hemodynamic recordings of severe aortic stenosis, with 60 mm Hg transvalvular gradient. Scale is 0 to 200 mm Hg. Degenerative calcific aortic stenosis was noted at operation. LV = left ventricle, Ao = aorta.

stroke volume and low forward output, with consequent systemic hypotension. This situation can create a downward spiral of progressive hemodynamic deterioration that may eventuate in cardiac arrest. This downward spiral leading to cardiac arrest is also commonly seen during induction of anesthesia, when loss of vasomotor tone diminishes cardiac preload. The cardiac surgical resident must be in alert attendance during anesthetic induction in patients with critical aortic stenosis. Patients with aortic stenosis are nearly impossible to resuscitate because of the "built-in" impediment to flow out of the left ventricle.

On the other hand, volume overload in the patient with severe aortic stenosis will lead to pulmonary congestion because of diastolic ventricular stiffness. Thus there exists a very narrow window of optimal filling pressures. In the setting of critical illness, a pulmonary artery catheter is of major assistance in volume regulation. There is very little benefit that can be accomplished via administration of medications in severe aortic stenosis, where the *mechanical* abnormality requires a *mechanical* (surgical) correction. Vasodilators, nitrates, and even the intra-aortic balloon pump have very little role in critical aortic stenosis.

Operative Correction

Critical aortic stenosis requires prompt surgery. Apart from control of volume and heart rate as temporizing maneuvers, medical therapy has very little to offer. We prefer coronary arteriography, prior to valve replacement, in order to guide the placement of coronary artery bypass grafts in case of concomitant coronary occlusive disease.[8] Percutaneous aortic valvuloplasty is only of temporary utility, appropriate only for very elderly patients who are not acceptable surgical candidates or who require urgent noncardiac surgery;[9-11] results do not last, for no amount of "stretching" of the valve by balloon can undo nature's process of calcific obliteration of the valve lumen. Replacement of the valve with a biological or mechanical prosthesis is essential if the dismal natural history of critical aortic stenosis is to be averted. Life expectancy following surgery is restored. Percutaneously delivered aortic valves are under clinical investigation in the United States, and may represent another option for extremely elderly or frail patients in the future.

✚ MITRAL STENOSIS

Etiology

In adults, mitral stenosis most often exists on a rheumatic basis, although more than 50% of such patients do not recollect a bout of rheumatic fever. Rheumatic involvement strikes the mitral valve with greatest frequency, the aortic valve with less frequency, and the tricuspid valve with even less frequency. Pulmonic valve involvement is rare.

Clinical Presentation

Typically, patients with severe mitral stenosis present with progressive dyspnea on exertion, eventuating in rest symptoms. Fatigue may be a prominent feature, reflecting limitation of forward cardiac output. Hemoptysis may occur from resultant pulmonary hypertension. A substantial minority of patients present with pulmonary congestion and right heart failure without clear etiology, and occult mitral stenosis must always be considered in such instances.

The patient with severe mitral stenosis in the critical care setting may appear with an irregular pulse and borderline blood pressure with signs of right and left heart failure. A malar flush may be seen, and the left ventricular impulse will not be strong. Many patients have a loud first heart sound and an opening snap on cardiac examination, and auscultation in the left lateral decubitus position reveals the presence of a low-pitched diastolic rumble characteristic of mitral stenosis. Cyanosis, hepatomegaly, and edema are ominous portents and correlate well with severely stenosed mitral valves.[12]

Mitral stenosis may remain occult until presentation with a stroke. In fact, an old dictum states that a young woman presenting with an acute stroke has mitral stenosis until proven otherwise. (Mitral stenosis is more common in the young and especially in females.)

Diagnostic Methods

The EKG may demonstrate atrial fibrillation or sinus rhythm with left atrial enlargement. The chest x-ray will be notable for left atrial enlargement ("double density") and pulmonary congestion. Echocardiography, first developed to diagnose mitral stenosis, remains the principle imaging modality for this disorder. Mitral valve leaflets appear thickened and restricted in their motion. The left atrium is enlarged. Doppler interrogation can allow an accurate estimation of valve area. In a number of patients, this technique reveals mixed mitral valvular disease, that is, stenosis and regurgitation.

Hemodynamic Profile

Pulmonary capillary wedge pressure (reflecting left atrial pressure) will be found to be elevated. A gradient will be found between the pulmonary capillary wedge pressure and the left ventricular end-diastolic pressure, representing the restriction of flow across the stenotic mitral valve (Figure 14.15). Calculated valve area is directly proportional to the measured cardiac output and inversely proportional to the transvalvular gradient. **Severe mitral stenosis exists if the area is less than 1.0 cm².** In chronic cases, elevated left heart filling pressures will lead to pulmonary artery hypertension and right heart overload, although there is an element of reversibility once mechanical treatment of mitral stenosis is carried out.[12]

Pharmacologic Management

Mitral valvular stenosis is a disorder of left ventricular filling and therefore requires careful optimization of volume status. **To optimize cardiac output in mitral stenosis, heart rate, particularly ventricular rate if the patient is in atrial fibrillation, must be controlled to allow for adequate filling in diastole.** Digitalis,

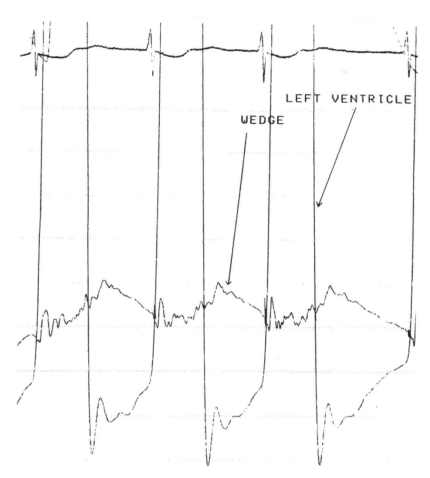

FIGURE 14.15

Hemodynamic recording of severe mitral stenosis in an 80-year-old patient with past rheumatic heart disease. Note gradient between pulmonary capillary wedge and left ventricular pressures in diastole. Valve area was 1.0 cm². Scale is 0 to 40 mm Hg.

Source: Courtesy of Jerome E Williams Jr, MD, and Joseph J Brennan Jr, MD, Yale University School of Medicine.

β-blockers, or calcium antagonists can be employed. A pharmacologic or electrical attempt to convert the patient to sinus rhythm may be appropriate. Anticoagulation is recommended to prevent systemic thromboembolism. Supplemental oxygen and the judicious use of diuretics are favored if pulmonary congestion is present. Transesophageal echocardiography to rule out atrial thrombus should be considered prior to elective cardioversion in patients with chronic atrial fibrillation; this is done to detect thrombi in the left atrial appendage that might be embolized by cardiovesion to sinus rhythm (when the atrium begins to beat again).

Operative Correction

In patients who do not have significant mitral regurgitation and whose valves are not significantly affected by leaflet rigidity, thickening, calcification, or subvalvular stenosis, percutaneous mitral valvulotomy has proved effective and durable.[9-10;13] (In contradistinction to aortic stenosis, the pathology in mitral stenosis is, in selected cases, anatomically suited to dilatation by balloon.) In cases not suitable for balloon dilatation, mitral valve replacement is required. This is especially the case for patients with mixed disease, stenosis and regurgitation.

⊞ A WORD ABOUT β-NATRIURETIC PEPTIDE[14-18]

β-natriuretic peptide (BNP) is a fairly recently appreciated marker for congestive heart failure. BNP is a cardiac neurohormone secreted from the cardiac ventricles in response to pressure or volume overload. This hormone naturally serves to augment renal excretion of salt and water—to help the body compensate for heart failure. As can be seen in Figure 14.16, BNP is elevated in heart failure (both acute and chronic) and can be used to supplement clinical judgment

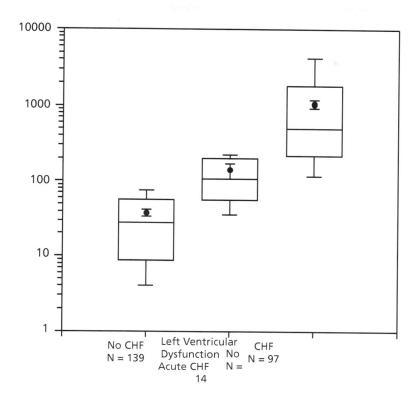

FIGURE 14.16

β-type natriuretic peptide levels of patients diagnosed with CHF, baseline left ventricular dysfunction, and without CHF. BNP = β-type natriuretic peptide; CHF = congestive heart failure.

Source: Reprinted with permission from Dao Q, Krishnaswamy P, Kazanegra R, et al. Utility of B-type natriuretic peptide in the diagnosis of congestive heart failure in an urgent-care setting. *J Am Coll Cardiol.* 2001;37(2):379-385.

in both the emergency department and the ICU. A level greater than 100 pg/mL is diagnostic of heart failure. The house officer should be aware of this fairly new test; the house officer should not, however, use BNP measurement as a crutch to replace careful, directed physical diagnosis for heart failure.

REFERENCES

1. Grossman W. Profiles in valvular heart disease. In: Grossman W, Baim DS, eds. *Cardiac Catheterization, Angiography, and Intervention.* 5th ed. Philadelphia: Lea & Febiger; 1995:735-756.

2. Setaro JF. Cardiac physiology. In: Bone RC, Dantzker DR, George RB, Matthay RA, Reynolds HY, eds. *Pulmonary and Critical Care Medicine.* St Louis: Mosby Year Book; 1993.

3. Remitz MS, Quagliarello V. Endovascular infections arising from right-sided heart structures. *Clin Cardiol.* 1992;10:137-149.

4. Cohn LH, Birjiniuk V. Therapy of acute aortic regurgitation. *Clin Cardiol.* 1991;9:339-352.

5. Zotz RJ, Dohmen G, Genth S, Erbel R, Meyer J. Diagnosis of papillary muscle rupture after acute myocardial infarction by transthoracic and transesophageal echocardiography. *Clin Cardiol.* 1993;19: 665-670.

6. Tcheng JE, Jackman JD, Califf RM, Stack RS. Managing myocardial infarction complicated by mitral regurgitation. *Primary Cardiol.* 1993;19:40-48.

7. Passik CS, Ackermann DR, Pluth JR, Edwards WD. Temporal changes in the causes of aortic stenosis: a surgical pathologic study of 646 cases. *Mayo Clin Proc.* 1987;62:119-128.

8. Rahimtoola SH. Perspective on valvular heart disease: update II. In Knoebel SB, Dack S, eds. *An Era in Cardiovascular Medicine.* New York: Elsevier; 1991:45-70.

9. Block PC, Palacios IF. Aortic and mitral balloon valvuloplasty: the United States experience. In: Topol EJ, ed. *Textbook of Interventional Cardiology.* Philadelphia: WB Saunders; 1990:831-848.

10. McKay RG. Balloon valvuloplasty. In: Grossman W, Baim DS, eds. *Cardiac Catheterization, Angiography and Intervention.* 4th ed. Philadelphia: Lea & Febiger; 1991:511-533.

11. Waller BF, McKay C, Van Tassel JW, Taliercio C, Howard J, Green F. Catheter balloon valvuloplasty of stenotic aortic valves. Part I. Anatomic basis and mechanisms of balloon dilation. *Clin Cardiol.* 1991;14:836-846.

12. Setaro JF, Cleman MC, Remets MS. The right ventricle in disorders causing pulmonary venous hypertension. *Clin Cardiol.* 1992;10: 165-183.

13. Carroll JD, Feldman T. Percutaneous mitral balloon valvotomy and the new demographics of mitral stenosis. *JAMA*. 1993;270:1731-1736.

14. Pepine CJ. In: Pepine CJ. *Diagnostic and Therapeutic Cardiac Catheterization*. Baltimore, MD: Williams & Wilkins; 1998:536.

15. Troughton R, Frampton C, Yandle T, Espine E, Nicholls M, Richards A. Treatment of heart failure guided by plasma aminoterminal brain natriuretic peptide (N-BNP) concentrations. *Lancet*. 2009:344:1126-1130.

16. McCullough PA, Nowak RM, McCord J, et al. B-type natriuretic peptide and clinical judgment in emergency diagnosis of heart failure: analysis from breathing not properly (BNP) multinational study. *Circulation*. 2002;106:416-422.

17. Dao Q, Drishnaswamy P, Kazanegra R, et al. Utility of B-type natriuretic peptide in the diagnosis of congestive heart failure in an urgent-care setting. *J Am Coll Cardiol*. 2001;37:379-385.

18. Jensen KT, Carstens J, Bedersen EB. Effect of BNP on renal hemodynamics, tubular function and vasoactive hormones in humans. *Am J Physiol Renal Physiol*. 1998;274:F63-F72.

SUGGESTED FURTHER READING

Stout KK, Verrier ED. Acute valvular regurgitation. *Circulation*. 2009;119:3232-3241.

A superb review of the regurgitant lesions, strongly recommended.

Leitner J, Wu W-C. Management of aortic valve disease: review questions. Self-assessment in cardiology. Turner White Communications, Inc. Wayne, PA.

Go ahead. Test yourself.

Kern, MJ. *The Cardiac Catheterization Handbook*. 4th ed. Philadelphia:: Mosby. Philadelphia; 2003.

For those who wish a more in-depth analysis of catheterization features.

Kern MJ, Deligonul U, Gudipati C. Hemodynamic and ECG data. In: Kern MJ, ed. *The Cardiac Catheterization Handbook*. St. Louis: Mosby Year Book; 1991:98-201.

Yang SS, Bentivoglio LG, Maranhao V, Goldberg H. Assessment of ventricular inflow and outflow obstruction. In: Yang SS, Bentivoglio LG, Maranhao V, Goldberg H, eds. *From Cardiac Catheterization Data to Hemodynamic Parameters.* 3rd ed. Philadelphia: FA Davis; 1988:122-151.

POSTOPERATIVE BLEEDING

This chapter looks specifically at postoperative bleeding in the cardiac patient. No attempt is made to review the entire topic of bleeding and coagulation mechanisms, which is covered well in basic surgical texts.

✚ PREVENTION

The key to minimizing postoperative bleeding is care during closure of the chest. Strict attention must be paid to all cannulation sites, suture lines, anastomoses, and vein graft branches. Noncardiac mediastinal and chest wall structures must be thoroughly assessed for hemostasis. The pericardium and the diaphragm are frequent sites of bleeding. The thymus often contains arteries and veins of sufficient caliber to cause troublesome bleeding. The innominate vein and its branches are frequent bleeding sites. The strap muscles at the apex of the incision must be given careful attention. The periosteum of the sternum must be thoroughly cauterized. The bone marrow itself is not often a cause of trouble, because bleeding stops reliably when tight, well-aligned approximation of the bone edges is achieved. Sites where sternal wires pass around or through the bone are notorious for bleeding; these must be assessed meticulously before the bone is approximated.

With a little experience, the senior house officer involved in closing the chest learns to assess rapidly and accurately all these possible bleeding sites while carrying out chest closure. Despite careful attention by expert personnel during closure, however, postoperative bleeding will occur occasionally.

It is known that cardiopulmonary bypass impairs coagulation mechanisms in many ways. These have been investigated extensively.[1-4] Major mechanisms elucidated include platelet destruction, impairment of function of surviving platelets, interference at several sites with the clotting cascade factors, disseminated intravascular coagulation, hyperfibrinolysis, and the so-called heparin rebound effect (see later).

In the present era, an overwhelming proportion of patients are on some form of anticoagulation preoperatively, be it Coumadin, aspirin, Persantine, Integrilin (epftibatide), Plavix (clopidogrel), abciximab (ReoPro), or other similar anticoagulants or antithrombotics. These agents certainly encourage bleeding. Economic and emotional factors often encourage operation before these drugs have fully worn off. Certain of these agents permanently disable platelets, so that 10 to 14 days will be required until all the disabled platelets in the circulation are replaced by the body.

Nonetheless, bleeding occurs much less frequently than it did in earlier eras, largely for three reasons:

1.   Many centers utilize the activated clotting time (ACT) or a similar test to titrate protamine administration at the completion of cardiopulmonary bypass.[1] In earlier times, heparin and protamine doses were determined by empirical formulas. The heparin dose was usually 300 U/kg of body weight initially, with 100 U/kg added about every hour during bypass. Protamine was usually administered at 1 mg

for every 100 U of total heparin given. Clotting studies, run in the main laboratory, often delayed objective assessment for hours.

The ACT can be done in the operating suite within minutes. ACT tests during bypass allow omission of routine heparin doses if heparin effect persists. ACT tests post bypass allow precise titration of protamine administration; if the ACT remains prolonged after the initial dose of protamine, an additional dose can be administered. The ACT has been shown to reduce postoperative bleeding significantly.[1]

Presently, many ICUs have an ACT machine on the premises, making this assessment immediately available to the house officer for his management of coagulation and bleeding.

2. In recent years, it has been realized that many patients will bleed if systolic arterial blood pressure (BP) is not strictly controlled. Also, recent years have brought the realization that cardiac output is well maintained, or even improved, at low normal blood pressures. **For hemostasis, as well as for afterload reduction, we maintain systolic arterial BP at less than 125 to 130 mm Hg in all postoperative cardiac patients.** It is very common to see dramatic increases in chest tube output during even brief hypertensive crises (as with BPs of 180 to 200 mm Hg); bleeding returns to normal as BP is controlled.

3. At many centers, a unit of the patient's own blood is routinely harvested via the aortic cannula before going on cardiopulmonary bypass. This is stored and transfused after coming off bypass. The platelets in this unit of blood will be the patient's own and will not have been traumatized by cardiopulmonary bypass. These platelets can greatly improve hemostasis.

✚ ASSESSMENT

Now, what constitutes abnormal postoperative bleeding? The house officer should realize that significant blood drainage does occur after major cardiac surgery. It is difficult to state numerical guidelines for universal use. Some patients may have almost no drainage in the collection chamber on arrival in the ICU; others may have several hundred milliliters; all may go on to be perfectly dry overnight.

Most patients will have drainage less than 100 mL/h. In general, drainage after arrival in ICU should not exceed 250 mL/h for more than 4 hours.[2] Hourly drainage beyond this limit should be brought to the attention of more senior personnel. **After 4 hours, drainage should be considerably less, preferably less than 100 mL/h.**

Even more important than the absolute volume of drainage is the trend over time. The house officer should be very concerned about a patient who drains 150, 200, 250, and 300 mL over successive hours. On the other hand, the patient who drains 250, 250, 200, and 150 mL is unlikely to have difficulty.

A basic principle that must be understood is that **even widely patent, large-bore chest tubes do not drain the mediastinum totally dry.** Some experienced clinicians feel that there is always as much clotted or undrained blood in the chest as there is drained blood outside. This occurs because of puddles, clots, and loculi. For these reasons, the house officer must be acutely aware that **tamponade can occur despite the presence of properly functioning chest tubes.**

If there is any concern about hemodynamic embarrassment from bleeding, the chest x-ray may be used to assess mediastinal size. Although difficult for the beginner, assessment of "degree of fullness" of the mediastinal shadow can be performed reliably by the experienced clinician. Here again, trends over time are important. At our center, we obtain a chest x-ray for assessment of the mediastinal shadow (and other structures) immediately postoperatively as well as the following morning, even if chest tube drainage is low. Some centers perform an additional chest x-ray at 4 hours postoperatively, specifically to check for any evidence of mediastinal widening that might indicate sequestered bleeding.

When bleeding does occur, its origin may be hematologic or surgical. The origin is hematologic if it is caused by inadequacy of circulating clotting factors. The origin is surgical if clotting factors are adequate but a mechanical defect exists, such as an open vein branch, bleeding suture line, oozing sternal wire, or other specific bleeding site.

A coagulation profile including prothrombin time (PT), partial thromboplastin time (PTT), and platelet count will detect most abnormalities of the circulating clotting factors. For routine, uncomplicated, non-prolonged cases, clotting factors are usually normal—especially when the ACT is used to guide heparin and protamine administration. With long pump runs (more than 3 hours) and very sick patients, clotting factors may indeed become depleted. Also, while platelet number may be normal after relatively short pump runs, platelet function will not be; in fact, platelet dysfunction is inevitable after cardiopulmonary bypass.

If the PTT alone is prolonged, this indicates persistent heparin effect. Many surgeons believe in a "heparin rebound" phenomenon, whereby a patient initially well neutralized with protamine may become re-heparinized in the early hours after cardiac surgery.[3] One factor may be that, as perfusion improves post surgery, vascular beds that were constricted are re-recruited into the circulation, bringing heparinized blood into circulation. Another cause of inadvertent re-heparinization is transfusion of the cell saver blood harvested intra-operatively; this always contains some residual heparin, which, some surgeons believe, is not completely removed in the cell "washing" process. In any case, another ACT may be done to confirm heparin excess. If only the pump team performs the ACT and that team is unavailable after hours, the conventional thrombin time (TT) test can be performed by the laboratory and is reasonably specific for heparin effect. Additional protamine is required for heparin rebound. In a patient bleeding early after cardiac surgery, many surgeons prefer to give some additional protamine (eg, 50 mg) empirically. If it is late after return from the operating room (say, beyond 4 or 6 hours), there is not much justification for additional protamine, as any heparin in the body can be expected to have been fully metabolized. (The half-life of heparin is 60 to 90 min.)

If PT and PTT are prolonged, circulating clotting factors are depleted. Protamine alone will not suffice. Clotting factors must be repleted, usually using fresh frozen plasma (FFP). Often 2 to 4 U of FFP must be administered. **The house officer must be aware that the effectiveness of transfused FFP will lapse within hours,** requiring re-administration, if the body's endogenous production remains deficient. The house officer should also be aware that **FFP is not benign;** it has been associated with noncardiogenic pulmonary edema in postoperative cardiac patients[5] and, of course, presents problems of potential transmission of infectious agents. **One should not administer FFP to correct clotting studies unless the patient shows excess bleeding.**

✚ TREATMENT

At our center, we often use a paradigm of interventions for the patient with serious bleeding in the early hours after cardiac surgery.

Strict BP Control

In the face of serious bleeding, we control BP even more strictly than usual. We often drop BP to 100 mm Hg systolic by afterload reduction (see Chapter 7, Continuous Infusion Agents). In certain cases, we may even use **controlled hypotension**—dropping systolic BP to 95, 90, or even 85 mm Hg for a brief period. The house officer must consult with a senior physician before using controlled hypotension, as this technique may impair cerebral, myocardial, or renal blood flow. At times, however, 30 or 60 min with mildly low BP may fully and permanently control bleeding.

Raising the Head of the Bed

Venous bleeding may respond dramatically to the simple maneuver of raising the head of the bed to a 30° to 45° angle. The innominate vein and its branches distend tensely when the patient is supine but often collapse fully as the head is raised. (The house officer should watch for this in the operating room.) Before raising the head of the bed, the house officer must ascertain that this is not contraindicated for some other reason. For example, if the intra-aortic balloon pump is in place, it may not be safe to raise the head, as the catheter tip may be made to impinge on the aortic arch, or the balloon may be made to kink at the groin. Likewise, after truly "open" procedures, many surgeons prefer to keep the patient supine for a number of hours to allow any residual intracardiac air to dissolve; raising the head might allow bubbles to migrate into the cerebral circulation. (Coronary bypass usually does not require opening the heart chambers; aortic and mitral valve surgery and left ventricular aneurysm or ascending aortic aneurysm resection do require opening of cardiac chambers, with resultant introduction of air into the heart.)

Air issues are less cogent in the present era because of the widespread use of CO_2 flooding of the operative field. CO_2 is heavy, so it fills the pericardial well. This means that any residual air in the heart is likely to be composed of CO_2. This is beneficial because CO_2 diffuses quickly across membranes, much quicker than atmospheric nitrogen. So any air bubbles entering the cerebral or coronary circulation in the present era are likely to absorb quickly.

Positive End-Expiratory Pressure

Some surgeons believe that positive end-expiratory pressure (PEEP) serves to tamponade mediastinal bleeding by virtue of pressure by the lungs themselves against oozing mediastinal tissues. There is evidence for and against the efficacy of PEEP in this setting.[6-9] If the patient is not especially sensitive hemodynamically, we do use PEEP for bleeding patients in our unit. PEEP can be added in increments of 2.5 cm H_2O, from the standard 5.0 cm H_2O used for all patients up to 12.5 cm H_2O. Assessment for hemodynamic embarrassment from PEEP is made with each increment. We usually do not go beyond 12.5 (or 15 at most) cm H_2O of PEEP for control of bleeding. This use of PEEP to control bleeding is now supported by studies in the literature.

Aminocaproic Acid

Some surgeons believe that once excess mediastinal hemorrhage has occurred, with formation of clots in the pericardium, localized accelerated fibrinolysis can take place. For this reason, many use the antifibrinolytic agent epsilon aminocaproic acid (Amicar) to control this process. When we use Amicar, we give 5 g IV over 1 hour followed by 1 g IV hourly for 4 hours.[10] Amicar may be harmful in disseminated intravascular coagulopathy, and this disorder should be reasonably ruled out before administration of this agent.

Protamine

In the bleeding patient, we usually give an additional dose of protamine while awaiting clotting studies to look for heparin effect. We usually give 50 mg IV over 10 min. **Protamine can drop BP and must be given slowly.**

Clotting Factors and Platelets

Clotting factors and platelets are given as required to correct confirmed deficiencies. We occasionally transfuse platelets despite normal counts if the run of cardiopulmonary bypass has been long and we suspect abnormal qualitative function of circulating platelets.

If the paradigm of discrete interventions described above is instituted early when a bleeding tendency becomes apparent, many patients will be rendered dry—permanently so. It is important to realize, however, that no such manipulations will compensate for a major mechanical defect that causes bleeding. If substantial bleeding continues, if the trend is for increasing bleeding, if there is hemodynamic embarrassment, or if a major mechanical defect is suspected, prompt reexploration is indicated. Timely reexploration and evacuation of clots often controls bleeding even when no discrete bleeding site is found. Timely reexploration can avoid hours of chasing bleeding with blood transfusions and clotting factors, which further debilitate the patient. The house officer will come to see that patients who have been reexplored come along well postoperatively, usually just as well as patients who do not have this complication.

Several additional points deserve emphasis. The experienced surgeon can tell quite well which patients will need to be reexplored. One criterion that some surgeons use can be assessed as well by the house officer. The level of blood in the chest tubes should oscillate with each heartbeat but should not advance with each heartbeat. **A fluid level in the chest tubes that advances inexorably with each heartbeat implies serious bleeding that will not respond to conservative measures and requires prompt reexploration** (see Figure 15.1). Note that advancing fluid level with each respiration is acceptable. We have found this criterion quite useful.

Another basic principle is that **if bleeding has not occurred over the first night following cardiac surgery, it will almost never occur subsequently.** By this time, cannulation sites and suture lines are well sealed by clot and fibrin. In fact, we liberalize our upper BP criterion to 150 to 160 mm Hg from the first postoperative morning on. By the second postoperative morning, even further liberalization is permissible.

The house officer should be aware as well that, on occasion, especially with turning of the patient, sudden drainage of several hundred milliliters may occur without active bleeding in progress; this may reflect a pool of old blood coming into communication with the chest drainage system. This is seen most frequently when a pleural space has been entered and left in continuity with the mediastinum.

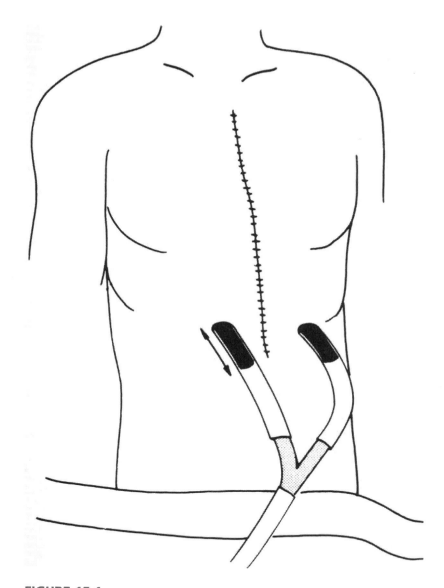

FIGURE 15.1

The chest tube observation criterion for assessment of postoperative bleeding. A level that rises inexorably with each heartbeat signifies bleeding of surgical significance that is likely to require reexploration.

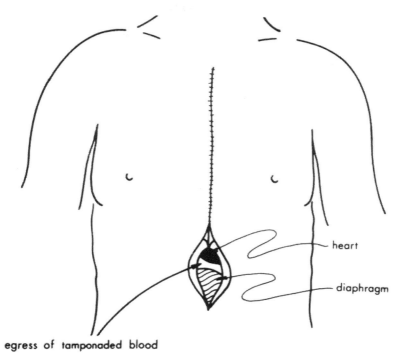

egress of tamponaded blood

FIGURE 15.2

Decompression of postoperative cardiac tamponade by opening the lower portion of the sternotomy incision and the linea alba.

Finally, the house officer should be prepared to handle massive mediastinal hemorrhage when it does occur. Rapid transfusion of blood should be carried out to replace losses. Losses will exceed measured drainage because of sequestration in the mediastinum. Tamponade should be treated with volume and possibly inotropic agents, as outlined in Chapter 16.

Massive hemorrhage may need to be handled surgically, even in the ICU. **In the postoperative patient, tamponade can be released in most cases by opening the subxyphoid part of the incision and removing the sutures from the linea alba** (Figure 15.2). This allows free drainage of the pericardium and usually restores vital signs very well. Further surgical intervention can be carried out in the operating room once vital signs have been restored.

When the linea alba is opened, of course, free bleeding to the outside may occur; this may be massive. In an occasional case, opening the linea alba may not suffice to release tamponade. Moreover, in certain cases, massive hemorrhage may have resulted in cardiac arrest, requiring open resuscitation. In all these circumstances, the house officer should be prepared to open the chest fully, even in the ICU, if required.

An ICU caring for cardiac patients should have a thoracotomy set available at all times. In addition, light and suction will be required. The skin is prepped quickly with antiseptic solution, the skin and subcutaneous sutures are divided, and the sternal wires are cut quickly with a wire cutter and removed. The chest is spread manually and the retractor is placed. Clots are evacuated manually and blood is suctioned.

Almost all bleeding sites can be controlled by manual pressure. The house officer should avoid the strong temptation to clamp bleeding sites; traumatic clamps can cause irrevocable damage to vascular structures. The fingertip is excellent for controlling aortic bleeding. A sponge packing controls most atrial suture lines. Bleeding grafts can be pinched by finger. When the acute emergency has been controlled, the patient can be transferred to the operating room, where, with proper lighting, suction, equipment, and personnel, definitive repair can be carried out.

Whenever possible, the house officer should await more senior personnel before carrying out the surgical interventions described in the preceding paragraphs. In the rare case when a true emergency exists and a more senior surgeon is unavailable, however, the house officer should not hesitate to intervene as indicated. Such interventions will be life-saving.

Aprotinin

Postoperative bleeding is such a common and troublesome problem that surgeons have long hoped for a panacea—a magic medication or technique that could prevent bleeding problems. An important medication of this type entered the scene just when the last edition of this book was published: aprotinin.[11-14] This drug entered and exited the formulary between editions of this book, but the story is relevant to the house officer even today. This drug is an inhibitor of the proteolytic enzymes plasmin and kallikrein involved in lysis of clots. Aprotinin was administered intravenously just before cardio-pulmonary bypass and then continuously during bypass. (One dosage regimen was 2 million IU initially, followed by 500,000 IU/h.) This drug had been investigated extensively in Europe, with the finding of dramatic reduction in the incidence and amount of bleeding after cardiac operations. The mechanism of this dramatic beneficial effect remained incompletely elucidated; inhibition of the fibrinolytic system and a direct augmentation of platelet function were postulated. Unfortunately, a tendency toward excess thrombosis with use of aprotinin was reported, at times involving the bypass grafts and even extracardiac vascular beds.[12] These observations first tempered enthusiasm and then led to withdrawal of the drug by the FDA. This was a controversial decision. Surgeons have never seen another intervention that produces as "dusty" a surgical field as aprotinin. It was almost a panacea, especially for major, prolonged cases and for thoracic aortic surgery.[11] There is hope that aprotinin analogs that replicate aprotinin's dramatic effectiveness without its putative toxicities may come out of drug development.

We are gaining experience with factor VII[15-17] for control of coagulopathic bleeding after cardiac surgery. We give smaller doses than recommended in drug formularies. We usually give 2 to 4 mg of factor VII. We see nearly immediate normalization of

TABLE 15.1 Measures at the House Officer's Disposal to Control Early Postoperative Bleeding

Physical interventions
- **Warming** (to improve enzymatic aspects of coagulation and thrombus formation)
- Push patient's temp to normal
- Use Bair Hugger
- Warm inhaled air (humidifier @100°F)
- Wrap the head in warm blankets
- Warm all IV fluids

BP control
- Keep systolic BP low (90 to 100 mm Hg)
- Use propofol or other means of sedation as first line of therapy for BP
- PEEP (to put some pressure on bleeding sites)
- Raise PEEP to 8 or 10 cm, if hemodynamics are unharmed
- Evacuation of clot (to allow tissue-to-tissue apposition)
- Strip chest tubes to maintain patency

Drugs to avoid
- Hetastarch (Hespan), as this volume expander creates an acquired von Willebrand defect
- Nitroglycerine, as this drug is a platelet inhibitor

Drugs to give
- Amicar
   5 gm bolus followed by 1 gm per hour drip postoperatively for 4 hours
- Protamine
   50 mg empirically
- Vitamin K
   10 mg IV
- DDAVP
   if patient has renal insufficiency or if patient was on antiplatelet drugs immediately preoperatively

Blood components to consider
- Platelets: empiric use if bleeding, as CPB alters platelet function in all cases
- Fresh frozen plasma: also empiric if bleeding, as clotting factors depleted with CPB or cell saver
- Packed red cells: if bleeding and Hct is under 30 (as 90% of clot is made of red cells)

Secondary components to consider, in this order
- See Annals of Thoracic Surgery 2009;88:1666.)
- Cryoprecipitate: if considerable TX has occurred or if fibrinogen < 150 (7 mL/kg)
- Factor VII (rFVIIa, Novoseven, dose is 20 mg/kg)

Various other interventions to consider
- Keep Ca++ on high side (some blood product anticoagulants bind Ca++)
- Treat acidosis (blood clots best when pH is normal)

coagulation parameters and cessation of non-surgical bleeding. We use smaller than generally recommended doses, as excess coagulation has been reported, and we do not want to chance graft or valve thrombosis. Also, factor VII is expensive. Perhaps this drug will replace aprotinin in effectiveness and in the surgeon's heart.

Table 15.1 supplies the house officer with a comprehensive list of measures he or she can take to control early postoperative bleeding.

REFERENCES

1. Verska J. Control of heparinization by activated clotting time during bypass with improved postoperative hemostasis. *Ann Thorac Surg.* 1977;24:170-173.
2. Cordell A. *Hematologic Complications of Intrathoracic Surgery.* Boston: Little, Brown; 1979:27-34.
3. Gollub S. Heparin rebound in open heart surgery. *Surg Gynecol Obstet.* 1967;124:337-346.
4. Edmunds LH Jr. Managing fibrinolysis without aprotinin. *Ann Thorac Surg.* 2010 Jan;89(1):324-331.
5. Hashim SW, Kay HR, Hammond GL, et al. Noncardiogenic pulmonary edema following cardiopulmonary bypass: an anaphylactic reaction to frozen plasma. *Am J Surg.* 1983;145:508-513.
6. Lai C, Chen J, Wu H, Wen J, Yang Y. Successful conservative management with positive end-expiratory pressure for massive hemothorax complicating pacemaker implantation. *Resuscitation.* 2007;75: 189-191.
7. Sedrakyan A, Wu A, Sedrakyan G, Diener-West M, Tranquilli M, Elefteriades J. Aprotinin use in thoracic aortic surgery: safety and outcomes. *J Thorac Cardiovasc Surg.* 2006 Oct;132(4):909-917.
8. Ilabaca PA, Ochsner JL, Mills NL. Positive end-expiratory pressure in the management of the patient with a postoperative bleeding heart. *Ann Thorac Surg.* 1980 Sep;30(3):281-284.
9. Murphy D, Finlayson D, Craver J, et al. Effect of positive end-expiratory pressure on excessive mediastinal bleeding after cardiac operations: A controlled study. *J Thorac Cardiovasc Surg.* 1983;85: 864-869.

10. Package insert. Amicar. Lederle Laboratories; Pearl River, NY.

11. Sedrakyan A, We A, Sedrakyan G, Diener-West M, Tranquilli M, Elefteriades J. Aprotinin use in thoracic aortic surgery: safety and outcomes. *J Thorac Cardiovasc Surg.* 2006 Oct;132(4):909-917.

12. Cosgrove DM, Huric B, Lytle BW, et al. Aprotinin therapy for reoperative myocardial revascularization: a placebo-controlled study. *Ann Thorac Surg.* 1992;54:1031-1036.

13. Boldt J, Knothe C, Sickman B, Fill S, Dapper F, Hempelmann G. Platelet function in cardiac surgery: influence of temperature and aprotinin. *Ann Thorac Surg.* 1993;55:652-658.

14. Tatar H, Cicek S, Demirdilic U, et al. Topical use of aprotinin in open heart operations. *Ann Thorac Surg.* 1993 Mar;55(3):659-661.

15. Grottke O, Henzler D, Rossaint R. Activated recombinant factor VII (rFVIIa). *Best Pract Res Clin Anaesthesiol.* 2010 Mar;24:95-106.

16. Warren OJ, Darzi AW, Athanasiou T. Recombinant activated factor VII in cardiac surgery—first do no harm. *J Cardiothorac Surg.* 2007;2:50.

17. Heise D, Brauer A, Quintel M. Recombinant activated factor VII (Novo 7) in patients with ventricular assist devices: case report and review of the current literature. *J Cardiothorac Surg.* 2007;2:47.

SUGGESTED FURTHER READING

Edmunds LH Jr. Managing fibrinolysis without aprotinin. *Ann Thorac Surg.* 2010;89:324-331.
Superb insights from an authority in the field.

16

CHEST TRAUMA

The general physiologic management of abdominal and extremity injuries is usually straightforward. The acute critical derangement is hypovolemia. Later, sepsis may supervene. Cardiac and thoracic injuries, however, do not present such a clear physiologic picture. This chapter will clarify the physiologic abnormalities in chest injuries and their management. The emphasis will be on acute management by the nonspecialist that is required to preserve the patient's life until the specialist can intervene. We will not go into the details of operative management of specific thoracic and cardiac injuries. Many of the conditions discussed can arise directly in the ICU setting without trauma per se, and the same principles of assessment and management apply.

The House Officer's Guide to ICU Care: Fundamentals of Management of the Heart and Lungs, 3rd ed. © 2013 John A. Elefteriades, Curtis Tribble, Alexander S. Geha, Mark D. Siegel, and Lawrence S. Cohen, eds. Cardiotext Publishing, ISBN: 978-1-935395-68-3.

Rutherford[1] has listed **six general categories of physiologic abnormality following chest trauma that are acutely life-threatening, and we have added a seventh:**

1. Airway obstruction
2. Flail chest
3. Sucking chest wound
4. Massive hemothorax
5. Tension pneumothorax
6. Cardiac tamponade
7. Air embolism.

These are the conditions that can take the patient's life within the first few minutes after arrival in the emergency room. Note that these are categories of physiologic abnormality, not specific injuries. Each category may follow any of a number of specific injuries, and a given injury may bring about several of these abnormalities. For example, massive hemothorax may be the result of an aortic transection from a motor vehicle accident, a gunshot wound of the lung parenchyma, or a knife wound of an intercostal vessel. Likewise, cardiac tamponade may result from an atrial knife wound, a blunt ventricular rupture, a coronary artery laceration, or other specific injury.

The discussion of these six entities will be organized as follows. First, we will define each condition. Next, we will discuss the physiology of how each condition hurts the patient. Then we will discuss how to diagnose each condition within minutes—based solely on vital signs, brief physical examination, and one single radiographic procedure. Finally, we will cover how to manage each condition within minutes.

The one diagnostic procedure required is the chest x-ray (CXR). Hematocrit, blood gases, electrocardiogram, and other studies may prove useful, but the chest x-ray is indispensable in every case.

✚ DEFINITIONS
Airway Obstruction

Airway obstruction is self-explanatory. Injuries to the chest can disrupt the airway in its course through the upper mediastinum. The lumen may be obstructed or the trachea or bronchi may be transected, with loss of continuity. These can be devastating injuries (Figure 16.1A).

Flail Chest

Flail chest is a disruption of the continuity of the rigid thoracic cage, with paradoxical movement of the disrupted segment. Since the thoracic cage in the transverse plane is a rigid oval, with ribs attached posteriorly at the spine and anteriorly at the sternum, flailing requires that at least one rib be broken in at least two places (Figure 16.1B). If one rib were broken in one place only, it would still be attached anteriorly and posteriorly. Usually, a number of adjacent ribs are broken in multiple spots, so that a segment of chest wall is free to be sucked in during inspiration and pushed out during expiration, while the intact chest cage moves in the opposite direction during each phase.

Sucking Chest Wound

A sucking chest wound results from a loss of integrity of the chest wall, so that air is free to move in and out of the pleural space to the atmosphere (Figure 16.1C). A chest tube (before it is hooked to the suction device) represents a sucking chest wound. The to-and-fro rush of air with breathing is one sign that the surgeon looks for to confirm that the tube is well situated in the pleural space.

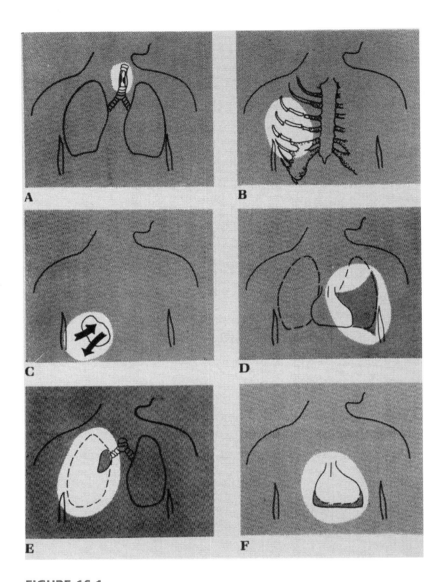

FIGURE 16.1

Schematic representation of the six major physiologic categories of injury that can take the patient's life within the first few minutes of chest trauma. **Panel A:** Airway obstruction. **Panel B:** Flail chest. **Panel C:** Sucking chest wound. **Panel D:** Massive hemothorax. **Panel E:** Tension pneumothorax. **Panel F:** Cardiac tamponade.

Massive Hemothorax

Hemothorax is the presence of blood in the pleural space; massive hemothorax is the presence of large amounts of blood in the pleural space (Figure 16.1D). Massive hemothorax is differentiated from simple hemothorax because a small hemothorax is not acutely life-threatening.

Tension Pneumothorax

Pneumothorax is the presence of air in the pleural space; tension pneumothorax is the presence of air under pressure. An ordinary pneumothorax is not acutely life-threatening, whereas tension pneumothorax may be (Figure 16.1E).

Cardiac Tamponade

Cardiac tamponade refers to impairment of cardiac function by fluid under pressure in the pericardial space. In the context of trauma, the offending fluid is blood. In nontraumatic conditions, transudates, exudates, purulent fluids, and chyle can cause tamponade (Figure 16.1F).

✚ PHYSIOLOGY OF CARDIORESPIRATORY EMBARRASSMENT

Much experimental work has gone into elucidating the physiology of chest injuries.[1-4] Both historical and modern theories have been summarized by Rutherford.[1] The explanations presented here are purposely oversimplified. By conceiving the injuries as described, however, the house officer will be led to appropriate therapeutic interventions.

Airway Obstruction

Airway obstruction injures the patient via hypoventilation and elevation of pCO_2. Obstruction of the airway impairs movement of air to and fro in the tracheobronchial tree; that is, it impairs minute volume. As is discussed in Chapter 1 (Ventilators and Respiratory Management), CO_2 rises as minute volume falls; O_2 is often preserved until minute volume falls very low. The patient with traumatic airway obstruction will be hypoventilated; in late stages, he or she may be hypo-oxygenated as well.

Flail Chest

The physiology of flail chest is similarly complex. Here, although the pleural space is not open, tidal volume is wasted in moving the chest wall in and out. This movement of the chest wall represents a wasted tidal volume equal to the area in square centimeters of the defect multiplied by the length of its to-and-fro travel (similar to the volume of displacement in a cylinder in an automobile engine, equal to bore times stroke). This volume is lost from each breath, and **in flail chest, as in sucking chest wound, the patient is overwhelmed by the work of breathing and dies hypoventilated.**

Sucking Chest Wound

Many mechanisms have been proposed to explain the distress seen with sucking chest wounds; none is totally satisfactory.[1] It is safe to say that distress can occur even without development of tension pneumothorax, that simple loss of function of the ipsilateral lung is not the critical defect, and that **some disturbance of the thoracic bellows appears likely.** Tidal volume is wasted moving air in and out of the pleural space, which, unlike the alveolus, is not a respiratory exchange membrane. The bigger the defect, the greater the ventilatory burden. Even a young, robust patient can succumb if the defect is large. **The patient who succumbs to a sucking chest wound dies hypoventilated, with a high pCO_2.**

Massive Hemothorax

The physiology of massive hemothorax can be confusing; many house officers believe that the patient succumbs because the blood impinges on the lung, impairing its respiratory function. This is not the mechanism. A young, otherwise healthy patient will usually not be symptomatic if one entire pleural space is filled with fluid. Such a patient manages to ventilate adequately with the opposite lung. Pneumonectomy can be done, even in elderly patients with poor lung function, and they are not rendered dyspneic at rest. (This situation is not entirely analogous, for in pneumonectomy the pulmonary artery is interrupted as well, preventing the shunting of blood through a collapsed lung.) In any case, **the patient with a massive hemothorax dies by exsanguination into the pleural space, not by restriction of pulmonary function. Nearly an entire blood volume can be lost into one hemithorax.**

Tension Pneumothorax

Tension pneumothorax does not kill the patient by eliminating function of the affected lung. Again, the patient could survive well with just the opposite lung functioning. Rather, **the patient with tension pneumothorax dies from circulatory embarrassment.** The superior vena cava (SVC) is relatively fixed to the adjacent organs. The inferior vena cava (IVC) is fixed to the liver. When pressure develops in one chest, the heart is displaced toward the opposite side. If displacement is great enough, it is thought, the venous return through the SVC and IVC can be impaired. Stroke volume and cardiac output suffer because of inadequate blood return to the heart. Shock may supervene.

Cardiac Tamponade

The house officer may have difficulty conceptualizing the physiology of cardiac tamponade. The pericardial space is relatively inelastic. It is unwilling to stretch beyond a finite volume. As this volume is exceeded, pressure builds in the pericardial space. This pressure is transmitted to the myocardium and to the ventricular chambers. Under normal circumstances, the right ventricle (RV) fills because the right atrial (RA) pressure, usually about 5 cm H_2O in a normal

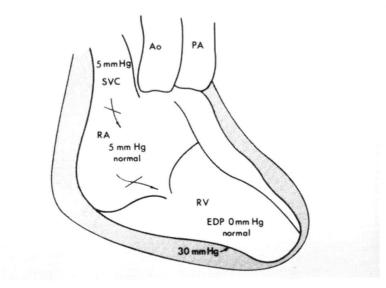

FIGURE 16.2

Pathophysiology of cardiac tamponade. Normal right heart filling pressures are shown. Blood in the pericardium creates an abnormally positive pressure in the pericardial space. This pressure is transmitted to the ventricular cavity. All gradients for filling of the ventricular cavity are lost. The heart cannot pump because the heart cannot fill. (Consideration, for purposes of clarity, is limited to the right heart.)

heart, exceeds the RV diastolic pressure, usually near zero in a normal heart. It is this RA-to-RV gradient that fills the ventricle. The RA is in turn filled because of SVC-to-RA and IVC-to-RA gradients. In tamponade, if, say, a pressure of 30 cm H_2O develops in the pericardial space and is transmitted to the RV, blood from the lower-pressure RA will not enter or fill the RV (Figure 16.2). Thus **in cardiac tamponade, the heart cannot pump because the heart cannot fill.** The patient dies hypotensive in cardiogenic shock.

It will be seen that these physiologic concepts have important therapeutic correlates. These will become clear in the discussion of how to treat these disorders. These explanations, although to some extent oversimplified, have been chosen because they lead to appropriate conclusions regarding acute treatment of these life-threatening injuries.

✚ DIAGNOSIS

Because the traumatic conditions described are acutely life-threatening, their diagnosis must be made rapidly. This discussion will focus on how to diagnose these conditions within minutes, based on vital signs, physical examination, and CXR only. No more sophisticated or time-consuming laboratory tests will be used.

Airway Obstruction

Airway obstruction is an obvious clinical diagnosis. The patient tries to move air but cannot. The respiratory muscles act, but the chest does not expand. Good air movement cannot be felt or heard at the nose and the mouth. One of the major benefits of a rotation on an anesthesia service is that it teaches the house officer to recognize airway obstruction: a stage of obstruction is part of every general anesthetic induction.

Flail Chest

Flail chest is a diagnosis of inspection. Many times, flails are missed because concerted inspection of chest wall motion is omitted. It is important that severely traumatized patients have all clothing removed. With attention to the chest, a flail will be apparent as a segment of chest wall that moves in with inspiration and out with expiration—out of synchrony with the remainder of the chest. This paradoxical movement can be appreciated also on palpation, and rib fractures and tenderness can also be found. Flail chest is not a sophisticated diagnosis; rather, with good observation, it is an obvious one.

Sucking Chest Wound

Sucking chest wound is a diagnosis made by listening—not through a stethoscope, but with one's ear. Once heard, the sound of air rushing in and out of the pleural space with each breath is unmistakable. It is the same sound that is made through a chest tube before the tube is connected. Again, this is not a sophisticated diagnosis. Usually, it is obvious from listening that a patient has a sucking chest wound the moment he or she is brought into the trauma room. From that point on, it is just a matter of removing the patient's clothing to identify the site of the chest wall defect.

Massive Hemothorax and Tension Pneumothorax

Massive hemothorax and tension pneumothorax share one physical finding and are disparate in another. The physical finding they share is decreased breath sounds. The physical finding in which they are disparate is resonance to percussion: hemothorax is dull, and pneumothorax is hyperresonant. The dullness of hemothorax may not be easy to appreciate in a noisy, hectic trauma room. The severely injured patient will be supine; the dullness of the hemothorax will be, accordingly, posterior only.

The diagnosis of massive hemothorax or tension pneumothorax will be confirmed by CXR, which is available within minutes in emergency wards. Tension pneumothorax is obvious by CXR (Figure 16.3). In addition to collapse of the lung, one sees displacement of the mediastinum, overexpansion of the ipsilateral intercostal spaces, and depression of the ipsilateral diaphragm. Hemothorax, even massive hemothorax, may be a subtle CXR diagnosis (Figure 16.4). Most house officers are accustomed to interpreting upright CXRs. On an upright CXR, a pleural effusion shows its characteristic meniscus-type layering shadow on posteroanterior and lateral views. On upright studies, a massive hemothorax would appear just like a large pleural effusion. In the severely traumatized patient, however, the CXR will likely need to be obtained supine.

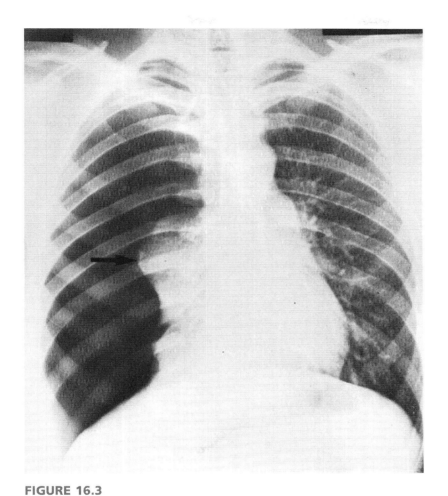

FIGURE 16.3

CXR in tension pneumothorax.

On a supine CXR, a massive hemothorax will show only as a diffuse increase in density of the affected hemithorax. A liter of fluid may be just detectable to the astute observer. Two liters of fluid may be subtle. It is important to be alert that in the traumatized patient, a homogeneous increase in density of one side of the chest probably represents major hemothorax. If the patient stabilizes before treatment is required, upright and lateral CXRs may clarify the diagnosis.

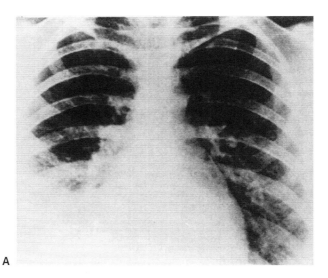

A

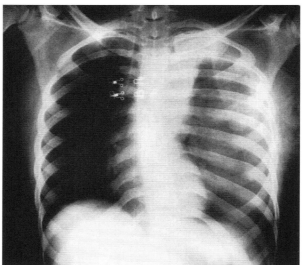

B

FIGURE 16.4

CXR in hemothorax. **Panel A:** Upright. Note meniscus of fluid in right hemithorax. **Panel B:** Supine. Note diffuse increase in density representing fluid in left hemithorax.

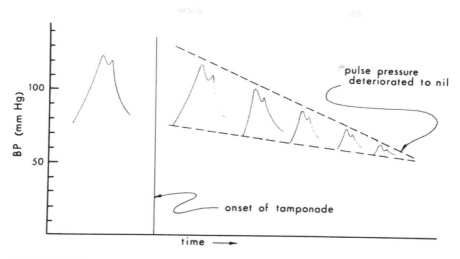

FIGURE 16.5

Progressive deterioration of pulse pressure in cardiac tamponade.

Cardiac Tamponade

Cardiac tamponade may be a more subtle diagnosis. The house officer should be aware of the classic triad (Beck triad) of findings in tamponade: decreased pulse pressure, distant heart sounds, and jugular venous distention. Pulse pressure refers to the difference between systolic and diastolic pressures. In tamponade, the blood pressure may vary from mildly to severely decreased. In particular, the pulse pressure suffers even before the systolic pressure reaches critically low levels. Figure 16.5 presents typical tracings of arterial pressure that might be seen in the ICU in a patient with progressive tamponade.

Fine points of cardiac auscultation are difficult to appreciate in a noisy, hectic trauma room. Usually, however, in patients with cardiac tamponade, the heart sounds will be very distant or even inaudible.

Jugular venous distention is easy to appreciate. It is important to remember that straining and agitation or overtransfusion can cause jugular venous distention, even in a patient who does not have tamponade. It takes only minutes to pass a central venous pressure (CVP) line and in this way ascertain CVP precisely. (It is not even necessary to use a manometer. The stopcock tubing will fill with blood when held upright in the air when the patient has tamponade.)

A word should be said about pulsus paradoxus and tamponade. Pulsus paradoxus refers to the inspiratory decrease in systolic blood pressure with breathing. A decrease of up to 15 mm Hg may be seen in normal subjects. Larger decreases are said to be characteristic of tamponade. To ascertain the degree of pulsus paradoxus requires excellent blood pressure–taking abilities and practice. The house officer should develop this skill. However, in the noisy emergency room, it may be difficult to ascertain the degree of paradox. It may be time-consuming also. Furthermore, a prominent pulsus paradoxus is an inconsistent finding in traumatic tamponade.[5] For these reasons, with trauma, we rely less on determinations of pulsus paradoxus than we do in less acute circumstances. For example, in the setting of daily monitoring of chronic low-grade tamponade from uremic pericardial effusion on the medical ward, measuring pulsus paradoxus is indicated and useful.

A word should be said about the CXR in tamponade. The house officer often expects a large heart shadow in the patient with traumatic tamponade; this is not usually seen. The pericardium is largely inelastic; if it were elastic, tamponade would not occur. Although the pericardium, and the heart shadow, may grow tremendously with chronic effusions, with acute tamponade the usual finding is a normal heart shadow. Occasionally (Figure 16.6), some straightening of the left heart border, obscuring the normal left pulmonary artery shadow, may be appreciated, giving the impression of "pressure" in the pericardial space.

Perhaps the most important point in diagnosis of tamponade is the patient's having sustained a penetrating injury in the region of

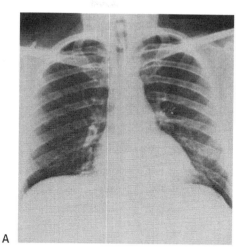

A

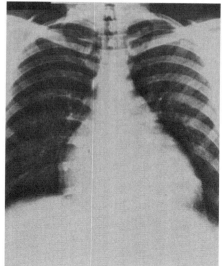

B

FIGURE 16.6

CXR in cardiac tamponade. Note the difference between normal left cardiac contour in **Panel A** and loss of angle in left cardiac contour in CXR of patient in tamponade in **Panel B.** In **Panel B,** contour appears full and tense.

Source: Reproduced with permission from Thompson T. *Primer of Clinical Radiology.* 2nd ed. Boston, MA: Little Brown; 1980.

the heart. If the patient has sustained a gunshot wound or knife wound near the heart and exhibits the classic triad of findings, chances are that he or she has tamponade. Keep in mind, however, that if the CVP is low in the hypotensive patient with chest trauma, the patient may well be hypovolemic without tamponade.

✚ TREATMENT
Airway Obstruction

Injuries of the intrathoracic great airways can be devastating. Unlike upper-airway obstruction, where tracheostomy may provide airway access beyond the injury, tracheostomy is not useful with injuries to the intrathoracic trachea and mainstem bronchi. Rigid bronchoscopy is essential in diagnosis and treatment. If there is distortion and obstruction of the airway, it may be possible to advance the bronchoscope beyond the injury and thus to carry out positive pressure ventilation beyond the injury. The airway may be transected without distorting obstruction. In these cases, pleural and connective tissues may conduct the tidal volume, allowing effective spontaneous ventilation. If all continuity is lost, again the rigid bronchoscope may allow instrumentation and ventilation of the distal tracheobronchial tree. Surgery is required after initial respiratory support, though many patients with such injuries succumb before specialized care is available. **For the house officer, the main task is prompt recognition of such injuries, so that the specialist can be called early.**

Flail Chest

Historically, flail chest has been treated by immobilization of the flail segment. This has been done by immobilizing in the "in" position (by sandbags or bricks) or in the "out" position (by grasping a rib with a towel clip attached to a weight hanging over a pulley). On occasion, internal fixation of rib fractures has been carried out surgically. This is fraught with difficulties and is usually unnecessary. **The modern treatment for flail chest is intubation and positive pressure ventilation.** When the lungs are expanded by positive pressure within the tracheobronchial tree, it makes no difference, physiologically, what the flail segment does. After 10 days to 2 weeks of ventilation, the chest wall begins to solidify, flailing diminishes, and the patient can be weaned to spontaneous ventilation and extubated.

Now, not every patient with flail chest requires intubation and positive pressure ventilation. Flails have different degrees of severity, and patients differ in the degree of embarrassment they can tolerate (ie, the amount of ineffective tidal volume they can afford to lose). If a particular flail is well tolerated in a patient, without distress and without hypoventilation, no specific treatment is required. It is important to remember that elderly patients, especially, may initially tolerate the flail but tire progressively from the respiratory embarrassment. It is important that such patients be watched carefully over the first several days, both by clinical observation and by arterial blood gas measurements.

In recent years, increasing attention has been drawn to the fact that in flail chest, significant pulmonary contusion more often than not accompanies the mechanical chest wall defect.[6,7] It has been learned that the underlying contusion may be as important as the chest wall defect, and perhaps more so in certain cases. It has been shown that the contused lung is very sensitive to fluid administration; vigorous fluid and crystalloid administration by the trauma team can lead to pulmonary edema in the contused lung segments, with resultant hypoxia. The EAST Group on Trauma has produced a superb monograph reviewing fully the historical and current evidence on pathophysiology of decompensation in flail chest.[8] Not only is contusion important, but potent inflammatory mechanisms (including cytokine liberation) are activated, which have adverse effects even on the contralateral, non-injured lung. Although avoidance of over-transfusion and "running the patient dry" are now accepted as important aspects of the care of patients with flail chest, most authorities would still agree that severe flails with respiratory embarrassment continue to require intubation and mechanical ventilation.

Sucking Chest Wound

The treatment for a sucking chest wound is an occlusive dressing. Vaseline gauze covered by sponges and tape works well. The occlusive dressing prevents the loss of tidal volume through the defect (the wasted ventilation of the pleural space discussed earlier in the section on physiology). Usually a closed (nontension) pneumothorax remains after placement of the occlusive dressing, but this does not represent a life-threatening condition. Astute medical technicians in battlefield circumstances have learned to have the injured patient with a sucking chest wound exhale fully immediately before placement of the occlusive dressing. This maneuver serves to minimize or eliminate residual pneumothorax. In the emergency room setting, a chest tube can be placed after application of the occlusive dressing to eliminate any residual pneumothorax.

Major chest wall defects eventually will need to be debrided and closed formally in the operating room. The treatment outlined earlier will prevent respiratory demise until formal treatment is undertaken.

Massive Hemothorax

House officers often consider placement of a chest tube to be the treatment for massive hemothorax. Although the chest tube is certainly helpful, it will be recalled from the earlier discussion that loss of ipsilateral lung function is not the key physiologic element in massive hemothorax. Rather, the key feature is **hypovolemia**—the patient exsanguinates. **Thus the treatment of massive hemothorax is volume replacement—specifically, administration of blood.** Although not usually critical, restoration of ipsilateral lung function by emptying the pleural space is also beneficial. Placement of a chest tube is therefore helpful and allows evaluation of the amount of blood lost and the ongoing rate of bleeding. The house officer should not be shocked if large amounts of blood are evacuated immediately. It is not uncommon for one drainage device to fill immediately. This volume usually represents blood already shed. The key criterion in further management is the ongoing rate of bleeding. **If bleeding continues at more than 200 mL/h for 3 hours, operative intervention should be considered.** The specialist can address this question. The critical aspect of initial care by the house officer is volume replacement.

It is important to note that the **overwhelming majority of knife wounds of the lung and a large majority of gunshot wounds of the lung do not require surgical treatment.** The pulmonary arterial circuit is a low-pressure system. When the lung is expanded to the chest wall after tube placement, the irritated visceral and parietal pleural surfaces appose and adhere. Between the low pressures involved and the tamponading by apposed tissues, most pulmonary parenchymal injuries stop bleeding without exploration. Air leaks from the parenchyma can almost always be controlled by chest tube placement and apposition of pleural surfaces.

The house officer should always be alert to the possibility of air embolism with such injuries (see below). Along with bleeding, air embolism may underlie a presentation of such injuries with a shock state.

Tension Pneumothorax

The treatment for tension pneumothorax is chest tube placement. This is fairly straightforward. House officers often have heard of instrumenting the chest with a needle or plastic intravenous cannula. Although these maneuvers may occasionally be helpful, placement of a chest tube takes little more time and is far superior. Every house officer should know how to place a chest tube, as each will perform procedures that can be complicated by tension pneumothorax (especially thoracentesis and placement of

central venous lines). Key concepts regarding chest tubes are covered in Chapter 17.

Cardiac Tamponade

The management of cardiac tamponade is not as straightforward. It
is useful to consider first the *medical* treatment of tamponade, that
is, treatment without needles, tubes, and surgery. We will, for the
moment, "tie the surgeon's hands." Here the mechanism by which
tamponade hurts the heart must be remembered. In tamponade,
the heart cannot pump because the heart cannot fill. To get the
heart to pump, one must get it to fill. To get the heart to fill, one
must provide a gradient from the cavae to the RV. As the RV pressures are high from pressure transmitted from the pericardial space,
CVP must be raised quite high. **Thus the medical treatment of
tamponade is volume administration.**[5] The house officer should
be cautioned that nurses and inexperienced physicians may look
skeptically on giving volume to a patient whose CVP is already
high. When blood pressure is failing in tamponade, one must drive
the CVP as high as possible to fill the heart and get the heart to
pump. Pulmonary edema is not an issue. Blood is not even reaching
the left heart, let alone backing up in the pulmonary circuit. Acute
right-sided CVP elevation is not dangerous. Were it to continue,
edema, ascites, and hepatic engorgement might develop, but with
acute tamponade and shock, the patient's life is at stake and a brief
elevation of CVP is a small price to pay. Often crystalloid replacement to drive CVP up is successful in restoring some effective circulation in tamponade.

Inotropes are not part of the usual treatment of tamponade because they do not address the underlying physiology, which is failure of the heart to fill. Furthermore, young patients in shock
probably will have great release of endogenous catecholamines.
Nevertheless, in desperate circumstances, inotropic support can be
instituted. Although β-agonism is probably unnecessary, some

α-agonism may raise systemic pressures, albeit at the expense of organ perfusion, and allow better coronary perfusion. This could improve cardiac performance.

Please keep in mind also that these patients often need to be intubated. This may have an adverse impact on hemodynamics, as positive pressure ventilation decreases venous return to the heart. Venous return is already deficient in tamponade.

Patients who develop tamponade after cardiac surgery may not have the healthy heart of the young traumatized patient. These patients may benefit from inotropic support before mechanical correction of postoperative tamponade is achieved.

The medical interventions discussed are important, but they represent essentially temporizing measures; the defect in tamponade is a mechanical one that requires a mechanical correction. We will discuss now what can be done after the surgeon's hands are "untied."

Pericardiocentesis is the first step in the surgical management of acute traumatic tamponade. The subxyphoid approach is illustrated in Figure 16.7. As is well appreciated, because of the inelastic nature of the pericardium, removal of even a small volume of blood can significantly lower intrapericardial pressures and produce dramatic improvement in vital signs. Pericardiocentesis in this setting is not easy and not always effective. Blood is likely to be thick and partially clotted; it may not draw back through the needle. The heart, coronary arteries, lungs, and liver may be injured.

Most authorities agree that a patient who requires pericardiocentesis for acute traumatic tamponade should be taken for operation to control the injury. The alternative—waiting to see if bleeding recurs—represents an unnecessary and possibly dangerous delay that is unlikely to prevent surgery.

The house officer should be familiar with another technique that is available for decompressing the pericardium urgently. This is **subxyphoid pericardiotomy** (Figure 16.8). This procedure can be

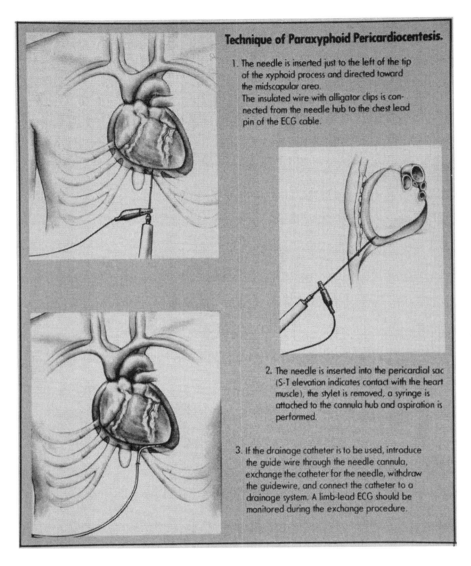

FIGURE 16.7

Subxiphoid pericardiocentesis. The needle is shown connected to a V lead of the EKG for detection of contact with the surface of the heart.

done on the emergency ward or in the operating room under local anesthesia (or without anesthesia if vital signs are failing). If vital signs are preserved, this procedure may be performed to prevent the deterioration seen with induction of general anesthesia. The procedure is done by making a midline vertical incision over the

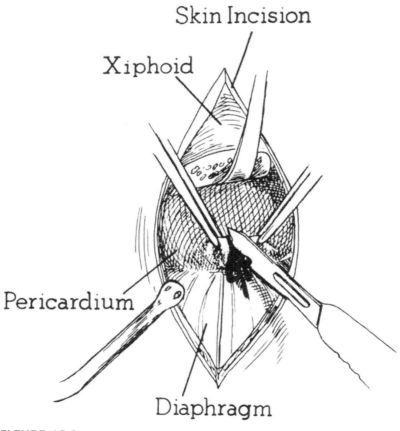

FIGURE 16.8

Subxiphoid pericardiotomy.

Source: Sabiston DC Jr, Spencer FC. Trauma to the Chest. *Surgery of the Chest.* 5th ed. Vol. 1:383-417. Philadelphia: Saunders; 1990. With permission from Elsevier LT.

lower sternum and the xyphoid process, excising the xyphoid process, and spreading the few intervening diaphragmatic fibers to visualize the pericardium. Then one picks up the pericardium and incises it. This provides immediate, thorough decompression of the pericardial space. A condition of tamponade can be converted in this way to a condition of cardiac injury without tamponade. Once this is performed, the patient will not die of tamponade. However, bleeding may be vigorous. With hemodynamic stability restored by the pericardiotomy, sternotomy or thoracotomy can then be done for definitive control of the injury.

In a postoperative patient who develops tamponade, opening the lower end of the wound and removing the sutures from the linea alba provides similar relief of tamponade under urgent circumstances (see Figure 16.2). Formal exploration and reclosure usually follow. The house officer on a cardiac service should prepare for and expect to need to perform this maneuver of opening the lower part of the sternum for postoperative cardiac tamponade.

✚ ADDITIONAL TOPIC: SYSTEMIC AIR EMBOLISM

The house officer must be familiar with the fascinating phenomenon of **systemic air embolism** following parenchymal lung injuries.[9] The pathophysiology of this condition is as follows (Figure 16.9). A parenchymal lung injury disrupts both *bronchi* and *pulmonary* veins. Air from the disrupted bronchi can enter the open pulmonary veins. (This is especially likely to occur if the trauma patient is on positive pressure ventilation. It is also especially likely if the patient is hypovolemic, as is often the case in major trauma. The positive pressure ventilation makes the air exiting the bronchi more likely to find routes of egress—into the pulmonary veins. The hypovolemia leads to lower pressure in the pulmonary veins—so that, instead of bleeding, these veins suck air liberated from the bronchi.) From the pulmonary veins, the air is carried into the left atrium,

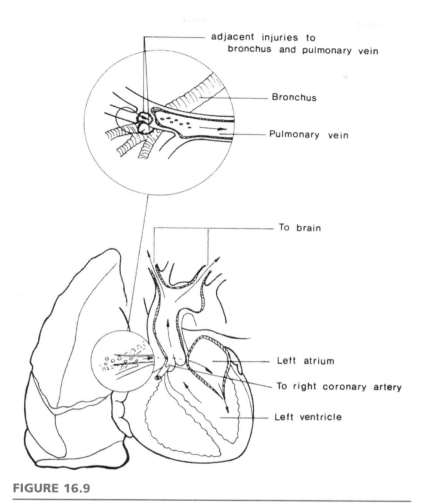

adjacent injuries to
bronchus and pulmonary vein

Bronchus

Pulmonary vein

To brain

Left atrium

To right coronary artery

Left ventricle

FIGURE 16.9

Schematic representation of systemic air embolism. (See text.)

and from there to the left ventricle. From the left ventricle, the air is ejected into the aorta and the systemic arterial tree, where it can cause ischemia by virtue of "air lock" in a specific vascular bed. If this air travels to the brain, it can cause a stroke. If it travels to the heart, it causes myocardial ischemia, often with cardiac arrest from ventricular fibrillation.

A common scenario is that the patient with a parenchymal lung injury, either stab or gunshot, enters the trauma room hypotensive, hypoxic, and agitated. On spontaneous ventilation, the pressure relationships do not produce air embolism. The patient is intubated for stabilization, and promptly arrests. The cause is often systemic air embolism. The institution of positive pressure ventilation has forced the air out of the bronchi and into the pulmonary veins. The right coronary artery, located just at the origin of the aorta, and directly anteriorly, where the air bubble tends to go by gravity, "traps" the bubble, leading to myocardial ischemia and ventricular fibrillation.

Air embolism to the heart usually goes to the right coronary artery because of its anterior location. This can produce heart block. The house officer should become immediately suspicious of air embolism when he sees heart block in a patient with penetrating chest trauma. The house officer should anticipate that more dire circumstances will occur soon, with rapid further deterioration due to myocardial ischemia. In the setting of heart block, the house officer should immediately call for senior backup, as the chest may well need to be opened and the patient may need to be placed on cardiopulmonary bypass.

Systemic air embolism can be seen also with iatrogenic trauma, as in needle biopsy of the lung, chest tube placement, and forceful irrigation of empyema tubes.

The house officer must maintain a high index of suspicion for systemic air embolism in traumatic chest injury. Air embolism is overwhelmingly underdiagnosed. The treatment is urgent thoracotomy. The patient is placed in Trendelenburg position to direct air away from the brain. The bronchovenous connection is interrupted by clamping the site of parenchymal injury or the hilum of the lung. To clamp the hilum, it is necessary to divide the inferior pulmonary ligament. Another alternative, described by Mattox,[10] is the "hilum twist" maneuver, which occludes the vessels and bronchus, thus discouraging continued air embolism.

At thoracotomy, air is vented from the aorta and the left ventricular apex. Open resuscitation is carried out. Formal lung resection is performed once hemodynamic stability is restored. Although systemic air embolism is almost invariably fatal, occasional survival with urgent thoracotomy has been obtained. Such thoracotomy must, of course, be carried out only by properly trained personnel. The house officer on duty needs to be aware of the syndrome and to have a high index of suspicion—so that he obtains the expert backup required.

The initial thoracotomy and open cardiac massage may be performed by a house officer with modest surgical training. The house officer can keep the patient alive with open cardiac massage, providing an opportunity for continued survival when senior staff arrive.

The house officer can help to prevent systemic air embolism by carrying out volume repletion before intubation. Avoiding high inspiratory pressures is also of benefit.

The phenomenon of *systemic* air embolism discussed here is to be contrasted with venous air embolism, in which air entering the great veins, usually from an open central line, travels to the lungs, causing an airlock in the pulmonary arteries with attendant cardiopulmonary collapse. Remember that a tiny amount of air can cause a devastating *systemic* embolism, whereas a large amount of air is required to cause circulatory collapse in venous air embolism.

✚ ADDITIONAL POINTS[12-15]

Although specifics of operative repair of particular cardiac and pulmonary injuries are beyond the scope of this text, a number of additional general guidelines deserve mention.

- **Stab wounds anywhere in the "thoracic mantle"** (see Figure 16.10) **should be suspected of producing cardiac injury.** The vulnerable area for cardiac injury depicted in Figure 16.10 is colloquially referred to in the present era as "the box."[11]
- **Gunshot wounds anywhere in the vicinity of the chest should always be suspected of producing cardiac injury** because of the unpredictable trajectory of bullets in the body.

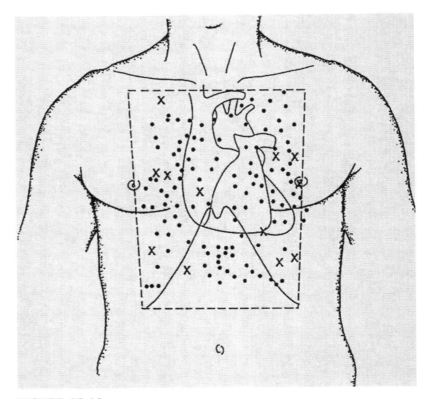

FIGURE 16.10

The "thoracic mantle," within which stab wounds should be considered to have produced cardiac injury unless proven otherwise.

Source: Reproduced with permission from Nagy K, Lohmann C, Kim DO, Barrett J. Role of echocardiography in the diagnosis of occult penetrating cardiac injury. *J Trauma.* 1995;38(6):859-862.

- **Finger control can stop bleeding from most wounds of the atria, ventricles, and aorta.** Application of clamps and instruments urgently under suboptimal circumstances is usually not necessary and can cause severe injury.
- **Because of the high position of the diaphragms in expiration, injuries anywhere below the nipples may produce intra-abdominal as well as intrathoracic injury.**
- **Emergency room thoracotomy is indicated only for *penetrating* cardiac injuries in patients *in extremis***

(without preserved blood pressure). For blunt injury, the dismal yield in survival does not justify emergency room thoracotomy. For patients with penetrating injury, especially when they present with sinus rhythm despite absent blood pressure, emergency room thoracotomy is not infrequently life-saving. For patients with preserved, albeit severely depressed, blood pressure, a trip to the operating room— with its better lighting and instrumentation—is much better than the difficult and dangerous emergency room thoracotomy.

- **The approach to transmediastinal gunshot wounds does not always mandate surgery.** If vital signs are unstable, immediate exploration is indeed required. If the patient is entirely stable, as is often the case, specialized, systematic evaluation of organs at risk may at times suffice. It is surprising how often the "educated" bullet traverses the mediastinum without producing major injury. Aortography (or CT scan, in the present era) is essential to rule out great vessel arterial injury. (There is no need to do any diagnostic studies to rule out occult venous injuries. If a venous injury is not actively bleeding, it will heal on its own.) Esophagography is essential to rule out esophageal injury. Bronchoscopy is essential to rule out central bronchial injury. Subxyphoid pericardial window (see earlier) can rule out intrapericardial bleeding. Cardiac echo may provide similar confirmation that there is no bloody pericardial effusion. Careful ICU observation, especially with echocardiographic exam, may suffice in place of pericardial window in selected patients.
- **The echocardiographic examination of the pericardial space is part of the modern FAST exam used by trauma teams.**[16] FAST stands for "Focused Assessment with Sonography in Trauma." This invaluable technique can detect blood not only in the pericardium, but also in the abdomen or chest.

If the house officer keeps in mind the basic physiology of these few categories of dysfunction after chest trauma and adheres to the treatment guidelines outlined, he or she can be assured of satisfactory early management of thoracic and cardiac injuries.

REFERENCES

1. Rutherford R. Thoracic injuries. In: Ballinger W, Rutherford R, Zuidema G, eds. *The Management of Trauma*. Philadelphia: WB Saunders; 1973:333-395.

2. Hood M. Trauma to the chest. In: Sabiston D, Spencer F, eds. *Gibbon's Surgery of the Chest*. Philadelphia: WB Saunders; 1983:291-317.

3. Symbas P. *Traumatic Injuries of the Heart and Great Vessels*. Springfield, IL: Charles C Thomas; 1972.

4. Trauma. In: Shoemaker W, Thompson W, Holbrook P, eds. *Textbook of Critical Care*. Philadelphia: WB Saunders; 1984:891-898.

5. Shoemaker W. Pericardial tamponade. In: Shoemaker W, Thompson W, Holbrook P, eds. *Textbook of Critical Care*. Philadelphia: WB Saunders; 1984:493-497.

6. Trinkle J, Richardson J, Franz J, et al. Management of flail chest without mechanical ventilation. *Ann Thorac Surg*. 1975;19:355-363.

7. Shackford S, Virgilio R, Peters R. Selective use of ventilator therapy in flail chest injury. *J Thorac Cardiovasc Surg*. 1981;81:194-201.

8. EAST Practice Management Workgroup for Pulmonary Contusion—Flail Chest. Practice Management Guideline for "Pulmonary Contusion—Flail Chest" June 2006. Available at http://www.east.org/tpg/pulmcontflailchest.pdf.

9. Elefteriades JA. Chest trauma. In: Kreis DJ, Gomez GA, eds. *Trauma Management*. Boston: Little, Brown; 1989.

10. Wall MJ, Maxson R, Mattox K. The pulmonary hilum twist as a damage control procedure. *Am J Surg*. 2003;186:49-52.

11. Nagy K, Lohmann C, Kim DO, Barrett J. Role of echocardiography in the diagnosis of occult penetrating cardiac injury. *J Trauma*. 1995;38(6):859-862.

12. Karrel R, Shaffer MA, Franaszek JB. Emergency diagnosis, resuscitation, and treatment of acute penetrating cardiac trauma. *Ann Emerg Med*. 1982;11:504.

13. Thompson T. *Primer of Clinical Radiology*. Boston: Little, Brown; 1980.

14. Sabiston DC Jr, Spencer FC. *Surgery of the Chest*. 5th ed. Philadelphia: WB Saunders; 1990.

15. Crandall M. Penetrating chest trauma. In: *Common Surgical Diseases*. 2nd ed. New York: Springer; 2008:45-47.

16. Hoffman B, Reardon R. Ultrasound Guide for Emergency Physicians: An Introduction. Available at http://www.sonoguide.com/FAST .html.

SUGGESTED FURTHER READING

Rutherford, R. Thoracic injuries. In: Ballinger W, Rutherford R, Zuidema G, eds. *The Management of Trauma*. Philadelphia: WB Saunders; 1973:333-395.

A particularly lucid account at just the right level of sophistication for the interested house officer. Lists the six devastating conditions discussed in this chapter.

EAST Practice Management Workgroup for Pulmonary Contusion—Flail Chest. Practice Management Guideline for "Pulmonary Contusion—Flail Chest" June 2006. Available at http://www.east.org/tpg/ pulmcontflailchest.pdf.

A superb, scholarly review of historical and recent scientific evidence on the pathophysiology and treatment of flail chest and associated pulmonary contusion.

Hoffman B, Reardon R. Ultrasound Guide for Emergency Physicians: An Introduction. Available at http://www.sonoguide.com/FAST.html.

An excellent, well-illustrated, lucid guide to the important FAST ultrasound technique.

Shoemaker W. Pericardial tamponade. In: Shoemaker W, Thompson W, Holbrook P, eds. *Textbook of Critical Care*. Philadelphia: WB Saunders; 1984:493-497.

A concise and clear account of this important condition.

CHEST TUBES

Junior house officers commonly require instruction on a number of aspects of chest tube use and care. Patients routinely come to the ICU from cardiac or thoracic surgery with chest tubes in place. Not infrequently, additional tubes may be required during the patient's ICU stay, for pneumothorax or hemothorax. The house officer must be comfortable with all aspects of chest tube placement and care in order to avoid errors in patient management.

✚ TUBE VARIABLES: SITE, TECHNIQUE, MATERIAL, SIZE

A question that often arises concerns where to place the chest tube. **In general, it is usually recommended that a tube placed for pneumothorax be directed anteriorly and superiorly and that a tube placed for hemothorax be directed posteriorly and inferiorly;** these sites are selected because air rises anteriorly and fluid falls posteriorly in a supine patient. The anatomic guidelines for anterior and posterior tube placement

The House Officer's Guide to ICU Care: Fundamentals of Management of the Heart and Lungs, 3rd ed. © 2013 John A. Elefteriades, Curtis Tribble, Alexander S. Geha, Mark D. Siegel, and Lawrence S. Cohen, eds. Cardiotext Publishing, ISBN: 978-1-935395-68-3.

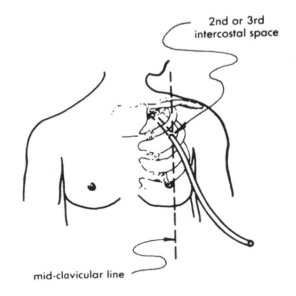

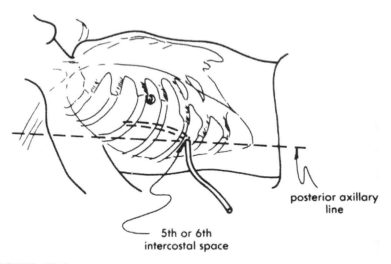

FIGURE 17.1

Standard sites for anterior (**top**) and posterior (**bottom**) chest tube placement.

are depicted in Figure 17.1. The anterior site of choice is the mid-clavicular line in the second or third intercostal space. (The angle of Louis marks the second intercostal space.) A tube placed more medially endangers the great vessels. A tube placed more cephalad endangers the subclavian artery and vein. A tube placed more caudad endangers the pulmonary hilum. The second or third interspace in the midclavicular line is uniformly and widely safe. The posterior site of choice is the midaxillary line in the fifth or sixth intercostal space. (Two finger-breadths below the nipple will approximate this level.) To place the tube more posteriorly would cause the supine patient to lie on the tube; this is uncomfortable and may kink or occlude the tube. To place the tube more caudad risks injury to the diaphragm and abdominal structures. The diaphragm, it will be recalled, can rise anteriorly almost to the nipple line during expiration. Furthermore, the costodiaphragmatic sulcus, the space of safety between the chest wall and the diaphragm, narrows quickly as one proceeds caudad.

Despite the preceding guidelines, in actual fact, **in the virgin chest**—without prior surgery or inflammatory adhesions, and with a free pleural space—**a tube placed at any site will evacuate air or fluid effectively.** The midaxillary line approach, especially, is universally applicable for air or fluid.

When the pleural space is not free—that is, when there exist adhesions from prior surgery, trauma, or inflammation—tube placement must be selected carefully. This will usually require the guidance of an experienced chest surgeon or interventional radiologist. If a pneumothorax occurs in a free chest, the lung comes down from the chest wall symmetrically along its perimeter. If a region of lung does not come down symmetrically, this suggests a tethering to the chest wall by adhesions (Figure 17.2). Fluid in a free chest forms a meniscus between the lung and the chest wall, giving a characteristic chest x-ray (CXR) appearance (Figure 17.3).[1] A localized fluid shadow implies that the fluid is loculated in a scarred

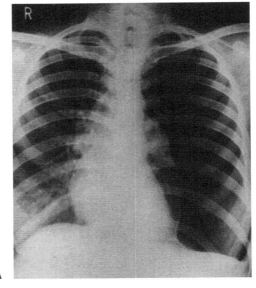

A

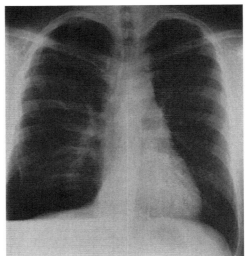

B

FIGURE 17.2

Chest x-ray in free (**A**) and nonfree (**B**) pneumothorax. In **Panel A,** pneumothorax is on patient's left. In **Panel B,** pneumothorax is at base and at apex on patient's right. In nonfree pneumothorax, tethering of the lung to the chest wall prevents uniform symmetrical collapse.

Source: Panel A is reprinted with permission from Sutton D. *Radiology and Imaging for Medical Students.* 6th ed. Edinburgh and New York: Churchill Livingstone; 1994.

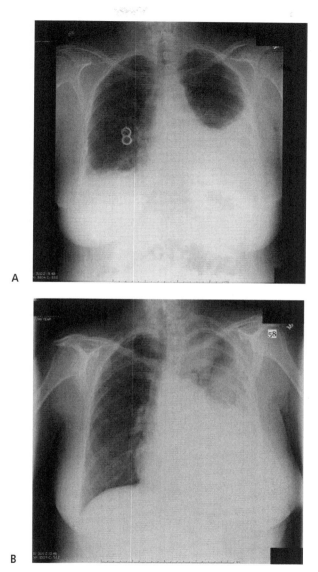

FIGURE 17.3

Chest x-ray in free (**A**) and loculated (**B**) pleural effusion. Loculated effusion is contained in one area against the chest wall.

pleural space. A nonuniform contour of a pneumothorax or locula-tion of a hemothorax should raise a red flag for the house officer. **To place a tube by rote in standard fashion (anteriorly or in the posterior axillary line) in a pleural space with adhesions risks injury to adherent underlying lung.** The site for placement must be selected carefully on the basis of three-dimensional reconstruc-tion of the anatomy, using posteroanterior and lateral CXRs or es-pecially a CT scan. The house officer may be best off studying the anatomy in detail, selecting a site, and then placing a radiopaque marker (a paper clip works well) at that site. Repeat two-dimen-sional x-rays will confirm appropriate selection of the proposed tube site or suggest adjustment of selection. **Above all, a tube must not be placed unless there is an underlying space, either air or fluid, at that site.** Several times yearly on a busy chest service, a tube is forcefully placed into the parenchyma of the lung because these important points are not appreciated.

Another frequent question concerns whether the tube should be placed via a trocar or by following a tract created by blunt finger dissection and a Kelly clamp. The house officer should gain experi-ence with each method under careful bedside supervision. Although the trocar system may allow the experienced surgeon more accurate direction of a smaller tube into complex pleural spaces, the blunt, Kelly clamp approach is more widely useful for the house officer, as the large-bore tubes required for operative and trauma patients can be placed only by this means. (Small trocar tubes can be important for babies and small children.)

The patient will feel pain when air or fluid is removed from the pleural space after tube placement. The pain of which the patient complains, although worrisome, usually signifies the approximation of visceral and parietal pleurae that is the desired end result of evac-uation of air or fluid from the pleural space.

It is important that appropriate anesthesia be provided for chest tube placement. We use lidocaine liberally. Good anesthesia of the skin (with a prominent wheal) goes a long way toward patient comfort. It is important to infiltrate the area around the rib over which the tube will be placed, and also the underlying pleura—and be liberal. We suggest that at least 20 or 30 cc of lidocaine be applied to the tissue layers. It is important, for stable patients, to supplement with some intravenous or intramuscular pain or sedative medications. Guidance on this point can be found in Chapter 22 (Sedation and Analgesia).

Tube type and size must be selected. Two major materials may be chosen: plastic or silicone (silastic). Clear plastic tubes are easy to use and effective. These tubes come in the large sizes necessary postoperatively or for trauma. The plastic tubes, moreover, always incorporate radiopaque markers. Silicone tubes are even more resistant to occlusion by clot or fibrin (this almost never occurs) and have become very popular for use at the time of open heart surgery.

House officers frequently select a tube too large or too small for the intended purpose. Large tubes are more difficult to place and more uncomfortable for the patient. Small tubes cannot handle heavy drainage of thick material. Some general guidelines for selection are as follows. The patient with a spontaneous pneumothorax and only air in the pleural space needs only a small tube: a 16F is excellent for this purpose. This tube will not be too uncomfortable to place but can be relied upon to evacuate air as long as required. For trauma or for a frank postoperative hemothorax, a 32F tube is appropriate. Even clots pass well through a tube this large. For an effusion that is not frankly bloody, an intermediate size, say 24F or 26F, is appropriate. A tube this size will properly drain an effusion, even a thick one, without entailing severe discomfort during placement.

✚ DRAINAGE SYSTEMS: BOTTLE SYSTEMS AND DISPOSABLE DRAINAGE UNITS

The end of the chest tube cannot be left open to air, because atmospheric pressure in the pleural cavity would cause pneumothorax. Various drainage systems are available, from simple to complex. These will be reviewed in some detail, for misconceptions abound and errors are frequent. The bottle systems are described mainly for their value in clarifying physiologic principles; their clinical use is historical in the present era.

The Heimlich Valve

Perhaps the simplest drainage system is the Heimlich valve (Figure 17.4). This is a rubber flutter valve that allows only unidirectional movement of air and fluid (out of the chest). Care should be taken to insert the valve in the proper direction. Air or fluid can force the rubber leaflets apart for egress from the chest. When egress has occurred, the rubber leaflets approximate, preventing entry of air into the chest. Inspiration further approximates the leaflets, maintaining negative intrathoracic pressure.

This simple device can be very useful under emergency circumstances, such as on the battlefield. Under such circumstances, this device can allow treatment of pneumothorax or hemothorax without complex equipment. However, the device itself is messy, as no collection system is incorporated. Furthermore, monitoring air

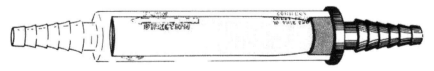

FIGURE 17.4

The Heimlich valve.

or fluid leak is difficult. In the hospital, other devices are more useful. It is possible to discharge patients with a Heimlich valve, especially for pneumothorax without pleural effusion. Other, more modern, miniature apparatus have been developed that approximate a Heimlich valve with an additional small collection chamber. Various commercial brands are available that permit discharge from the hospital with the tube in place.

Bottle Systems

The **one-bottle system** represents the next level of sophistication above the Heimlich valve (Figure 17.5). In this system, a length of tubing connects the chest tube itself to a glass or plastic straw passing through a stopper into a large glass bottle. Another glass rod vents the inside of the bottle to air. Sterile water is added to a level of several centimeters above the end of the drainage straw. This level provides the so-called water seal.

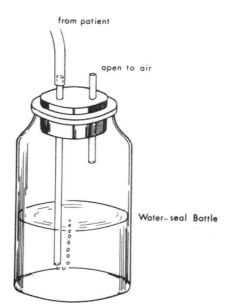

from patient

open to air

Water–seal Bottle

FIGURE 17.5

The one-bottle system.

Air and fluid can still drain easily from the pleural space with the tip submerged. However, the pleural space remains sealed, as air cannot enter the submerged tip of the straw. With inspiration, water may be lifted several centimeters up the straw, but no air can enter.

This simple system is remarkably versatile and effective. Almost any thoracic operation can be accommodated by this one-bottle system. Indeed, this very system was still preferred at a specialty chest hospital in the United Kingdom where one of the authors trained—for even the most complex thoracic operations.

Fluid drainage can be monitored by graduating the bottle and marking on a tape along its side. Subtracting the original amount of fluid used for water seal from the total contents at a particular time gives the amount of fluid drained.

An air leak is easily detected: Bubbles are seen exiting from the drainage straw. The greater the bubbling, the greater the air leak from the chest.

The drainage straw acts as a manometer, allowing continuous, instantaneous monitoring of intrapleural pressure. With inspiration, water is drawn up into the tube. The height of water drawn above the level in the bottle equals, in centimeters of water, the negative pressure in the chest. When an air leak exists, water is drawn up only with inspiration. As the air leak seals, negative pressure supervenes throughout the respiratory cycle. (It will be recalled from physiology that a negative inspiratory pressure of 10 to 15 cm H_2O normally exists in the pleural space.) **As the pulmonary parenchyma seals more effectively with time after a thoracic operation, the water column rises higher and higher in the straw.** The one-bottle system provides the surgeon this wealth of information about intrathoracic events.

The concept of tidal fluctuation is important as well. When a chest tube is first placed, the level of water in the drainage straw fluctuates widely with each breath (Figure 17.6); this fluctuation is called the *respiratory tidal*. The overall height of the water level

pressure

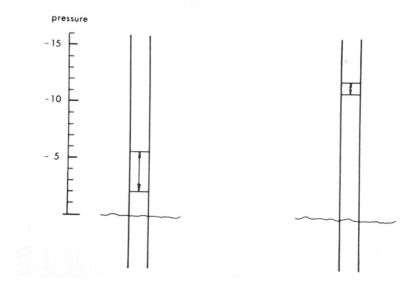

- 15

- 10

- 5

FIGURE 17.6

Respiratory tidal fluctuation of the water seal level. The wide, low tidal at the left is characteristic of the early period following thoracotomy. The narrow, high tidal at right is characteristic of the late period following thoracotomy, indicating sealing of pleural space.

rises with parenchymal sealing as time passes after a thoracic operation; also, **with time, the respiratory tidal decreases.** This reflects apposition and sticking of visceral and parietal pleurae around the tube, excluding the tube from free communication with the pleural space. This occurs only as the leakage of fluid and air abates; it is a good sign, indicating that tubes can be removed soon. All this additional information about intrathoracic events is provided as well by the water seal manometer in the one-bottle system. Assessment of these events becomes second nature with experience.

The one-bottle system does have a disadvantage: Because effluent fluid collects in the bottle, the water level rises with time. The rising level provides a stronger water seal, for intrapleural air must reach a higher pressure before it bubbles through and is evacuated.

If the fluid level is allowed to rise unchecked, a pneumothorax may result. It is best to change the bottle at intervals to maintain a water seal only 2 to 3 cm in height.

The **two-bottle system** (Figure 17.7) adds a collecting bottle in series between the patient and the water seal bottle. Function is entirely identical to the one-bottle system except that the interposed collection bottle prevents the undesired rise in water seal height as drainage collects. Fluctuations in the water seal straw have exactly the same significance as with the one-bottle system.

The **three-bottle system** adds one more elaboration (Figure 17.8). The vent of the water seal bottle is connected to suction, but via a third, suction control bottle. (Suction could be applied directly to the water seal bottle vent if accurately controlled suction were

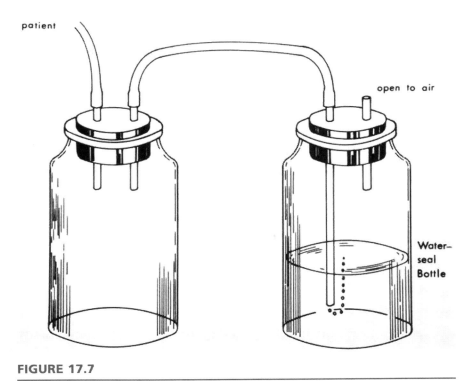

FIGURE 17.7

The two-bottle system.

available; this is not usually the case.) Because hospital wall suction is excessively strong and can cause significant tissue injury, a foolproof suction control is mandatory. This foolproof control is provided by the third bottle. The vent of the water seal bottle is connected to a straw passing into the suction control bottle. Another straw passes out of the suction control bottle to the wall suction. A third straw passes into the bottle with its tip resting below an adjustable level of water. The level of water is specified by the physician. This level limits the suction applied to the chest tube. For example, if 15 cm of saline is placed in the bottle, negative pressure applied will be 15 cm regardless of the amount of wall suction applied. Any wall negative pressure greater than 15 cm will merely draw air in through the open straw. The third bottle should always be bubbling; otherwise, less than the specified amount of suction is

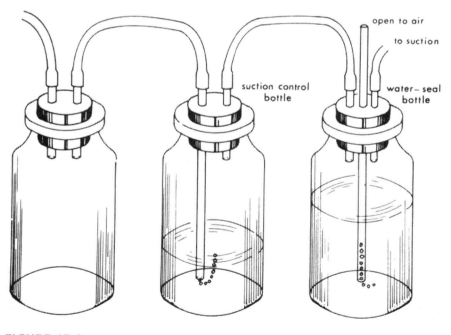

open to air

to suction

suction control
bottle

water–seal
bottle

FIGURE 17.8

The three-bottle system.

being applied from the wall. The house officer must recognize that this bubbling represents not an air leak but just suction control. Air leak, as with the one- and two-bottle systems, is read only in the water seal bottle. The simple addition of this third bottle eliminates the danger of parenchymal injury from excess wall suction.

Disposable Systems

A variety of disposable systems, which house an entire three-bottle system in one plastic enclosure, are available (Figure 17.9). The house officer should recognize that these disposable units are just a three-bottle system in a compact, convenient, disposable, non-breakable configuration. Each has a collection, a water seal, and a suction control chamber. The house officer should become familiar with the particular disposable system used at his or her hospital and identify each of the three key elements. In the water seal chamber, air leak, pleural pressure level, and respiratory tidal can be followed and carry the same meaning as in the bottle systems. In the suction control chamber, a variable amount of fluid can be added to achieve a specified level of suction. As in the three-bottle system, the suction control chamber should always be bubbling.

✚ MANAGEMENT PARTICULARS

Suction or Water Seal

Although suction is used routinely at many centers, **almost all patients can be handled perfectly well with simple water seal.** For almost all patients, application of suction is superfluous. Even a major pneumothorax can be evacuated through water seal in just a few respiratory cycles. Even the moderate air leaks that follow lobectomy are easily handled by simple water seal. Only those patients with massive air leak require suction; **suction does remove air more effectively than water seal when the leak is massive.** Inadequacy of water seal to relieve pneumothorax completely will be apparent from incomplete expansion of the lung on the CXR

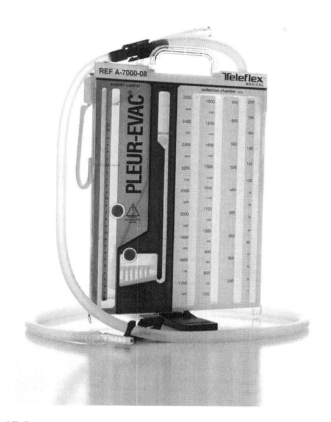

FIGURE 17.9

A commonly used disposable collection system.

Source: Reproduced with permission from Teleflex Medical Inc.

obtained after lobectomy or following tube placement for spontaneous or traumatic pneumothorax. The remaining rim of air can be evacuated by addition of suction to the system.

Nonetheless, at most hospitals, suction is used routinely. Though not strictly necessary in most cases, it is not at all detrimental. The house officer can usually expect to see this policy unless he or she specifies otherwise.

Clamping of Tubes

Despite common misconceptions, with one exception, **chest tubes and apparatus should never be clamped.** Nursing protocols at many hospitals have perpetuated the myth that during transport the patient's chest tube system should be clamped. This offers no benefit and may be dangerous for the patient with an ongoing air leak. With the system clamped, the patient with an air leak may develop a tension pneumothorax. **The proper state for transport of a chest tube patient is water seal.** On water seal, no tension pneumothorax can develop; rather, air under pressure in the pleural space will drain freely through the water seal.

The one exception to the rule not to clamp is during evaluation in preparation for tube removal (see below).

Suction Control

Despite common misconceptions, **increasing the amount of wall suction, to increase bubbling in the suction control chamber, does not increase effectiveness of the pleural drainage system;** this merely serves to draw more atmospheric air through the suction control water level and to cause more noise. The proper way to increase effective suction is to add water to the suction control chamber. This transmits more of the wall suction to the patient before entraining atmospheric air. Usually 15 to 20 cm H_2O is used routinely. When required, this can be increased to 25 to 30 cm H_2O.

In *very* rare cases, multiple tubes attached to multiple suction devices may be required to accommodate the most massive air leaks. In this case, surgical control of the bronchial or parenchymal defect may be required.

Assessment of Severity of Air Leak

The severity of air leak can be evaluated by the amount of bubbling in the water seal chamber of the chest drainage apparatus. In particular, **the severity of the air leak is reflected by the proportion**

of the respiratory cycle during which bubbling occurs. In the spontaneously respiring patient, a mild air leak will cause bubbling during peak expiration only; it is during expiration that airway pressures are maximal. With a moderate leak, bubbling occupies the entire expiratory phase. With a severe air leak, bubbling occurs during the inspiratory phase as well as during all of the expiratory phase. With massive leaks, bubbling is continuous.

In patients on positive pressure ventilation, these relationships are reversed. A mild leak expresses itself as bubbling during inspiration; on the ventilator, inspiration is a positive pressure phenomenon. During expiration, bubbling ceases except with more severe leaks.

The house officer should recognize that **air leak is normal following major pulmonary resections;** it does not imply surgical error. Rather, leak is expected from all areas where lung parenchyma is divided, especially at sites of incomplete fissures. As explained in Chapter 19 (Problems Following Noncardiac Thoracic Surgery), these parenchymal leaks uniformly stop within a day or two of pleural apposition.

The question often arises whether an air leak is actually coming from the patient or from a leak in the tubing system. If the tubing and connections between the patient and the drainage device are not tight, air can enter the system, giving the spurious appearance of an air leak. This question can be resolved in a straightforward manner. Finding a continuous leak, without significant variation in bubbling with the respiratory cycle, serves as a clue that air may be entering the system. (Only very large true air leaks would show this pattern.) The question is resolved by temporarily clamping the chest tube at the patient's chest wall. If the leak is false (ie, caused by air entering the system from outside), bubbling continues. If the leak is true (ie, coming from the patient), bubbling ceases. When a false leak is confirmed, connections and tubing are examined and defects corrected. When true leak is confirmed, drainage is resumed as previously.

Occasionally, the defect causing a false leak may be not in the tubing system but between the chest tube proper and the patient's chest wall. In this circumstance, the suction in the apparatus draws air into the chest (between the tube and its tract in the chest wall) and then evacuates it through the tube. Disappearance of the leak on water seal may suggest this circumstance. Confirmation is provided when the leak disappears permanently with placement of an occlusive pursestring suture or occlusive Vaseline gauze dressing around the tube entrance site.

Tubing Care

The rubber or silastic tubing that connects the chest tube to the drainage device is frequently improperly or inadequately managed, especially on wards that handle chest tubes infrequently. Often the tubing is found occluded by the patient's own weight. In the presence of a significant air leak, of course, this can cause a tension pneumothorax. A less blatant but more common error is to allow a loop in the tubing (Figure 17.10). If water collects in the loop to a height greater than the suction control limit (usually set at 15 to 20 cm H_2O), the tube will be effectively sealed—just as if it were clamped! This also can cause pneumothorax and tension pneumothorax. **The tubing from patient to drainage device must always remain horizontal or descending, never ascending or looping.** A level, horizontal loop that lies flat on the mattress is permissible.

Also, in general, the tubing and drainage device should not be raised above the patient's level, for reverse drainage is possible.

Stripping of Tubes

Some surgeons and some ICUs practice stripping of tubes. Some use the powdered hand or even a mechanical device for this purpose. Others feel that stripping can promote bleeding. It has, in fact, been demonstrated experimentally that stripping can produce very high negative pressures in the chest. These negative pressures

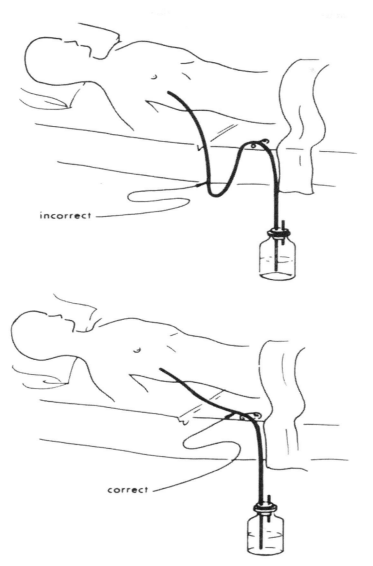

FIGURE 17.10

An ascending segment of tubing or loops in the tubing (**top**) leading to the collection bottle will cause a fluid trap that disables the system. The proper method is to keep the tubing always level or descending (**bottom**).

could dislodge normal, useful clots at potential bleeding sites. Institutional policies vary, but we prefer "walking" the drainage fluid through the tube rather than forceful stripping.

Tube Removal

In general, **mediastinal chest tubes placed following cardiac surgery can be removed when drainage falls to less than 100 mL over 8 hours.** When this criterion is met, the chance of significant subsequent accumulation of blood or fluid is remote. This criterion is usually met by the morning of the second day after surgery.

For tubes placed following pulmonary surgery, both air and fluid drainage criteria must be met. Most surgeons insist on leaving tubes in place at least 24 or 48 hours beyond the last time that any air leak was noted. The reason for this delay is to allow continued strong apposition of visceral and parietal pleurae under the influence of suction to achieve secure "sticking" of these layers. Following noncardiac chest surgery, the fluid criterion is somewhat more stringent than following cardiac surgery: most surgeons will not remove tubes until drainage is less than 100 or 150 mL/24 h. The intent is to minimize the likelihood of accumulation of a significant postoperative pleural effusion. These criteria are, to some extent, traditional and arbitrary. Recent studies suggest that the traditional criteria may be too conservative.

Occasionally, the presence of the tube itself can promote serious drainage. In this case, the experienced chest surgeon may make the decision to remove tubes despite drainage that exceeds the preceding criteria.

On rare occasions, cardiac or thoracic surgery may produce a chyle leak (with associated chylothorax). This is seen as a milky color to the drainage. The milky color may not appear for 2 or 3 days, as the red color of blood admixture may overwhelm the white. A milky, chylous appearance should be called to the attention of senior personnel; the tube should generally not be removed in the face of active chylous drainage. Inexperienced personnel may express a concern that the chylous drainage is infected, because of its white color. In matter of fact, chyle almost never gets infected, as it contains extremely abundant leukocytes.

For tubes placed following spontaneous pneumothorax, as for tubes placed after pulmonary surgery, it is customary to allow 24 or 48 hours beyond the last noted air leak for optimal seal. Occasionally, we will clamp the tube for several hours prior to anticipated removal when we want to rule out intermittent bubbling. This low level of leak may not be detectable even with frequent monitoring of the water seal chamber. With the tube clamped, however, even a small leak will manifest a pneumothorax within several hours on CXR. If no pneumothorax is realized, intermittent bubbling has been ruled out, and the tube may be removed safely.

When a tube is removed, the tract must be sealed in some way until the body tissues close. The body's own seal is usually complete within 48 hours. Until that time, two alternatives are available. Some surgeons place a pursestring, or "U," stitch around the chest tube site; this is in addition to the tube securing stitch and is tightened as the tube is withdrawn. Alternatively, a Vaseline gauze and dry sponge dressing may be taped tightly in place over the opening as the tube is withdrawn. This dressing can be removed in 48 hours.

In spontaneously respiring patients, tubes are withdrawn during forced expiration; this prevents air entry into the chest. **In patients on mechanical ventilation, tubes are withdrawn during positive pressure inspiration,** for the same reason. In either setting, tubes must be pulled sharply and quickly, to prevent air entry. A safe rule is that when multiple tubes are present and attached to the same drainage device, they may be clamped, cut, and removed separately.

The house officer usually obtains a CXR after tube removal to ascertain that no air has been let into the chest. When tubes are purely mediastinal, as following cardiac surgery, this is probably unnecessary. Even with cardiac surgery, however, tubes may be placed in the pleural space if the pleura is entered during the operative procedure. Unless the house officer is certain that tubes are exclusively mediastinal, not pleural, it is best to obtain a CXR. Again, local custom will dictate.

The house officer should realize that even if air is let in during tube removal, there is no need to panic. This air has come from the outside, not from the bronchial tree or the lung parenchyma. There is no reason to expect a worsening of the pneumothorax. Rather, with time, spontaneous resolution will occur. The house officer should review the CXR with more senior personnel to determine if the iatrogenic pneumothorax is small enough to be tolerated by the patient until spontaneous resolution; if not, another tube will need to be placed.

Tube-related infection? No less an authority than Dr. von Hippel, who literally wrote the book on chest tubes and chest bottles, has stated that he has never seen an infection related to a chest tube. So von Hippel recommends that one never rush removal of a tube out of concern for its inducing infection. The authors concur.

✚ SUBCUTANEOUS, CERVICAL, AND MEDIASTINAL EMPHYSEMA

Subcutaneous emphysema, with its characteristic "bubbly" ("crisped rice-like") sensation on palpation, may occur when a pneumothorax decompresses itself into the soft tissues (as via a chest wall injury or a chest tube site). This can be seen especially when the pleural space is obliterated by prior surgery or inflammation, so that the lung parenchyma leaks air but cannot fall away from the chest wall. This condition can progress rapidly but, though unsightly, is not dangerous. If an intrapleural air space exists, a chest tube should be placed and will prevent further accumulation. If subcutaneous emphysema has become massive or threatens to do so, small skin incisions can be made infraclavicularly, with spreading of soft tissues by clamp. Regular "milking" of subcutaneous air through the incisions by the nurses will permit early resolution.

Cervical emphysema—and its radiographic counterpart, mediastinal emphysema—can be seen whenever a parenchymal leak dissects along the bronchial tree into the mediastinum. Injury to the bronchus itself is occasionally the cause. (See Chapter 16, Chest Trauma.) Cervical and mediastinal emphysema are rarely of physiologic importance. In rare cases, when great pressure develops, a tamponade-like effect on the heart may occur. If deterioration in vital signs is felt to be occurring on this basis, total decompression can be obtained by performing an "almost tracheostomy."[2] Dissection is carried out as for tracheostomy, but the trachea itself is not opened. This vents all cervical continuations of the mediastinal tissue planes, decompresses the heart, and restores vital signs.

By understanding these guidelines, modifying them according to local practice, and gaining some hands-on experience, the house officer should become comfortably capable in chest tube management.

REFERENCES

1. Sutton D. *Radiology and Imaging for Medical Students.* 6th ed. Edinburgh and New York: Churchill Livingston; 1994.
2. Von Hippel A. *Chest Tubes and Chest Bottles.* Springfield, IL: Charles C Thomas; 1970.

SUGGESTED FURTHER READING

Rexilius BG. *Chest Drainage and Suction.* Philadelphia: FA Davis; 1977.
Von Hippel A. *Chest Tubes and Chest Bottles.* Springfield, IL: Charles C Thomas; 1970.
These two texts, the first by a registered nurse and the second by a surgeon, are excellent short volumes that cover in greater detail the principles that have been condensed in this chapter. Both are highly recommended.

MANAGEMENT OF ACUTE PULMONARY DISEASE

✚ RESPIRATORY FAILURE

The purpose of the respiratory system is to oxygenate the blood and to remove carbon dioxide. Respiratory failure exists when oxygenation and/or carbon dioxide removal are inadequate. **Respiratory failure is defined as present when pO_2 is less than 60 mm Hg or pCO_2 is greater than 50 mm Hg.** These criteria identify presence of life-threatening respiratory dysfunction. Oxygenation may fail alone (hypoxia), CO_2 removal may fail alone (hypercapnia), or both respiratory functions may fail together (hypoxia and hypercapnia). Further deterioration in pO_2 or pCO_2 beyond these failure criteria may lead to cardiac and/or cerebral dysfunction and death on that basis. Also, once respiratory failure begins, rapid progression of abnormalities in pO_2 and pCO_2 may be seen, with consequent cardiopulmonary arrest. In fact, any hypercarbia significantly outside of the normal CO_2 range (up to pCO_2 46 mm Hg) should arouse concern. (Of course, many patients with chronic lung disease live long-term at levels of

The House Officer's Guide to ICU Care: Fundamentals of Management of the Heart and Lungs, 3rd ed. © 2013 John A. Elefteriades, Curtis Tribble, Alexander S. Geha, Mark D. Siegel, and Lawrence S. Cohen, eds. Cardiotext Publishing, ISBN: 978-1-935395-68-3.

pO_2 and pCO_2 beyond the preceding criteria; these criteria for ventilatory failure apply to acute respiratory decompensation in patients without preexisting hypoxia or hypercarbia.)

Dyspnea and tachypnea are the usual clinical signs that signal respiratory failure and lead to the arterial blood gas (ABG) determinations that confirm the diagnosis. Cyanosis may also be clinically apparent. Cardiac abnormalities (arrhythmia, hypertension) and neurologic abnormalities (confusion, obtundation, restlessness) may also signal respiratory failure and warrant ABG determination.

Rate and depth of respiration are important in the evaluation of hypercarbia. Slow, shallow respiration, as seen during sleep or from sedation by pain medications, implies that CO_2 retention may well be simply on the basis of suppression of respiratory drive, a transient and usually nonthreatening condition. Hypercarbia in face of tachypnea and dyspnea has a much more ominous significance: This implies that CO_2 removal is failing despite maximal respiratory effort. Mild to moderate hypercarbia may also be seen as a compensation for metabolic alkalosis, in which case it is a normal phenomenon and not an expression of respiratory failure. (See "The Acid-Base Nomogram" in Chapter 23, Additional Topics.) This situation is seen most commonly in the ICU after very aggressive diuresis, with induction of the so-called hypokalemic, hypochloremic alkalosis of volume contraction.

Common causes of acute hypoxic respiratory failure in the ICU include atelectasis, pneumonia, pneumothorax, pulmonary edema, and pulmonary embolism. Common causes of acute hypercarbic respiratory failure include excess sedation, bronchospasm, atelectasis, pleural effusion, retained secretions, and respiratory muscle fatigue. In general, hypoxia implies perfused but underventilated alveoli, and hypercarbia implies ventilated but underperfused alveoli. (See Chapter 1, Ventilators and Respiratory Management.)

Treatment of respiratory failure is, of course, directed toward the underlying cause, which is determined in large part on the basis of physical examination and CXR. This treatment may include diuresis for pulmonary edema, broncholitics for bronchospasm, pulmonary toilet for retained secretions or atelectasis, and specific mechanical treatment for pneumothorax or effusion. Oxygen supplementation is, of course, indicated. **If immediate improvement is not seen with these measures, respiratory support by intubation and mechanical ventilation should be effected promptly—before a vicious cycle of deterioration ensues.** (The management of mechanical ventilation is reviewed in Chapter 1, Ventilators and Respiratory Management.) Intubation and mechanical ventilation are not infrequently required in the postoperative cardiac surgical patient, who may have atelectasis, effusion, an element of pulmonary edema, and muscle weakness. **The house officer should, when more experienced help is not available, always err on the side of early preemptive intubation for incipient respiratory failure.** Failure to do so, especially in the postinfarct or postoperative surgical patient, may result in cardiac arrest, from which recovery may be difficult. The period of mechanical ventilation, once instituted, allows time for correction of the underlying precipitating abnormalities. It has been demonstrated that once CO_2 retention occurs, the respiratory muscles are literally "exhausted";[1] the patient is unlikely to recover from this downward spiral until after a week or so of mechanical support. (This is just like the week or so it takes a marathoner to recover from muscle fatigue.) Hypoxia and hypercarbia exacerbate this fatigue by interfering with nutritive balance of the respiratory muscles themselves. The take-home message is do not let a struggling patient fail completely before resting him or her on mechanical respiratory support.

✚ ACUTE BRONCHOSPASM

Acute bronchospasm is commonly seen in ICU patients. After cardiac surgery, fluid overload and irritation of the airways related to intubation and retained secretions make patients vulnerable to bronchospasm. After acute myocardial infarction, a component of pulmonary edema may contribute to bronchospasm. Recognition of the bronchospastic attack is based on auscultation, usually occasioned by a call to the house officer to report that the patient is dyspneic. In some cases, watching the patient breathe can reveal air trapping that might not be clearly audible on auscultation. **During an attack of acute bronchospasm, significant hypoxia and/or significant hypercarbia on assessment of ABG indicate a serious situation with potential for rapid deterioration.** Immediate treatment is required.

General modalities for treatment of acute bronchospasm in the ICU patient include the following:[2]

Oxygen administration. Oxygen administration not only improves oxygen saturation, but also corrects the hyperventilation occasioned by acute bronchospasm, leading to less dyspnea and less work of breathing.

Diuresis. Especially after acute myocardial infarction or cardiac surgery, fluid overload with pulmonary edema causes airway edema, which narrows the small bronchi and may cause or exacerbate airway obstruction and bronchospasm. Lasix (40 mg IV) is almost always appropriate. When the emergency is corrected, attention to maintaining a net negative fluid balance over the next few days is important as well.

Steroids. We have found IV steroid administration to be extremely beneficial, especially for the bronchospasm frequently seen following extubation after cardiac surgery. Airway inflammation is improved promptly. We use hydrocortisone (100 mg IV q 8 h × 48 h). Even after cardiac surgery, a brief course of steroids does not lead to infectious complications. We find that by the end of the 48-hour treatment period, the irritation of the airways and the clearance of secretions have improved markedly. We have found steroid treatment to be much better tolerated than theophylline administration in cardiac patients with bronchospasm.

Inhaled bronchodilators. Inhaled bronchodilators have become the treatment of choice for acute bronchospasm. The respiratory therapist will be able to offer a variety of inhalation treatments that can be given by nebulizer or inhaler (including isoproterenol, metaproterenol, albuterol, and combinations of drugs), which will deliver bronchodilators topically into the airways to augment treatment of acute bronchospasm. Intravenous epinephrine or isoproterenol may also be useful. (See Chapter 7, Continuous Infusion Agents)

β-agonists. β-agonists relax the bronchial smooth muscle. We have found terbutaline (0.25 to 0.5 mg sc q 4 h) to be a well-tolerated adjunct for relief of bronchospasm. We have not seen undue tachycardia or supraventricular or ventricular ectopy following treatment, and we actually prefer β-agonists to theophylline treatment in the post-MI or postoperative cardiac surgical patient.

Theophylline. Theophylline, once the mainstay agent for treating acute bronchospasm, has fallen into disfavor (appropriately) because of its very narrow therapeutic window; that is, side effects are common with doses sufficient to serve a beneficial clinical effect.[3] We use IV aminophylline only as a last resort in post-MI and postoperative cardiac surgical patients, because in these settings supraventricular and ventricular ectopy is commonly induced by such treatment. We find that atrial fibrillation is almost invariably seen shortly after initiation of aminophylline treatment in the postoperative cardiac surgical patient. Moreover, the actual effectiveness of aminophylline as a bronchodilator has come into question. When we do use aminophylline, we err on the low side of recommended doses (5 mg/kg load over 20 min and 0.5 mg/kg/h maintenance), aiming for levels toward the low end of the therapeutic range (which is 10 to 20 mg/cc). Oral administration is better tolerated after acute MI or cardiac surgery, and despite our posture of avoiding IV aminophylline, we do at times treat even postinfarction and postoperative patients with oral theophylline (Theodur 200 to 300 mg p.o. q 12 h).

Mechanical ventilation. Because acute bronchospasm can deteriorate quickly, leading to life-threatening hypoxia and/ or hypercarbia and cardiopulmonary arrest, the house officer should maintain a low threshold for intubation and positive pressure ventilation in the setting of acute bronchospasm. Mechanical ventilation restores gas exchange immediately, providing time for institution of the other therapeutic modalities in a safe and timely fashion.

✚ MASSIVE HEMOPTYSIS

Massive hemoptysis is defined as the expectoration of 600 cc or more of blood within a 24-hour period. Such severe hemoptysis constitutes an emergency of the first order. Tuberculosis (with tuberculous cavity or penetrating hilar lymph node), chronic infection (bronchiectasis, lung abscess), and neoplasm are common causes of massive hemoptysis. **Death in hemoptysis occurs usually not from exsanguination, but from asphyxiation,** a principle that has important therapeutic correlates. In other words, the patient drowns before he exsanguinates. Aortobronchial fistula from infected aortic grafts and pseudoaneurysms are rare but dramatic additional potential causes of massive hemoptysis. Also, massive hemoptysis can occur from pulmonary artery perforation caused by a Swan-Ganz catheter (usually from overdistention of a pulmonary artery radicle during a "wedging" maneuver).

General supportive measures include the following: Hemostatic competence must be ensured. All anticoagulant mediations must be discontinued. Aspirin-containing medications can be important culprits, as can Plavix. Serious coagulation deficits can be corrected with fresh frozen plasma or platelets. The patient is positioned upright if neurologically intact or with the bleeding side down (decubitus position) if neurologically impaired, to prevent spilling of blood into the nonbleeding lung. Cough suppression with codeine is effected to minimize mechanical disturbance of the bleeding lesion and local clot. Blood transfusion may be indicated if the hematocrit is low. (In extreme cases, cardiopulmonary bypass and ECMO can be applied to save a life in a situation of massive hemoptysis that does not respond to more conventional treatments.)

It is important to localize the site of bleeding. An alert patient often "senses" that the bleeding is coming from the right or the left side. The chest x-ray may be very helpful; the underlying lesion responsible for the hemoptysis (tumor, cavity) may be visible, or the "ground glass" appearance of aspirated blood in the parenchyma may localize the bleeding site. It is important to recognize that information from the x-ray may not be definitive; specifically, an endobronchial lesion different from the one apparent by chest x-ray may be the culprit, or aspirated blood may have drained to and opacified a lobe different from the one causing the bleeding.

Immediate bronchoscopic examination during the acute bleeding episode is key, as definitive localization of the bleeding site may be possible. We prefer rigid bronchoscopy because of the superior ability to clear endobronchial blood and clot in order to visualize the actual point of origin. Flexible bronchoscopy may suffice if rigid bronchoscopy is not available. Bronchoscopy of any type after the bleeding has ceased is often not definitive.

Because massive hemoptysis is life-threatening and tends to recur even after a specific episode has terminated, surgical treatment (usually by lobectomy) is the treatment of choice. Application of surgical treatment, however, presupposes that (1) the bleeding site has been identified definitively and (2) the patient is a suitable candidate for thoracic surgery. Often these conditions are not met. The site of bleeding may not be entirely clear. The patient often has significant underlying lung disease, and the acute hemoptysis may make precise assessment of pulmonary function inaccurate or unsafe. In the case of definitive localization of the site of hemoptysis and satisfactory general candidacy for operation, lobectomy constitutes definitive treatment.

Two general options are available for patients not deemed suitable candidates for operation: bronchial occlusion and bronchial artery embolization. Bronchial occlusion can be effected either by inflation of a balloon catheter in the mainstem bronchus of the bleeding lung or by intubation with a double-lumen tube (which allows ventilatory separation of the two lungs). (Double-lumen tubes can be dangerous if staff is not familiar with their use.) Bronchial occlusion accomplishes two goals: it prevents aspiration of blood into the "good" lung, and it produces tamponade of the bleeding bronchus by trapping shed blood in the ipsilateral bronchial tree. At times, with bronchial occlusion, the whole lung on the affected side opacifies fully with shed blood. This almost always terminates the bleeding. Adequate oxygenation and ventilation are carried out using the "good" lung only. After 48 to 72 hours, the bronchial blocker or double lumen tube is removed, allowing resumption of ventilation of the "bad" lung. The infiltrates usually clear in days to weeks, often without further hemoptysis.

Because massive hemoptysis usually originates pathologically from the high-pressure bronchial (not the low-pressure pulmonary) arteries, angiographic localization and bronchial artery embolization are feasible. This technique is fairly effective.[4] The complication of paraplegia from inadvertent occlusion of the spinal artery, which may arise from the bronchial artery, can be devastating.

PULMONARY EMBOLISM[5-9]

Pulmonary embolism is an extremely common cause of death in hospitalized patients, seen in up to one of every four patients undergoing autopsy. Prevention is key. Although many adjuncts have been used—including subcutaneous heparin, Dextran, pneumatic calf compression, and anti-embolism stockings—early and aggressive ambulation following myocardial infarction or cardiac surgery is essential for the prevention of pulmonary embolism.

An important principle is that **the hemodynamic disturbance from pulmonary embolism is caused not only by the occlusion of pulmonary artery radicles by the embolus itself, but also by the release of vasoactive amines into the pulmonary circulation, with consequent pulmonary artery vasoconstriction.** The vasoactive amines are released from the platelets involved in the continued thrombus deposition and destruction in, on, and around the main embolism. It is this vasoconstriction that raises pulmonary vascular resistance and pulmonary artery pressures, causing right heart strain, with elevation of central venous pressure and hemodynamic embarrassment up to and including cardiogenic shock. (The house officer should keep in mind that in standard pneumonectomy, one-half of the pulmonary vascular bed is acutely interrupted, usually without adverse hemodynamic sequelae. This observation emphasizes the pathologic importance of the vasoactive amine-induced pulmonary vasoconstriction that arises from pulmonary embolism but not from surgical pneumonectomy.)

Recognition of pulmonary embolism rests on maintaining a high index of suspicion. Cough, dyspnea, hypoxia, and pleuritic chest pain are well-known symptoms. These phenomena are seen even in the absence of pulmonary embolism in many postoperative cardiac surgical patients. If the symptoms seem at all out of the ordinary, we maintain a low threshold for diagnostic intervention.

Pulmonary embolism is extremely unlikely if the arterial pO_2 is not depressed. Some degree of hyperventilation usually accompanies the hypoxia of pulmonary embolism, leading to an arterial blood gas pattern of hypoxemia and hypocarbia (hyperventilation) in pulmonary embolism. This pattern is not, however, specific enough to rule in a pulmonary embolus.

Ventilation-perfusion scanning, once the diagnostic procedure of choice, has been supplanted by CT scanning in the diagnosis of pulmonary embolism. The CT is highly accurate for this disorder. Also, the cardiac echo, readily available at the bedside in coronary and postcardiac surgical ICUs, may detect thrombi still residing in right-sided cardiac chambers or in the main pulmonary arteries. The echo can supply other information relative to the diagnosis of pulmonary embolism,[7] such as estimates of pulmonary artery pressure and of right ventricular strain. echo can also provide useful information about alternative diagnostic entities besides embolism in the acutely deteriorating patient, such as myocardial infarction, left ventricular dysfunction, aortic dissection, and pericardial effusion with tamponade. **Cardiac echo promises to play a larger role in the future in suspected pulmonary embolism.**[8]

In the ICU setting, the question often arises whether an acute episode of hypotension or drop in cardiac output may be caused by pulmonary embolism. The Swan-Ganz catheter is very helpful in this regard. **It is very unlikely that hypotension is caused by acute pulmonary embolism if the central venous pressure and pulmonary artery systolic pressure are not acutely and markedly elevated.** Elevation of pulmonary artery pressure to the range of 50 to 60 mm Hg systolic and 30 to 40 mm Hg mean may be seen in acute massive pulmonary embolism. This helpful observation allows the house officer to focus his or her attention on other etiologies for hypotension without wasting precious time in the investigation for pulmonary embolism. Remember, however, that **the normal right ventricle cannot generate pressures higher than 60 mm Hg systolic with acute pulmonary embolism;** right heart failure ensues before pressure rises above this range with acute phenomena. This is in contradistinction to states of chronic pulmonary hypertension, where the hypertrophied right ventricle can generate systemic or even suprasystemic pressures.

The vast majority of patients with pulmonary embolism are adequately treated with intravenous heparin. Hemodynamics improve quickly, as the heparin terminates the cycle of clot formation and release of vasoactive amines. A loading dose of 5,000 to 10,000 U of heparin is used, followed by a continuous infusion of 800 to 1,200 U/h to maintain a PTT about one and a half to two times control. Coumadin is added orally after several days, and heparin is discontinued when, about 7 to 10 days postembolism, the PT is therapeutic (one and a half to two times control).

In patients with severe hemodynamic compromise, thrombolytic therapy (streptokinase or rTPA) may be considered.[9] These agents, which actually lyse fresh clots, lead to quicker hemodynamic improvement. In postoperative cardiac patients, however, thrombolytic therapy is usually (but not always) contraindicated because of risk of bleeding from fresh operative sites and suture lines.

In patients who manifest refractory hemodynamic embarrassment or hypoxia despite mechanical intubation and positive pressure ventilation, inotropic support, and anticoagulation with heparin and/or thrombolysis, emergency surgical performance of pulmonary embolectomy may be indicated.[5] Although the operative risk may be high, reflecting the desperate condition of many of these patients, hemodynamics may be restored immediately in selected patients and salvage effected. Patient selection is key; patients without organ complications from cardiogenic shock and without cardiac arrest and ongoing CPR actually do quite well in the present era. Although originally performed by Trendelenburg without the heart-lung machine, pulmonary embolectomy is currently performed on cardiopulmonary bypass. (See Figures 18.1 and 18.2.)

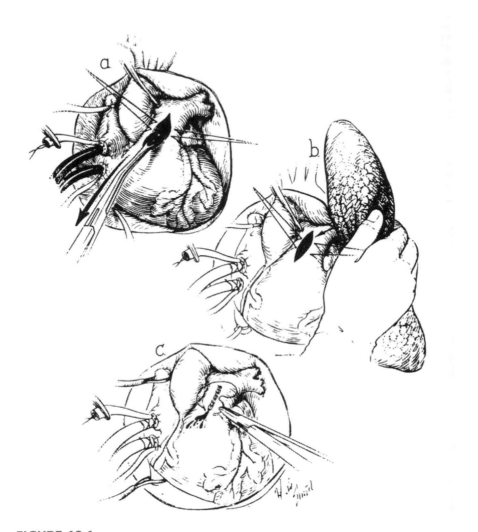

FIGURE 18.1

The technique of pulmonary embolectomy. The procedure is most commonly performed on cardiopulmonary bypass, although on occasion when the heart-lung machine is not available, the original nonbypass Trendelenburg procedure is performed. A longitudinal incision is made in the proximal pulmonary artery and clot is removed both directly (**A**) and by compression of the lung (**B**). The pulmonary artery is then closed (**C**).

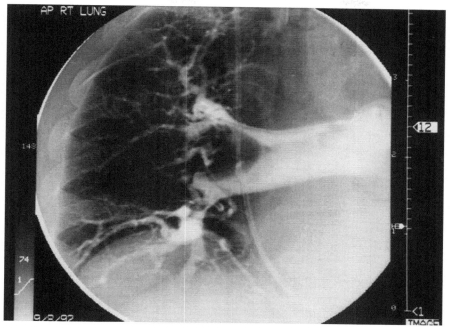

FIGURE 18.2

Pulmonary arteriogram in a case of massive pulmonary embolism requiring operative pulmonary embolectomy on cardiopulmonary bypass because of refractory hypoxia and shock. The patient did well, with immediate correction of hypoxia and hemodynamic embarrassment.

REFERENCES

1. Aubier M. Respiratory muscle fatigue. *Intensive Care Med.* 1989;15 (Suppl 1):S17-S20.
2. Swadron SP. Boston Scientific Assembly (October 5-8, 2009). Challenging cases in pulmonary medicine. *Contemporary Cardiology.* 2nd ed. New York: Springer (Humana Press); 2007;147-160.
3. Littenberg B. Aminophylline treatment in severe, acute asthma: a meta-analysis. *JAMA.* 1988;259:1678-1684.
4. Magilligan DJ Jr, Ravipoti S, Zayat P, Shetty PC, Bower G, Kvale P. Massive hemoptysis: control by transcatheter bronchial embolization. *Ann Thorac Surg.* 1981;32:392-400.

5. Anyanu AC, Aklog L. Surgical pulmonary embolectomy. *Contemporary Cardiology*. 2nd ed. New York: Springer (Humana Press); 2007;147-160.

6. Lee L, Kavinsky CJ, Spies C. Massive pulmonary embolism: review of management strategies with a focus on catheter-based techniques. *Expert Rev Cardiovasc Ther*. 2010;8(6):863-873.

7. Magilligan DJ Jr, Ravipoti S, Zayat P, Shetty PC, Bower G, Kvale P. Massive hemoptysis: control by transcatheter bronchial embolization. *Ann Thorac Surg*. 1981;32:392-400.

8. Torbicki A, Tramarin R, Morpurgo M. Role of echo/doppler in the diagnosis of pulmonary embolism. *Clin Cardiol*. 1992;15:805-810.

9. Cuccia C, Campana M, Frajnzoni P, et al. Effectiveness of intravenous rTPA in the treatment of massive pulmonary embolism and right heart thromboembolism. *Am Heart J*. 1993;126:468-472.

SUGGESTED FURTHER READING

Swadron SP. Boston Scientific Assembly (October 5-8, 2009). Challenging cases in pulmonary medicine. *Contemporary Cardiology*. 2nd ed. New York: Springer (Humana Press); 2007;147-160.
An excellent, well-illustrated reference, covering both bronchospasm as well as massive hemoptysis (and other emergencies as well).

Hyers TM, ed. Pulmonary embolism and hypertension. *Clin Chest Med*. 1984;5:383-554.
An entire text devoted to the subject of pulmonary embolism—authoritative, complete, and interesting to read.

Knott-Craig, CJ, Oostuizen JG, Rossouw G, Joubert JR, Barnard PM. Management and prognosis of massive hemoptysis: recent experience with 120 patients. *J Thorac Cardiovasc Surg*. 1993;105:394-397.
An up-to-date review in a large number of patients, which looks not only at results in terms of survival to hospital discharge, but at subsequent survival as well.

19

PROBLEMS FOLLOWING NONCARDIAC THORACIC SURGERY

Five major categories of problems can occur acutely following chest surgery, including thoracotomy, lung biopsy, lobectomy, and pneumonectomy:

- **Bleeding**
- **Arrhythmias**
- **Space problems**
- **Volume loss in remaining lung tissue**
- **Congestive heart failure**

Each of these categories requires the understanding and awareness of the house officer.

The House Officer's Guide to ICU Care: Fundamentals of Management of the Heart and Lungs, 3rd ed. © 2013 John A. Elefteriades, Curtis Tribble, Alexander S. Geha, Mark D. Siegel, and Lawrence S. Cohen, eds. Cardiotext Publishing, ISBN: 978-1-935395-68-3.

✚ BLEEDING

Major bleeding can follow lobectomy or pneumonectomy. Not only may a ligature come off a pulmonary artery or vein, but the fragile pulmonary artery may tear at the site of an intact ligature (from continued beat-by-beat trauma). Bleeding from a major vessel will usually result in rapid compromise of vital signs. A dramatic volume of bleeding through the chest tubes will usually be evident.

Urgent reoperation may be necessary. Rarely, reoperation in the ICU may be necessary. Such interventions may on occasion be life-saving. **Almost all sites of bleeding can be controlled by manual compression** until expert surgical assistance and proper lighting and equipment are available. Blind application of traumatic nonvascular clamps must be avoided.

Aside from bleeding from major vessels, considerable oozing may occur from denuded parenchymal surfaces, especially when incomplete fissures are opened bluntly or when adherent, inflamed pleural surfaces are separated. The surgeon will achieve meticulous hemostasis in the operating room. Still, several hundred milliliters of bleeding per hour may occasionally be seen early after thoracic surgery. The house officer should alert senior personnel of such bleeding but must not panic. As parenchymal surfaces appose to the parietal pleura, bleeding from raw tissues will stop. Ensuring full expansion of the lung is important for this reason.

As will be discussed later, pneumonectomy is often performed without indwelling chest tubes. Bleeding is more common after pneumonectomy, because there is no parenchymal surface to appose onto the pleura. Without a chest tube in place, significant bleeding may not be obvious. If deterioration of vital signs or falling hematocrit suggest bleeding, a chest x-ray (CXR) will allow assessment of fluid volume on the side of pneumonectomy. Normally after pneumonectomy, the space fills with fluid over days to weeks (Figure 19.1). **A rapid rise in fluid level in the pneumonectomy space in the first hours postoperatively suggests bleeding.**

✚ ARRHYTHMIAS

The same supraventricular arrhythmias that follow cardiac surgery may follow thoracic surgery. Their management is detailed in Chapter 2.

Usually the thoracic surgical patient has a healthier heart than the cardiac surgical patient. The former usually tolerates supraventricular tachycardia better, allowing the house officer a longer safety margin in treatment.

Traditionally, many surgeons prophylactically digitalize the elderly patient who undergoes lobectomy or pneumonectomy. Many surgeons use a cutoff of 60 or 65 years of age. Much debate has been carried out over the years regarding the benefits and risks of prophylactic digitalization. The main benefit is that the digitalized patient who goes into atrial fibrillation does so at a controlled rate. The risk is that, especially with potassium fluxes, digitalis toxicity may be seen. This issue was more germane in earlier years, when digitalis was the only available agent. Now that intravenous β-blockers and calcium antagonists are available, immediate control of rate when atrial fibrillation occurs is attained more easily than before; this affords time for "after-the-fact" digitalization.

The house officer will be informed regarding whether prophylactic digitalization or β-blockers are utilized for thoracic patients at his or her institution.

✚ SPACE PROBLEMS

After lobectomy, a variety of compensatory mechanisms allow the space previously occupied by the excised lobe to be filled: the remaining lobe overexpands; the mediastinum moves to the operated side; the diaphragm moves up; the ribs move closer together. Most often, these mechanisms, combined with proper chest tube placement, result in the remaining lobe's completely filling the pleural cavity. **Occasionally, after lobectomy, the pleural cavity may not**

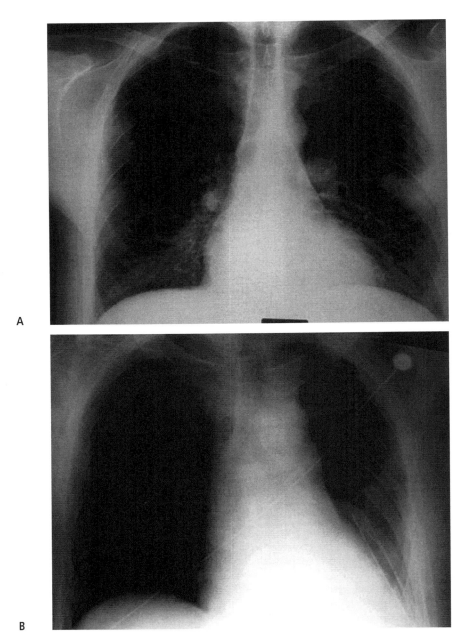

FIGURE 19.1

Chest x-rays showing progressive filling of the postpneumonectomy space by fluid with time. **Panel A:** Preoperative. Note lesion in the left mid-lung field. **Panel B:** Postoperative, with tubes in place emptying pleural space.

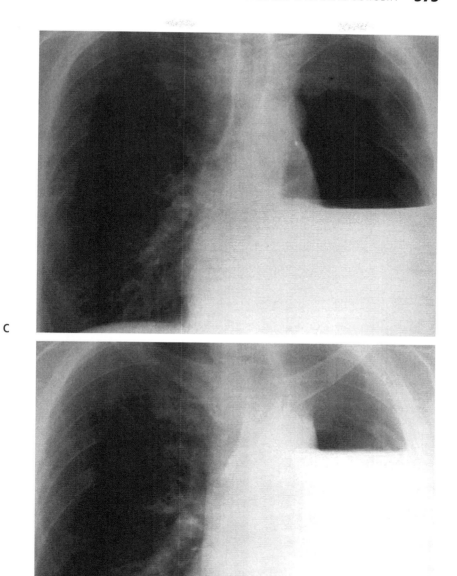

C

D

FIGURE 19.1

(*Continued*) **Panel C:** 5 days postoperatively. **Panel D:** 10 days postoperatively. Note rising fluid level in **C** and **D**. The pleural space will eventually fill entirely with fluid.

be filled entirely. The house officer must follow postoperative CXRs closely and call any remaining major space (pneumothorax) to the attention of senior staff. A number of manipulations of the drainage systems are available to overcome such a problem. These are carried out at the judgment and discretion of the surgeon.

Another reason incomplete expansion is important regards the postoperative air leak. **Air leak is normal after pulmonary surgery.** Parenchymal areas of adhesion and incomplete fissures will leak air of necessity following surgical mobilization. (The bronchial stump, of course, must be closed totally securely.) These parenchymal leaks will usually seal within hours of complete apposition of the lung to the chest wall. If an air space remains, adjacent parenchyma may not adhere to the visceral pleura and may continue to leak for days.

Special consideration must be paid to postpneumonectomy space problems. After pneumonectomy, the same mechanisms (mediastinal shift, diaphragmatic elevation, and narrowing of intercostal spaces) serve to minimize the empty space in the operated thorax. **The compensatory mechanisms cannot, however, totally obliterate the postpneumonectomy space, as no lung remains on the operated side.** Over days to weeks, that space will fill with fluid, which will eventually form an organized coagulum.

On the first night after thoracic surgery, postpneumonectomy space problems may cause major hemodynamic abnormality,[1-5] as a result of shifts in mediastinal position. Some surgeons believe that the mediastinum shifts toward the unoperated side most commonly, because fluid is secreted more rapidly than air is absorbed from the postpneumonectomy space. Other surgeons believe that the mediastinum shifts most commonly toward the operated side, because fluid secretion lags behind air absorption. Other factors may be relevant. When the patient is turned from the lateral decubitus position to the supine position at the completion of the resection, the diaphragm may be pushed up by intra-abdominal contents, with increase in pressure on the operated side and displacement of the mediastinum toward the unoperated side. On the other hand, at times air may be pushed through the chest wall closure into the soft tissues or the atmosphere, resulting in net negative pressure in the postpneumonectomy space and shift of the mediastinum to the operated side. It is best for the house officer to conclude that, **in particular cases, following pneumonectomy, significant mediastinal shift may occur toward either the operated or the unoperated side.**

Shift in either direction may cause major hemodynamic upset. Significant shift toward the operated side may occlude the great veins and impair cardiac filling. Shift toward the unoperated side may impair function of the sole remaining lung. Mediastinal shift has also been implicated as a cause of arrhythmias following pneumonectomy.

When hemodynamic instability occurs following pneumonectomy, mediastinal position must be assessed immediately. In fact, the house officer should monitor mediastinal position regularly to *prevent* excess deviation. Feeling for deviation of the trachea and percussing for location of the left ventricular apex may give some valuable clinical information regarding mediastinal displacement. Above all other tests, however, **it is the CXR that allows precise assessment of mediastinal position.** The CXR must be taken squarely anteroposterior or posteroanterior, as minor rotation of the x-ray may cause misleading contours. Usually, the mediastinal shifts are obvious if they are the cause of hemodynamic instability. In contralateral shift, the remaining lung will be seen to be severely compressed. In ipsilateral shift, the heart shadow may lie against the chest wall.

Mediastinal shift must be corrected when it is severe in extent or when it causes hemodynamic embarrassment. Most surgeons close the chest following pneumonectomy without an indwelling chest tube. Shift toward the unoperated side (by excess positive pressure in the pneumonectomy space) is corrected by aspirating air by needle and syringe until mediastinal position normalizes. Shift toward the operated side (by excess negative pressure in the pneumonectomy space) is corrected by injecting air by needle and syringe until mediastinal position normalizes. Aspirations or injections must be done with strict aseptic technique, as the empty pneumonectomy space infects easily. The house officer must discuss all manipulations with senior staff experienced in postpneumonectomy space problems.

Some surgeons do leave a tube to simple water seal following pneumonectomy. (This tube must *never* be placed to suction; this would cause high negative pressure and fatal ipsilateral mediastinal shift.) When this system is used, the tube is withdrawn from water seal once hourly to allow equilibration with atmospheric pressure. The level of water in the straw serves as a water manometer, allowing continuous assessment of intrapleural pressure. (See Chapter 17, Chest Tubes.) The ideal postpneumonectomy pressure is mildly negative (approximately 2 to 6 cm H_2O). (If a particular surgeon uses this chest tube system following pneumonectomy, the house officer must review in detail the surgeon's instructions for manipulations.) In this system, the tube is removed the morning after surgery.

A relatively new chest drainage system (a special postpneumonectomy Pleurevac from Deknatel, Inc) automatically controls pressure in the postpneumonectomy space; by virtue of two water seal chambers, this special device continually allows air to enter or exit the space to keep pressure within selected parameters. This system eliminates the need for the house officer to "lift the straw hourly from the water reservoir." This is an ingenious system that essentially eliminates postpneumonectomy hemodynamic instability related to mediastinal shift. This device takes over the house officer's responsibility reliably. Not all surgeons employ this device, however.

Hemodynamic compromise from mediastinal shift is unlikely after the immediate postoperative night. By the following morning, the circulatory system has usually adapted to minor shifts and the mediastinum begins to fix its position by edema and fibrosis. CXR position is still monitored daily, but adjustments rarely need be made.

✚ VOLUME LOSS

It is very common on the first, second, or third postoperative days to see significant or even total atelectasis in the lung tissue remaining after lobectomy.

Many factors encourage this atelectasis. Even an optimal resection may narrow, by edema, the remaining bronchial tree. Viscid secretions are exacerbated by premedication and anesthesia and may plug bronchi. (Mucinex (guaifenasin) may alleviate this sort of plugging.) Postoperative pain discourages deep breathing. The house officer must carefully assess and follow aeration of the remaining lobes. If aeration appears to be diminishing, pulmonary toilet must be intensified. Analgesics must be given to allow deep breathing and coughing. Incentive spirometer exercises must be emphasized. Endotracheal suctioning may be necessary.

If total atelectasis develops and does not respond overnight to intensive bronchopulmonary toilet measures, bronchoscopy should be carried out. Our preference is for rigid bronchoscopy, which permits excellent suctioning of secretions and plugs. Many use flexible bronchoscopy. A large-caliber bronchoscope with a large suction lumen is best for this purpose (a larger scope than the one used for diagnostic bronchoscopy). When total atelectasis occurs, of course, the house officer must follow arterial blood gases closely, as considerable shunting and hypoxia can occur. Once chest tubes are out and the patient is up and about, full expansion usually is maintained by normal respiratory excursion.

After pneumonectomy, of course, no lobe remains on the operated side. It is not uncommon, however, to see infiltrates on the side of the nonoperated, dependent lung. The house officer should expect to see these CXR changes, which reflect secretions draining into the dependent lung during the procedure. These infiltrates usually clear overnight.

There exists a specific syndrome called "post-pneumonectomy ARDS."[6-8] This occurs early after about 10% of pneumonectomy operations and carries a high mortality (> 50%). Risk factors for its development include high tidal volume ventilation of the one lung and prior pharmacotherapy with amiodarone. The house officer can recognize this syndrome by dyspnea, hypoxia, and infiltration of the remaining lung on CXR. Treatment is supportive.

✚ CONGESTIVE HEART FAILURE

Pulmonary resection decreases the vascular bed through which the right heart can pump; in effect, pulmonary vascular resistance is raised, increasing right ventricular afterload and pulmonary artery pressures. This is especially significant after pneumonectomy, where half the pulmonary vascular bed is removed. Though a normal healthy lung compensates for occlusion of a single pulmonary artery, this often is not the case in operated patients, whose remaining lung may be afflicted with preexisting pulmonary disease.[1]

Additionally, the lung remaining after pneumonectomy is liable to be flooded easily. It is best to run these patients "dry."[2,9] Pneumonectomy carries a considerable mortality. Right heart failure is one important factor. Right heart function is best followed by keeping track of central venous pressure. In fact, the Swan-Ganz catheter is almost contraindicated. It cannot safely be placed preoperatively, because it may go into the portion of the lung to be resected (unless fluoroscopic control is utilized). Placing the Swan-Ganz catheter postoperatively may carry the danger of disruption of the pulmonary artery stump by the advancing catheter. In any case, left heart function is usually normal; function of the right heart is well assessed by a simple central venous pressure catheter.

✚ PULMONARY EMBOLISM

Several important papers have focused specifically on thromboembolism following pulmonary resection.[10,11] With careful screening by pre- and postoperative venous duplex and ventilation-perfusion scanning, it was found that 25% of patients had deep vein thrombosis and/or pulmonary embolism following pulmonary resection. Thromboembolic disease was more common in patients with bronchogenic carcinoma (compared to other causes for resection), larger tumors (compared to small tumors), and larger resections (pneumonectomy or lobectomy compared to segmentectomy and wedge resection). The house officer should keep pulmonary embolism in mind in the post-thoracotomy patient, especially since the post-thoracotomy state may obscure the common manifestations of pulmonary embolism (pain, dyspnea, effusion, hypoxia).

✚ ADDITIONAL PROBLEMS

Two other conditions can cause major instability early after thoracic procedures. These will be covered briefly, for they are rare. Also, one important suggestion regarding on-the-table extubation after thoracic surgery will be made.

Lobar Torsion

Torsion of a remaining lobe may occur. This results from surgical division of normal stabilizing attachments (including incomplete fissures, pulmonary ligaments, and mediastinal pleural attachments). The surgeon will often fix the remaining lobe with sutures or staples to prevent torsion. When torsion does occur, severe toxicity results; the lobe will progress to gangrene if the condition is not recognized. A hazy appearance of the lobe on CXR may suggest torsion. Bronchoscopy may confirm the diagnosis, as a twisted lobar bronchus can be seen.[12] Urgent reexploration and resection of the affected lobe must be carried out immediately.

Cardiac Herniation

When the pericardium has been opened for intrapericardial pneumonectomy, herniation of the heart may occur through the defect. This unusual complication is lethal unless immediate operation and reduction are carried out. CXR may confirm the diagnosis, but there may not be sufficient time to obtain and develop the film. The key is prevention at the time of surgery by closing even small pericardial defects. An awareness of this disorder and an index of suspicion for it on the part of the house officer may be life-saving.

On-the-Table Extubation

One additional comment should be made concerning mechanical ventilation of the patient after pulmonary resection. Many chest surgeons, the authors included, feel it is important to extubate the patient as soon as possible after thoracic surgery, preferably on the operating table before transfer. Prolonged ventilation may be deleterious in a number of ways. Positive pressure puts extra strain on the bronchial stump and encourages parenchymal air leaks. Prolonged intubation stimulates tracheobronchial secretions and interferes with mucosal defense mechanisms of the bronchial tree. With careful selection of patients preoperatively, on-the-table extubation will be possible in the vast majority of cases.

REFERENCES

1. Young W, Perryman, R. Complications of pneumonectomy. In: Cordell A, Ellision R, eds. *Complications of Intrathoracic Surgery.* Boston: Little, Brown; 1979:257-266.
2. Kirsh M, Rotman H, Behrendt D, et al. Complications of pulmonary resection. *Ann Thorac Surg.* 1975;20:216-236.
3. Maier H. Pneumonectomy: methods of improving morbidity and mortality rates. *Surg Clin North Am.* 1962;42:1527-1536.
4. Von Hippel A. *A Manual of Thoracic Surgery.* Springfield, IL: Charles C Thomas; 1978-1979.

5. Langston H, Barker W. The adult thoracic surgical patient. In: Neville W, ed. *Intensive Care of the Surgical Cardiopulmonary Patient*. Chicago: Year Book; 1983:235-261.

6. Jeon K, Yoon JW, Suh GY, Kim J, Kim K. Risk factors for post-pneumonectomy lung injury/acute respiratory distress syndrome in primary lung cancer patients. *Anesth Intensive Care*. 2009;37:14-19.

7. Van Mieghem W, Coolen L, Malysse I, Lacquet LM, Deneffe, GJ, Demedts MG. Amiodarone and the development of ARDS after lung surgery. *Chest*. 1994;105:1642-1645.

8. Kutlu CA, Williams EA, Evans TW, Pasorino U, Goldstraw P. Acute lung injury and acute respiratory distress syndrome after pulmonary resection. *Ann Thorac Surg*. 2000;69:376-380.

9. Gibbon J, Gibbon M, Kraul C. Experimental pulmonary edema following lobectomy and blood transfusion. *J Thorac Surg*. 1942;12:60.

10. Kameyama K, Cheng-Iong H, Liu D, et al. Pulmonary embolism after lung resection: diagnosis and treatment. *Ann Thorac Surg*. 2003; 76:599-601.

11. Ziomek S, Read RC, Tobler HG, et al. Thromboembolism in patients undergoing thoracotomy. *Ann Thorac Surg*. 1993;56:223-227.

12. Brooks J. Complications following pulmonary lobectomy. In: Cordell A, Ellison R, eds. *Complications of Intrathoracic Surgery*. Boston: Little, Brown; 1979;235-256.

SUGGESTED FURTHER READING

Jeon K, Yoon JW, Suh GY, Kim J, Kim K. Risk factors for post-pneumonectomy lung injury/acute respiratory distress syndrome in primary lung cancer patients. *Anesth Intensive Care*. 2009;37:14-19.
An important read.

Spirn PW, Gross GW, Wechsler RJ, Steiner RM. Radiology of the chest after thoracic surgery. *Semin Roentgenol*. 1988 Jan;23(1):9-31.
Reading the chest x-ray after thoracic surgery is key.

Kirsh M, Rotman H, Behrendt D, et al. Complications of pulmonary resection. *Ann Thorac Surg*. 1975;20:216-236.
A clearly written and inclusive review with illustrative x-rays.

20

AORTIC EMERGENCIES

Thoracic aortic emergencies include acute aortic transection, rupture of thoracic aortic aneurysm, and acute aortic dissection. These are distinct entities often confused by house officers and practitioners alike. Much of this confusion stems from unfortunate terminology. Nonetheless, these conditions are among the most dangerous and challenging that the house officer faces in the coronary or surgical intensive care units. Before addressing specifically the role of the junior house officer in the management of aortic emergencies, certain general matters of orientation will be clarified.

⊞ TYPES OF AORTIC PATHOLOGY

Acute aortic dissection should be distinguished clearly from acute transections of the thoracic aorta and from chronic "arteriosclerotic" aneurysms of the thoracic or abdominal aorta (Figure 20.1).

The House Officer's Guide to ICU Care: Fundamentals of Management of the Heart and Lungs, 3rd ed. © 2013 John A. Elefteriades, Curtis Tribble, Alexander S. Geha, Mark D. Siegel, and Lawrence S. Cohen, eds. Cardiotext Publishing, ISBN: 978-1-935395-68-3.

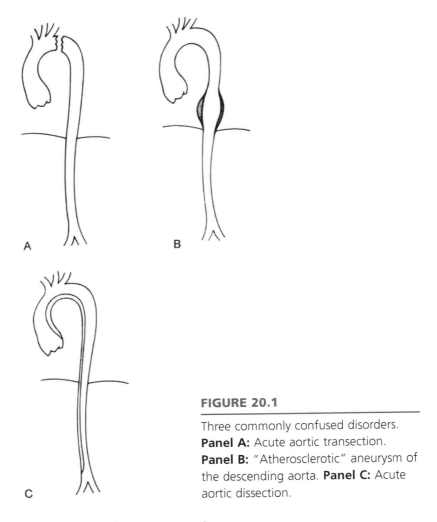

FIGURE 20.1

Three commonly confused disorders. **Panel A:** Acute aortic transection. **Panel B:** "Atherosclerotic" aneurysm of the descending aorta. **Panel C:** Acute aortic dissection.

Acute Aortic Transection

Acute transections of the thoracic aorta follow severe blunt trauma. The aortic wall is torn, often circumferentially, and at times transmurally. This condition is often immediately fatal because of exsanguination. Those who survive to reach the emergency center have the tear contained by the adventitia and pleural tissue overlying the aorta, preventing exsanguination. The aorta itself is intrinsically normal prior to the injury. The wall has normal strength. The layers of the wall do not split from each other for any significant distance—indeed, they cannot, because the basic consistency of the tissues is normal. This disorder is merely a tearing, not a dissection. It requires urgent repair through the left chest, which is often done with a special technique of bypass without an oxygenator, called left atrial to femoral artery bypass. This technique simply "borrows" some left atrial blood and distributes it to the lower body through a simple centrifugal pump. A short prosthetic graft is placed end to end to replace the aorta at the site of the tear (Figure 20.2); occasionally, the native tissues may be approximated primarily.

In the present era, aortic transections can be handled well with a carefully placed stent graft that goes across the site of the injury.[1] This approach can have advantages, as avoiding open surgery may often be beneficial due to the multi-trauma characteristics of these patients. Intra-abdominal injuries (liver, spleen) and myocardial and lung contusions, as well as closed brain injuries, are common associated findings.

A high index of suspicion for aortic transection is essential. This message has been well promulgated, and most house officers are well aware that they should suspect this injury in any victim of high-speed deceleration injury, especially in face of mediastinal widening or loss of clarity of the aortic knob or the stripe of the descending aorta on x-ray examination. The diagnostic investigation for this suspected disorder has gone through flux, as discussed in Chapter 12 (Thoracic Imaging in Acute Disease). Although aortography has in the past been the gold standard, CT angiography is currently the investigation of choice.

The treatment in suspected cases, or in documented cases before operative intervention is performed, is **strict blood pressure control.** In patients young and healthy except for the traumatic event, we keep blood pressure at 80 to 90 mm Hg systolic. In case operative intervention needs to be delayed, β-blockers can be added to decrease the strength of cardiac contraction.[2,3] This "anti-impulse" therapy with β-blockers and afterload reduction can stabilize many

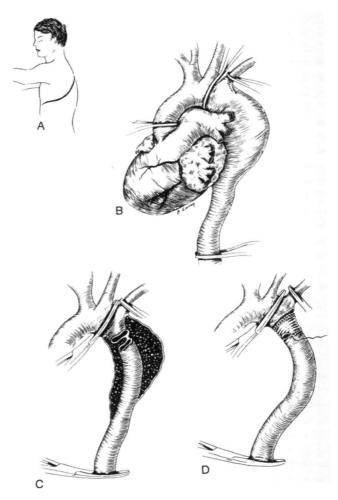

FIGURE 20.2

Operative procedure for acute aortic transection. A short Dacron graft is inserted at the site of transection just beyond the subclavian artery. **A.** Posterolateral thoracotomy incision. **B.** The injured aorta. **C.** The hematoma. **D.** The repair in progress.

Source: Reprinted with permission from Haimovici H. *Vascular Surgery: Principles and Techniques.* New York: McGraw-Hill; 1976.

of these patients for days until other injuries have been addressed or subsided, at which time stent or surgical treatment can be applied.

Chronic "Arteriosclerotic" Aneurysms

Chronic "arteriosclerotic" aneurysms of the thoracic and abdominal aorta result from weakening of the aortic wall and fusiform dilatation. The abdominal aorta distal to the renal arteries is most commonly affected. Rarely, the process may extend proximal to the level of the renal arteries. The thoracic aorta is less commonly involved than the abdominal aorta. When the thoracic aorta is involved, the aneurysm is usually in the descending aorta. Inside the fusiform dilatation, one finds organized, laminated thrombus. Although the aorta itself at the aneurysm is markedly abnormal, it has stretched concentrically, not dissected longitudinally. The layers of the aortic wall are normally adherent. Such dilatation of the aorta has long been considered to be of arteriosclerotic origin. This concept has recently been challenged, with an inherited molecular predisposition coming to light.[4,5] Nonetheless, dissection of one layer of the aortic wall from another is not part of this process. These aneurysms can rupture; they do not commonly dissect. Surgery is carried out electively when these aneurysms reach a size at which rupture becomes a significant danger. Most surgeons operate when the diameter of the descending aorta reaches 6 cm or begins to change rapidly. A prosthetic graft is used to replace the diseased aorta, with or without cardiopulmonary bypass (Figure 20.3). If the aortic arch is involved by such an aneurysm, cardiopulmonary bypass is required for the repair. When these aneurysms do rupture, bleeding may be contained by mediastinal pleural tissues or by the retroperitoneal tissues. When the emergency physician calls to report a "dissecting" abdominal aneurysm, he does not mean that at all, but rather an abdominal aneurysm that has ruptured but remains contained. The same applies for rupture of this condition in the thorax.

Acute Aortic Dissection

Acute aortic dissection refers to a specific condition in which the layers of the aorta are split from each other, with blood under pressure entering between the layers and propagating the split to

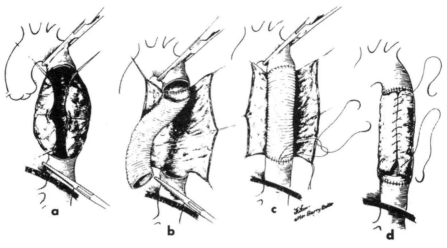

FIGURE 20.3

Operative procedure for "arteriosclerotic" aneurysm of the descending aorta. The aneurysm is opened and replaced by a long Dacron graft, which is then wrapped with the wall of the aneurysm. (Shown sequentially in **A** through **D**.)

Source: Reproduced with permission from Sabiston DC, Spencer FC. *Gibbon's Surgery of the Chest.* 4th ed. Philadelphia: WB Saunders; 1983.

various extents. This process begins with a tear through the intima and inner media at one specific site. Blood under pressure gains access within the media and forces its separation into layers.[6] The split occurs within the tunica media. The split is often brought on by extreme exertion or emotion.[6] The intima and inner media are forced inward. The outer media and adventitia are forced outward (Figure 20.4). This separation of layers is the "dissection." It is an acute process that occurs in a chronically degenerated aorta. At one instant, the dissection is not present. At the next instant, the initial tear occurs and the dissection propagates. The degeneration of the aortic wall that allows this to occur is a chronic process. Long-standing hypertension is thought to be the most important predisposing factor. Connective tissue disorders (especially Marfan's syndrome) are other predisposing conditions. With each hypertensive beat, the aorta is battered. The media in particular is weakened.

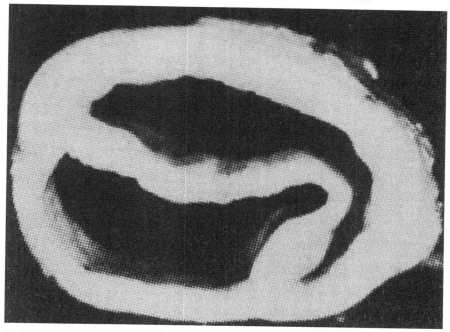

FIGURE 20.4

Gross pathology specimen of a descending aorta involved by acute aortic dissection. The true lumen is below and to the left, and the false channel is above and to the right.

Source: Reproduced with permission from Roberts, WC. Aortic dissection: Anatomy, consequences, and causes. *Am Heart J.* 1981:101;195. With permission from Elsevier.

After years of weakening, the media degenerates to the point where the initial tear and the dissection can occur.

It is the use of the term *dissecting aneurysm of the aorta* that fosters confusion with chronic "arteriosclerotic" aneurysms. It is best not to think of acute aortic dissection as an aneurysm at all. Until the acute phenomenon occurs, the aorta may or may not be aneurysmal. After the split occurs, although the aorta usually has widened acutely, it is the splitting of layers that has caused the widening that constitutes the crucial pathophysiologic event. It is best to term this acute phenomenon an "acute aortic dissection" rather than an "aneurysm" of any type.

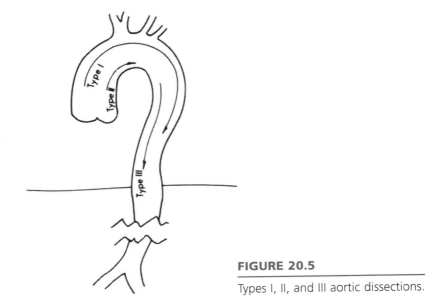

FIGURE 20.5

Types I, II, and III aortic dissections.

There are three basic types of acute aortic dissections (Figure 20.5). In types I and II, the initiating intimal tear occurs in the **ascending** aorta. In type I, the dissection propagates beyond the ascending aorta, often into the aorta arch, down the descending aorta, down the abdominal aorta, and into the iliacs. In type II, the dissection confines itself to the ascending aorta. In type III, the dissection begins in the **descending** aorta, beyond the left subclavian artery, and then propagates distally. The important point for the house officer is to be aware that **the initial tear in aortic dissection tends to occur in two very specific locations: about 4 cm above the aortic valve in ascending dissection, and just beyond the subclavian artery in descending dissection. Management guidelines are based strongly on the location—ascending or descending—of the initial tear. A common and increasingly popular classification describes all dissections involving the ascending aorta as Type A and all dissections involving only the descending aorta and below as Type B. This simple classification has advantages, as therapy is predicated on whether the dissection is Type A or Type B.**

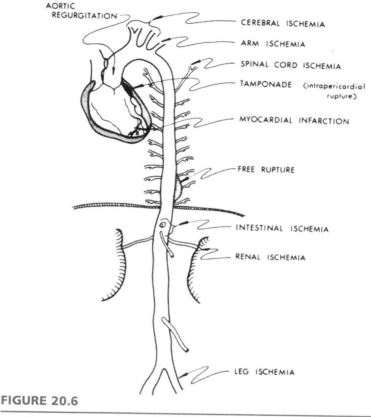

FIGURE 20.6

Specific major complications of acute aortic dissection.

✚ SEQUELAE OF AORTIC DISSECTION

Dissection can cause several general categories of harm to the patient (Figure 20.6).

Rupture

The force of pulsatile blood may break through the outer medial-adventitial layer, causing rupture of the aorta into the pericardium or, more rarely, into the chest or abdomen. Exsanguination can occur rapidly if the rupture is free. Bleeding may be contained to some degree by the fibrous tissue investing the descending thoracic and abdominal aorta, as well as the pleural or peritoneal tissues.

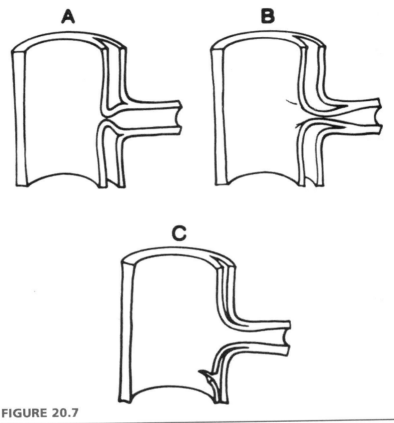

FIGURE 20.7

Schematic representation of the mechanism by which aortic dissection can "pinch off" an arterial branch of the aorta. **Panel A:** The dissection process with branch vessel occlusion. **Panel B:** Worsening of the pinching off of the branch as the dissection intensifies. **Panel C:** Relief of occlusion by the "fenestration" procedure. (See text.)

Tamponade

The pericardium attaches to the aorta several centimeters above the aortic valve along the ascending aorta. The ascending aorta lies freely in the pericardial cavity, surrounded by a thin layer of epicardium. For this reason, a dissection involving the ascending aorta can rupture into the pericardium. This can cause tamponade of varying severity.

Branch Occlusion

Flow through any of the branches of the aortic arch, descending aorta, or abdominal aorta may be occluded by the dissection. This occurs because pressure in the false lumen compromises the true lumen (Figure 20.7). Involvement of the innominate or carotid arteries can cause stroke. Involvement of the innominate or subclavian arteries can result in arm ischemia. Involvement of the thoracic intercostals can render the spinal cord ischemic, with resultant paraplegia. Involvement of mesenteric vessels can cause intestinal ischemia. Involvement of the renal arteries can cause renal failure and Goldblatt-type (renovascular) hypertension. Involvement of the iliac or femoral arteries can result in lower-extremity ischemia. Also, the coronary arteries themselves can become involved, resulting in myocardial ischemia or infarction.

Aortic Regurgitation

The dissection in the ascending aorta (in Type A) can "unseat" the aortic valve from its annulus, resulting in acute aortic regurgitation. This disorder is usually very poorly tolerated. Severe congestive heart failure or cardiogenic shock often follows quickly.

✚ SPECIFIC CARE

The role of the house officer in caring for patients with acute aortic dissection will be discussed under several headings: recognition, assessment, management decisions, preoperative care, operative management, and postoperative care.

Recognition

The burden of recognition usually falls on the medical house officer in the emergency department or the coronary care unit. The patient with an acute aortic dissecton has pain in the chest and/or the thoracic back. He or she is usually triaged with patients who have angina or myocardial infarction. The excruciating nature of the pain and the association with pain in the back should arouse suspicion that dissection may be occurring. Absence of EKG changes of ischemia may lead to further suspicion that the process is not myocardial ischemia. Ischemic EKG changes, however, do not necessarily rule out an acute aortic dissection, since coronary involvement can be a sequel of the dissection. A history of long-standing hypertension also should raise suspicion. The chest x-ray (CXR) is the key in differentiating patients with dissection from the many with ischemic pain. The shadows of the ascending aorta, the aortic knob, and the descending aorta will be widened and distorted when these segments are involved (Figure 20.8). Also, the physical findings of injury according to the four patterns described earlier—rupture, tamponade, branch occlusion, and aortic regurgitation—can be quite specific, as in the case of loss of a peripheral pulse or development of a new diastolic murmur. **A patient in whom the suspicion of acute dissection exists should undergo urgent imaging (by CT, MRI, or echocardiography).** (See Chapter 12, Thoracic Imaging in Acute Disease.)

The house officer should note that acute aortic dissection is **not** rare. **Acute dissection is, in fact, the most common acute catastrophe involving the human aorta,** occurring even more commonly than rupture of abdominal "atherosclerotic" aneurysms. It is lack of recognition that accounts for the impression that this disorder is unusual. Many patients presenting with chest pain and dying promptly in the emergency department are diagnosed as myocardial infarctions; careful autopsy series reveal that many of these patients have actually died from acute Type A aortic dissection.

Aortic dissection is a difficult diagnosis to make. In fact, only about half the cases are correctly diagnosed antemortem. These cases are highly litigated.[7] Key for the house officer is to have a high index of suspicion in any patient with chest, back, or abdominal pain or symptoms without other obvious cause. In fact, aortic dissection has been called "the great masquerader," because it can mimic disease of virtually any organ system, including brain, spinal cord, intestines, kidneys, extremities. This is because the blood

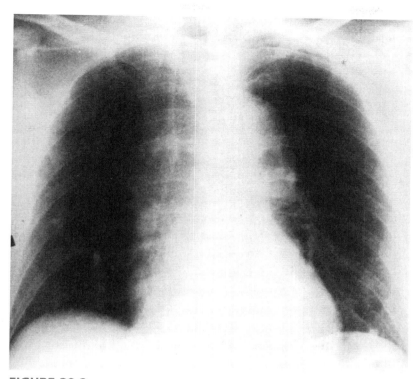

FIGURE 20.8

Presenting CXR of a patient with acute aortic dissection. The Type A dissection involved the ascending aorta, the aortic arch, and the descending aorta; widening of each of these aortic segments and blunting of their contours can be discerned.

supply to any of those organs can be interrupted by the dissection process. Advice to the house officer is as follows:

- Maintain a high index of suspicion for acute aortic dissection.
- Image liberally (CT, MRI, echo).
- Use the D-dimer test.

The D-dimer test is 99% sensitive for aortic dissection (but not at all specific). This test detects the thrombosis/thrombolysis process, which is always activated inside the false lumen by aortic dissection. Of course, D-dimer is also positive in deep vein thrombosis, pulmonary embolism, and myocardial infarction. However, **if the D-dimer is not elevated, the patient does not have an aortic dissection.**

Also, **keep in mind what we call the "triple rule-out CT scan."**[8] In a patient who appears very ill, without clear diagnosis, a chest CT can rule out the three major potential lethal diagnoses: myocardial infarction (coronary calcification will be visible on the CT scan), pulmonary embolism (clot in the pulmonary arteries will be visible on the CT scan), and acute aortic dissection (dissection layers will be clearly visible on CT imaging). (See Figure 20.9.) Thus, the triple rule-out CT can protect the house officer and patient from failure to recognize one of the three big killers.

Assessment

The house officer must assess the type of dissection: Is it ascending or descending? This can be usually done on the basis of symptoms, physical exam, and CXR. Ascending dissection presents with anterior

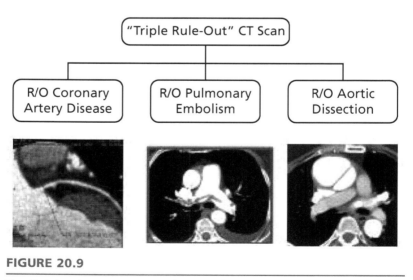

FIGURE 20.9

The "triple rule-out" CT scan. (See text.)

chest pain, while descending dissection presents with pain in the thoracic back. The house officer must ascertain as well which of the sequelae of dissection has occurred.

Intrathoracic rupture will cause a left hemothorax to appear on CXR. Intra-abdominal rupture will lead to peritoneal signs. Cardiac tamponade will present as described in Chapter 16, Chest Trauma. Occlusion of carotid or arm or leg arteries will be apparent from absent pulses and ischemia in the involved vascular distributions. Coronary occlusion will usually manifest on EKG. Renal occlusion will show as oliguria, anuria, or intractable hypertension. Intestinal ischemia is the most difficult to detect; peritoneal signs may not follow for many hours. If the patient is having any nausea or abdominal discomfort, or if there is abdominal distention, intestinal involvement is likely. Spinal cord ischemia shows as distal sensory/ motor disturbance.

Aortic valve involvement will produce symptoms and signs of congestive heart failure or pulmonary edema. It is critical to listen for the murmur of aortic regurgitation.

On the basis of history, physical exam, and CXR, the house officer should be able to formulate a good assessment of the type of dissection and the extent of its complications. Aortic imaging (by CT, MRI, or echo) will corroborate and amplify the impression from the physical examination. Clinical and radiographic assessment will allow decisions regarding whether surgery is indicated and, when necessary, which surgical procedure should be performed.

Management Decisions

Though management of acute dissections remains controversial and complex, the general principles regarding surgical management used at our institution can be simplified as follows. (Practice at some institutions may differ; this simplified paradigm is intended to provide the house officer with some orientation for decision making in this complex disorder.)

Ascending dissections require urgent surgery, if for no other reason than because the risk of fatal intrapericardial rupture exists. The process of intrapericardial rupture has often begun before the patient's presentation to the hospital. Some time usually intervenes between the onset of intrapericardial bleeding and flagrant tamponade with complete failure of cardiac function. More often than not, for ascending dissections, other complications, especially occlusion of important branch vessels and unseating of the aortic valve, would require intervention even if intrapericardial rupture did not occur. For this reason, ascending dissections represent surgical lesions.

Descending dissections are generally treated medically (see later) unless specific complications necessitate surgical intervention.[9-11] Some authorities disagree and consider these lesions surgical as well[12] (although those who espouse this approach are diminishing), and many experts in the present era recommend endovascular stent therapy. Free rupture of a descending dissection can usually be prevented by prompt and sustained blood pressure control. If vital branch vessels have been occluded by the dissection, however, surgery must be carried out. Barring unpreventable rupture or major vessel occlusion, descending dissections are medical lesions.

Preoperative Care

Specific preoperative care comprises two basic endeavors:

1. Blood pressure must be controlled.
2. Continued reassessment of extent of dissection and complications incurred must be carried out.

In patients being treated for dissection—before surgery, after surgery, or in place of surgery—blood pressure must be strictly controlled. Blood pressure must be reduced to the minimum levels that will sustain life and adequate organ function. Usually, we like to see systolic blood pressure of 100 mm Hg or

less. Higher pressures increase the likelihood that each heartbeat will rupture the thin adventitia or propagate the dissection further.

In the acute setting, continuous infusion of sodium nitroprusside (Nipride) is very effective in controlling blood pressure to any level desired. Particulars regarding use of continuous infusion agents are covered in Chapter 7. Nifedipine (10 to 20 mg) given sublingually can be very useful as an initial measure during transport or while the continuous infusions are being prepared.

Intravenous esmolol is given at intervals to help with blood pressure control. In fact, by impairing contractility and decreasing the rate of rise of systemic pressure with each heart beat, β-blockers are specifically indicated in treating aortic dissection; by this means, the forcefulness of each heartbeat is diminished. Blood pressure control (by nitroprusside) combined with β-blockers to decrease contractility is called "anti-impulse therapy" and has become the medical cornerstone of treatment of aortic dissection. (See Figure 20.10 for a depiction of the importance of both afterload reduction and β-blockers for a symbiotic reduction in the impulse of cardiac contraction.) Labetalol is a newer agent that is being used in dissection as an alternative to esmolol and nitroprusside;[13] labetalol has both vasodilating and β-blocking properties and can be used as a single agent in place of nitroprusside and esmolol. Labetalol can be given by continuous infusion; an initial bolus of 20 mg can be followed by an infusion of 2 mg/min. This drug has a long half-life (6 to 8 hours). Continuous infusion should be discontinued when control of heart rate and blood pressure are achieved to avoid cumulative toxicity. Table 20.1 shows the options available for intravenous therapy of acute aortic dissection.

When transition to chronic oral therapy is made, we usually use an afterload-reducing agent, such as hydralazine or an ACE inhibitor (angiotensin converting enzyme inhibitor) or ARB (angiotensin receptor blocker) and a β-blocker (such as metoprolol). Blood pressure limits are liberalized only slightly for chronic control.

TABLE 20.1 Options for Intravenous Therapy of Acute Aortic Dissection

Name	Category	Loading Dose	Maintenance Dose	Adverse Effects	Caution
Sodium nitroprusside	Vasodilator	0.3-3 mcg/kg/min, max limit for adult is 10 mcg/kg/min for 10 minutes	1-3 mcg/kg/min	Nausea, vomiting, agitation, muscle twitching, sweating, cutis anserina, thyrocytannate and cyanide toxicity, tachycardia	In patients with hepatic or renal dysfunction
Propranolol	β-blocker	1-3 mg (given at 1 mg intervals over 1 minute); can be repeated in not less than every 4 hours	1-3 mg every 4 hours	Hypotension, nausea, dizziness, cold extremities, reversible hair loss, bradycardia	In patients with bradycardia or history of CHF and bronchospasm; maximum initial dose should not exceed 0.15 mg/h (approx 10 mg)
Esmolol	β-blocker	500 mcg/kg bolus	Continuous 50 mcg/kg/min up to 200 mcg/kg/min	Hypotension, nausea, dizziness, bronchospasm, dyspepsia, constipation, increase in digoxin level	In patients with CHF, asthma, on concomitant CCB therapy
Labetalol	α- and β-blocker	20 mg over 2 mins then 40-80 mg every 10-15 mins (maximum 300 mg)	Continuous IV at 2 mg/min & titrate up to 5-10 mg/min	Vomiting, nausea, scalp tingling, burning in throat, dizziness, heart block, orthostatic hypotension	In patients with lung disease, concomitant CCB therapy
Diltiazem	CCB	0.25 mg/kg IV bolus (up to 25 mg)	5-10 mg/h by continuous infusion	Peripheral edema, nausea, vomiting	In patients on concomitant β-blockers
Enalapril	Vasodilator ACE inhibitor	0.625-1.25 mg bolus	0.625-5 mg every 6 hours	Precipitates fall in BP in high renin states, variable response, renal failure	In patients with high possibility of MI, renal dysfunction
Fenoldopam	Dopamine D1 receptor agonist	.03-0.1 mcg/kg/min initially	0.1-0.3 mcg/kg/min maximum 1.6 mcg/kg/min	Tachycardia, hypotension, headache, nausea, flushing, hypokalemia, elevation of IOP	In patients with glaucoma

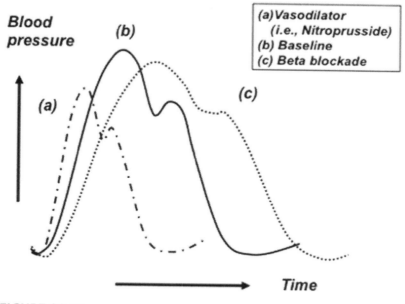

Blood pressure

(a) *Vasodilator*
   (i.e., Nitroprusside)
(b) *Baseline*
(c) *Beta blockade*

(a)

(b)

(c)

Time

FIGURE 20.10

Importance of both β-blockade and afterload reduction as "anti-impulse therapy" for acute aortic dissection. Note that Nitroprusside alone actually increased dp/dt; this can be dangerous in patients with actue aortic dissection. Note that β-blockade decreases dp/dt. The two together have a synergistic beneficial effect in decreasing both the blood pressure and the strength of cardiac contraction.

Source: Reprinted with permission from Sanz J, Einstein AJ, Fuster V. Acute aortic dissection: anti-impulse therapy. In: Elefteriades JA, ed. *Acute Aortic Disease*. New York: Informa Healthcare; 2007.

The house officer must be aware, especially in the acute setting, that inducing low or normal blood pressure in these patients with chronic, severe hypertension may, while treating the dissection, impair specific organ function. If the patient has cerebral, coronary, or renal artery disease, the reduced pressure head may prove insufficient for perfusion of those respective vascular beds. If mental obtundation or oliguria develops, the intravenous infusion should be titrated down to ensure adequate cerebral and/or renal perfusion.

Operative Management

The house officer should have some basic understanding of the methods of surgical correction of these complex disorders in order to care for the patient preoperatively and postoperatively. Again, for purposes of clarity, operative procedures will be simplified in this discussion, so that the house officer may concentrate on developing a fundamental perspective.

Ascending dissections are treated by replacement of the ascending aorta (Figure 20.11). The segment of aorta between the aortic valve and the aortic arch—the segment in which the intimal tear resides—is excised and replaced by a graft. This is done on cardiopulmonary bypass. Occasionally, for technical reasons, this operation must be done under deep hypothermia with circulatory arrest (DHCA)—a type of "suspended animation" in which the heart-lung machine is turned off for a period of time.[14-16] Replacing this specific segment of aorta accomplishes several important goals. Future rupture into the pericardium is prevented. The intimal tear is removed, so that blood under pressure no longer enters the false lumen through that tear. This usually suffices to restore blood supply to branches occluded by the dissection. If blood supply is not restored to a particular branch system, further treatment (as for descending dissection, discussed later) may be required. The ascending aortic replacement (depicted in Figure 20.11) does not eliminate the remainder of the dissected aorta; for this reason, lifelong blood pressure control is required afterward.

In ascending dissections, if the aortic valve has been unseated by the dissection, the valve is repaired or replaced at the time that the ascending aorta is replaced. This eliminates the acute aortic regurgitation that is often quickly fatal if not corrected.

For descending dissections, we have advocated what we call the *complication-specific approach*[17] (Figure 20.12). In this approach, if no complications occur, descending dissection is treated medically, with the aforementioned anti-impulse therapy. If complications do occur, an operation is carried out, with the specific operation

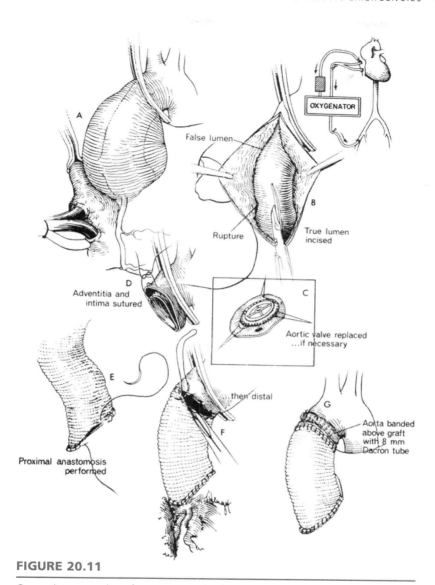

FIGURE 20.11

Operative procedure for acute aortic dissection involving the ascending aorta. Shown sequentially in **A** through **G**. Adventitial and intimal layers of dissection are reapproximated proximally and distally. The ascending aorta is replaced by a Dacron graft. The aortic valve is replaced if necessary (**C**).

Source: Reproduced with permission from Cooley, D. *Techniques in Cardiac Surgery*. 2nd ed. Philadelphia: WB Saunders; 1984.

Uncomplicated	Medical management

Complicated	Surgical management
• Rupture ⟶	Graft replacement
• Ischemia ⟶	Fenestration or stent
• Expansion ⟶	Graft replacement or stent

FIGURE 20.12

The complication-specific approach to descending aortic dissection. The thromboexclusion procedure is no longer in use, having been replaced by stent-grafting technique.

determined by the specific complication. Frank rupture is treated by replacement of the descending aorta by a Dacron graft. Impending rupture (manifested by rapid enlargement) is treated by aortic replacement or stent graft placement. If the complication is branch occlusion and organ ischemia (most commonly, occlusion of an iliac artery with leg ischemia), the "fenestration" procedure is performed,[18] accomplishing decompression of the false lumen and restoring blood flow to the affected organ (Figure 20.13). This procedure is quite effective in restoring lower-extremity perfusion; it is usually effective as well in restoring perfusion to kidneys and intestines. Endovascular creation of a fenestration is also possible. Stent therapy may be applicable for limb ischemia, as can crossover femoral-femoral artery bypass, in selected cases.

The objective of surgical treatment in descending dissection is to treat or prevent rupture and restore perfusion to vital organs; lifelong antihypertensive management is required from then on for residual dissected segments.

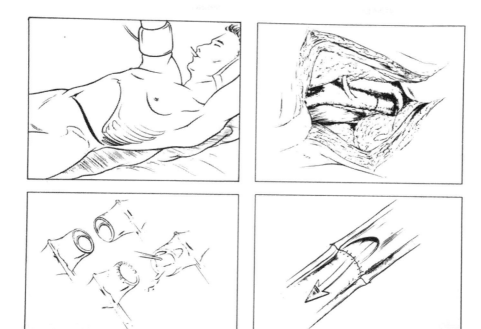

FIGURE 20.13

The fenestration procedure. **Upper left:** A flank incision is made. **Upper right:** The retroperitoneum is entered, and the abdominal contents reflected to the right, exposing the abdominal aorta. Note transverse line where aorta will be opened, below the renal arteries (note renal vein shown) and above the superior mesenteric artery (shown). **Lower left:** The aorta is transected. The intimal flap is resected from the top end (creation of "fenestra," or window). The two layers at the lower end are reapproximated by a simple suture. **Lower right:** The entire aorta is reconstituted by sewing the upper and lower ends together. No graft is required.

Source: Used with permission from Elefteriades JA, Hammond GL, Gusberg RJ, Kopf GS, Baldwin JC. Fenestration revisited: a safe and effective procedure for descending aortic dissection. *Arch Surg.* 1990;125(6):786-790. Copyright ©1990 American Medical Association. All rights reserved.

Postoperative Care

The preceding descriptions of the relevant surgical procedures make clear that **surgery does not cure the dissection.** Rather, **for both ascending and descending dissections, surgery is aimed at reversing or preventing life-threatening complications.** Because surgery does not eliminate the dissected aorta, postoperative care by the house officer must, as preoperatively, be directed toward the following:

1. Strictly controlling blood pressure.
2. Maintaining anti-impulse therapy (via supplemental β-blockade).
3. Continuously assessing adequacy of perfusion of branch organs.

Intestinal ischemia and infarction that were not apparent preoperatively may make themselves known postoperatively. Unfortunately, this intestinal ischemia may at times take the lives of survivors of the surgical procedure. (Sometimes, if suspicion of intestinal malperfusion comes to light early, the surgeon may opt to extend the sternotomy a bit into the linea alba at the time of the aortic replacement, permitting a "look-see" into the peritoneum for evidence of intestinal malperfusion).

REFERENCES

1. Oberhuber A, Erhard L, Orend KH, Sunder-Plassmann L. Ten years of endovascular treatment of traumatic aortic transection—a single centre experience. *J Thorac Cardiovasc Surg.* 2010;58:143-147.
2. Feldman M, Shah M, Elefteriades JA. Medical management of acute Type A aortic dissection. *Ann Thorac Cardiovasc Surg.* 2009;15: 286-293.
3. Shah M, Elefteriades JA. Medical management of acute Type A aortic dissection: Tales of turkeys, tygon tubing, and evolving paradigms. In: Safi HJ, McPherson DD. *Houston Aortic Symposium: Frontiers in Cardiovascular Disease.* Chicago, IL: Greenwood Publishing; 2009: 91-107.

4. Tilson MD, Stansel HC. Differences in results for aneurysm versus occlusive disease after bifurcation grafts: results of one hundred elective grafts. *Arch Surg.* 1980;115:1173-1175.

5. Tilson MD, Fieg EL, Harvey M. Malignant neoplasia in patients with abdominal aortic aneurysms. *Arch Surg.* 1984;119:792-794.

6. Hatzaras IS, Bible JE, Koullias GJ, Tranquilli M, Singh M, Elefteriades JA. Role of exertion or emotion as inciting events for acute aortic dissection. *Am J Cardiol.* 2007;100:1470-1472.

7. Elefteriades JA, Barrett PW, Kopf GS. Litigation in nontraumatic aortic diseases—a tempest in the malpractice maelstrom. *Cardiology.* 2008;109:263-272.

8. Elefteriades JA, Farkas EA. Thoracic aortic aneurysm: clinically pertinent controversies and uncertainties. *J Am Coll Cardiol.* 2010;55: 841-857.

9. Anagnostopoulos CE. *Acute Aortic Dissections.* Baltimore, MD: University Park Press; 1976.

10. Najafi H. Aortic dissection. In: Sabiston DC, Spencer FC, eds. *Gibbon's Surgery of the Chest.* Philadelphia: WB Saunders; 1983:956-967.

11. Little AG, Anagnostopoulos CE. Aortic dissections. In: Glenn WWL, Baue AE, Geha AS, et al, eds. *Thoracic and Cardiovascular Surgery.* Norwalk, CT: Appleton-Century-Crofts; 1983:1555-1565.

12. DeBakey ME, Lawrie GM, Crawford ES, et al. Surgical treatment of dissecting aortic aneurysms: 28 years experience with 527 cases. *Contemp Surg.* 1984;25:13-23.

13. Wilson DJ, Wallen JD, Vlachakis ND, et al. Intravenous labetalol in the treatment of severe hypertension and hypertensive emergencies. *Am J Med.* 1983;75(Suppl):95-102.

14. Griepp RB, Ergin MA, Lansman SL, Galla JD, Pogo G. The physiology of hypothermic circulatory arrest. *Semin Thorac Cardiovasc Surg.* 1991;3:188-193.

15. Gega A, Rizzo JA, Johnson MH, Tranquilli M, Farkas EA, Elefteriades JA. Straight deep hypothermic arrest: experience in 394 patients supports its effectiveness as a sole means of brain preservation. *Ann Thorac Surg.* 2007;84:759-766; discussion 766-767.

16. Stein L, Elefteriades JA. Protecting the brain during aortic surgery: an enduring debate with unanswered questions. *J Cardiothorac Vasc Anesth.* 2010;24:316-321.

17. Elefteriades JA, Hartleroad J, Gusberg RJ, et al. Long-term experience with descending aortic dissection: the "complication-specific" approach. *Ann Thorac Surg.* 1992;53:11-21.
18. Elefteriades JA, Gusberg RJ, Kopf GS, Hammond GL, Baldwin JC. Fenestration revisited: procedure of choice for descending aortic dissection with blood flow compromise. *Arch Surg.* 1990;125:786-790.

SUGGESTED FURTHER READING

Elefteriades JA. Beating a sudden killer. *Sci Am.* 2005;293:64-71.
A good introduction to current thoughts and issues in thoracic aortic disease, including causation and pathophysiology.

Elefteriades JA, ed. *Acute Aortic Disease.* New York: Informa Healthcare; 2007.
The house officer can pick and choose the chapters of most interest at his or her current stage.

Anagnostopoulos CE. *Acute Aortic Dissections.* Baltimore, MD: University Park Press; 1976.
Now a classic, this volume recounts the unraveling of the mysteries of this disorder in a fascinating narrative by an expert in the field.

ACUTE KIDNEY INJURY

Acute kidney injury (AKI) and acute renal failure (ARF) often compli-cate critical illness.[1-4] Reported rates vary widely, reflecting the many definitions employed; however, recent work suggests more than 50% of critically ill patients develop kidney injury. Incidence rises with age, co-morbidity, and organ dysfunction. AKI is associated with greater mortality, cost, length of stay, and duration of mechanical ventilation. Almost 5% of ICU patients require renal replacement therapy (RRT).[1-4] Although most recover function, up to 30% of those treated with acute RRT go on to need chronic RRT within 3 years.[2]

This section will focus on diagnosis, prevention, and treatment of AKI and ARF. Given the large number of acronyms used in this challenging field, a glossary is provided to help the reader (Table 21.1).

The House Officer's Guide to ICU Care: Fundamentals of Management of the Heart and Lungs, 3rd ed. © 2013 John A. Elefteriades, Curtis Tribble, Alexander S. Geha, Mark D. Siegel, and Lawrence S. Cohen, eds. Cardiotext Publishing, ISBN: 978-1-935395-68-3.

TABLE 21.1 Common Acronyms Used in Critical Care Nephrology

Acronym	Meaning
AKI	Acute kidney injury
AKIN	Acute Kidney Injury Network
ARF	Acute renal failure
ATN	Acute tubular necrosis
BUN	Blood urea nitrogen
CAVH	Continuous arteriovenous hemofiltration
Cr	Creatinine
CRRT	Continuous renal replacement therapy
CVVH	Continuous venovenous hemofiltration
CVVHD	Continuous venovenous hemodialysis
CVVHDF	Continuous venovenous hemodiafiltration
ESRD	End-stage renal disease
FENa	Fractional excretion of sodium
FEurea	Fractional excretion of urea
GFR	Glomerular filtration rate
IHD	Intermittent hemodialysis
PD	Peritoneal dialysis
RIFLE	Risk injury failure loss end-stage kidney disease
RRT	Renal replacement therapy
SLED	Sustained low-efficiency dialysis

✚ DIAGNOSIS OF AKI

Many criteria have been used to define AKI, creating a confusing literature. In recent years, the RIFLE criteria ("*Risk*," "*Injury*," "*Failure*," "*Loss*," "*E*nd-stage Kidney Disease") and a modified version, the AKIN criteria (*Acute Kidney Injury Network*), have been advocated and increasingly adopted (Table 21.2).[4,5]

TABLE 21.2 AKIN Classification and Staging System for AKI[5]

Stage[+]	Creatinine	Urine Output
1	Increase in serum Cr > 0.3 mg/dL or > 1.5-2x baseline	< 0.5 mL/kg/h for more than 6 hours
2	Increase in serum Cr > 2-3x baseline	< 0.5 mL/kg/h for more than 12 hours
3[*]	Increase in serum Cr > 3x baseline or serum Cr > 4.0 mg/dL with acute increase > 0.5 mg/dL	< 0.3 mg/kg/h for 24 hours or anuria for 12 hours

[+]Patients meeting either criterion in each stage are classified in that stage.
[*]Patients who receive RRT are automatically classified as Stage 3.

AKI is traditionally divided into three etiologic categories: pre-renal, intrinsic renal, and postrenal (Table 21.3).[1] Prerenal AKI results from decreased kidney perfusion, causing a reversible decrease in glomerular filtration rate (GFR) and increased BUN and creatinine (Cr). Common causes include volume depletion, congestive heart failure, and cirrhosis. If not corrected, prerenal AKI can lead to acute tubular necrosis (ATN). Postrenal AKI results from obstruction of the urinary collection system, for example due to tumors, calculi, or prostatic hypertrophy. Prompt relief of obstruction can completely reverse AKI. Intrinsic renal AKI results when the nephron's structures—the vessels, glomeruli, tubules, or interstitium—are damaged. The most common cause of intrinsic renal AKI is ATN, usually precipitated by sepsis, shock, or intravenous contrast. Prerenal and ischemic ATN cause 75% of ARF in the ICU.[1]

Early recognition may lead to interventions that reverse or mitigate AKI. Important findings like a sustained drop in urine output to less than 0.5 mL/kg/h or less than 400 mL/day should raise concern.[1,2] Severe AKI can occur with normal urine output, particularly with postrenal or intrinsic causes. The serum Cr only rises after injury has occurred and an increase as small as 0.3 mg/dL should be considered important. The total serum Cr can

TABLE 21.3 Classification of AKI[1]

Classification	Examples
Prerenal	Volume depletion Hemorrhage Congestive heart failure Cirrhosis Renal artery stenosis or occlusion Nonsteroidal anti-inflammatory drugs (NSAIDs) Angiotensin converting enzyme inhibitors (ACEI) Angiotensin II receptor blockers (ARBs)
Intrinsic Renal	Vascular (eg, vasculitis, malignant hypertension) Glomerulonephritis Interstitial nephritis (eg, drug-induced) Acute tubular necrosis Ischemic Nephrotoxic (eg, contrast, aminoglycosides, myoglobin)
Postrenal	Obstruction of collecting system Bladder outlet obstruction Bilateral ureteral obstruction

overestimate GFR, particularly before the Cr reaches a new steady state. Multiple factors besides clearance affect the serum Cr, including age, race, gender, muscle mass, medication, rate of production, and volume of distribution.

Important tests include a urinalysis, evaluation of urine chemistries, and often a renal ultrasound.[1] A urinalysis may suggest ATN, particularly if muddy brown casts or tubule epithelial cell casts are seen.[6] Casts may be absent in some cases of ATN, and the quantity of debris in the urine does not correlate with severity of injury. A renal ultrasound looking for hydronephrosis is necessary if obstruction is possible and should generally be performed when the etiology of AKI is in doubt.

Measurement of the fractional excretion of sodium (FENa) helps distinguish prerenal from intrinsic renal disease. Successful sodium reabsorption in the renal tubules is essential for volume homeostasis.

In the setting of renal hypoperfusion, for example due to dehydration, hypotension, or low cardiac output, normal renal tubules maximally reabsorb sodium to defend volume status. Sodium is reabsorbed disproportionately to creatinine, resulting in a low FENa, which is calculated as follows:

(Urine sodium × Plasma creatinine / Plasma sodium × Urine creatinine) × 100

A FENa < 1% supports a prerenal state, whereas a FENa > 2% suggests intrinsic renal disease. Unfortunately, an isolated FENa is of limited value and does not completely rule out intrinsic renal disease. As with all diagnostic tests, the FENa should be interpreted in the context of other available information.

✚ PREVENTION AND SUPPORTIVE TREATMENT

AKI is often preventable.[1-4] Key principles include avoiding nephrotoxins such as prolonged courses of aminoglycosides; intervening early, for example when urine output falls or Cr starts to rise; and carefully supporting blood pressure and renal perfusion. Diuretics can promote urine output but do not improve GFR; they may be counterproductive in the setting of volume depletion.[6-7] Low-dose ("renal dose") dopamine neither prevents nor treats AKI.[8]

IV contrast is an important cause of AKI, particularly in patients with chronic kidney disease, diabetes, advanced age, congestive heart failure, hypovolemia, and hemodynamic instability.[1,4,9] Although often relatively benign, contrast-induced nephropathy can cause significant morbidity, particularly in patients with poor baseline renal function—in severe cases leading to RRT and sometimes end-stage renal disease (ESRD). IV contrast should be avoided whenever possible; not all CT scans require contrast and safer tests, such as ultrasounds, may provide needed diagnostic information. When contrast is required, it should be used frugally. Adequate volume status before contrast administration is essential. In patients at risk, intravenous normal saline or bicarbonate should be strongly considered before and after the procedure to ensure adequate hydration. N-acetylcysteine (Mucomyst) may provide additional benefit.

Once AKI is discovered, it is essential to prevent further harm. Medications that are renally metabolized or excreted may require dose adjustments. The house officer must pay careful attention to electrolyte balance, particularly potassium concentrations in the setting of acidosis and oliguria. **Stop automatic sliding-scale potassium replacement as soon as you suspect acute renal failure may be imminent;** otherwise, you will be struggling 12 or 24 hours later with life-threatening hyperkalemia. Patients may have trouble excreting free water loads, so you must follow serum sodium concentrations closely. In the setting of a metabolic acidosis, careful bicarbonate supplementation may forestall the need for RRT. Diuretics may help treat volume overload, although higher doses, continuous infusions, or combination therapy (eg, furosemide and metolazone) may be needed. Nephrology input may be crucial—particularly if there is doubt about the etiology—if a renal biopsy is necessary, if the patient develops complex metabolic or electrolyte abnormalities, or if the need for RRT is anticipated.

Renal Replacement Therapy

The optimal approach to RRT in the ICU is controversial. A great deal of research has addressed indications, timing, modalities, and intensity, with much remaining inconclusive. Local practice style and expertise often determine management choices.

Indications and Timing

RRT should be initiated before patients develop florid complications such as uremic pericarditis, encephalopathy, and coagulopathy.[1,2] Absolute indications include severe metabolic acidosis, hyperkalemia, and hypervolemia unresponsive to supportive therapy

TABLE 21.4   Absolute Indications for Initiating RRT[1,10]

Indication	Specific Criteria
Azotemia	BUN > 100 mg/dL
Uremia	Encephalopathy, pericarditis, bleeding
Hyperkalemia	K > 6-6.5 mmol/L or ECG abnormalities
Hypermagnesemia	Mg > 4 mmol/L and/or anuria, absent deep tendon reflexes
Acidosis	pH < 7.00 to 7.15
Oliguria/anuria	Urine output < 200 mL/12 h or anuria
Fluid overload	Diuretic resistant edema or severe CHF
Drug overdose	Dialyzable toxin (eg, lithium)

(Table 21.4). In sensitive postoperative cardiac patients, we often move to RRT earlier than the criteria in Table 21.4. The optimal time to initiate RRT is unknown. The potential advantages of RRT need to be balanced against the risks of catheter placement, hemodynamic instability, and metabolic flux, as well as added cost and complexity.[10]

Modalities

Several RRT modalities are available.[2] Peritoneal dialysis (PD) is rarely initiated for acute renal failure in developed countries, although it can be continued in chronic PD patients with a working catheter in place. Hemodialysis (HD) can be given during intermittent sessions (IHD) or continuously (CRRT). Sustained low-efficiency dialysis (SLED) is similar to IHD, but sessions last several additional hours, allowing more gradual treatment sessions, which may be better tolerated when patients are hemodynamically tenuous.

The choice between IHD and CRRT is controversial.[1] Head-to-head comparisons have failed to show measurable outcome advantages with either approach.[2,11] The choice of modality largely depends on local expertise and experience.

CRRT is most commonly used in hemodynamically unstable patients, although IHD can be successful, even in patients on vasopressors. CRRT may be better tolerated, particularly when there is a need to remove large volumes of fluid; IHD is more likely to induce hemodynamic instability because relatively large quantities of solutes and fluids may be removed quickly. CRRT is more expensive and resource intensive.[1] By definition, CRRT immobilizes patients, which is a disadvantage if physical therapy is an option. This immobility is a special disadvantage in postoperative cardiac surgical patients.

Several different CRRT techniques are available, using different vascular access routes and modalities for solute clearance and fluid removal.[2] Both arteriovenous and venovenous circuits can be used, although the latter is far more common. With arteriovenous circuits, two catheters are placed, one in an artery, another in a central vein. Blood is pumped through the dialysis circuit under the pressure of arterial blood. Arteriovenous circuits impose risks to the artery, however, and are limited by the pressures patients can generate. Venovenous circuits are used far more commonly, using a double lumen catheter placed into a central vein such as the femoral, subclavian, or internal jugular. Blood is removed from one lumen and an artificial pump sends blood through the dialysis circuit. In general, venovenous CRRT is felt to be more efficient and safe and is generally the first choice when pumps are available.

The main intent of CRRT is to manage fluid balance, remove toxins, and correct electrolyte and acid-base abnormalities. Two modes are commonly employed: hemofiltration and dialysis. With all modes, fluid balance is determined by the quantity of fluid removed through the circuit and the amount returned as replacement fluid. Decisions to achieve negative, even, or positive fluid balance fall to the clinicians caring for the patient.

With continuous venovenous hemofiltration (CVVH), convection occurs across a semi-permeable membrane, removing water and solutes. In contrast, with continuous venovenous hemodialysis

(CVVHD), diffusion occurs across a semi-permeable membrane with solutes and water responding to osmotic forces resulting from concentration differences between the patient's blood and dialysate fluid. To maximize efficiency, dialysate is pumped in the direction opposite to blood flow. Dialysate composition can be prepared and used according to the patient's metabolic needs, for example using different concentrations of bicarbonate and potassium. For the most part, both modalities are acceptable and decisions should be driven by local expertise and availability of appropriate equipment.

The optimal intensity and frequency of RRT is unknown. Preliminary work suggested that more intense therapy improves outcomes, but subsequent studies have called that finding into question.[12-15]

As with initiation, the appropriate time to stop RRT is unknown. Recognizing recovery of renal function is challenging since volume status and metabolic parameters are largely determined by RRT. CRRT can generally be converted to IHD when patients stabilize hemodynamically. If return of renal function is suspected, it may be reasonable to carefully withhold RRT while watching for signs that resumption of therapy is necessary. In the majority of ICU survivors with acute renal failure, sufficient renal function will return and allow RRT to be discontinued; however, a significant number may progress to ESRD in the long term.[2]

REFERENCES

1. Lameire N, Van Biesen W, Vanholder R. Acute renal failure. *Lancet.* 2005;365(9457):417-430.
2. Pannu N, Klarenbach S, Wiebe N, Manns B, Tonelli M; Alberta Kidney Disease Network. Renal replacement therapy in patients with acute renal failure: a systematic review. *JAMA.* 2008;299(7):793-805.
3. Mehta RL, Pascual MT, Soroko S, et al. Spectrum of acute renal failure in the intensive care unit: the PICARD experience. *Kidney Int.* 2004;66(4):1613-1621.

4. Lameire N, Biesen WV, Vanholder R. Acute kidney injury. *Lancet.* 2008;372(9653):1863-1865.

5. Mehta R, Kellum J, Shah S, et al. Acute Kidney Injury Network: report of an initiative to improve outcomes in acute kidney injury. *Crit Care.* 2007;11(2):R31.

6. Clarkson M, Friedewald J, Eustace JA, Rabb H. Acute kidney injury. In: Brenner B, ed. *Brenner and Rector's the Kidney.* 8th ed. Vol. 1. Philadelphia: Saunders Elsevier; 2007:943.

7. Mehta RL, Pascual MT, Soroko S, Chertow GM, Group PS. Diuretics, mortality, and nonrecovery of renal function in acute renal failure. *JAMA.* 2002;288(20):2547-2553.

8. Jones D, Bellomo R. Renal-dose dopamine: from hypothesis to paradigm to dogma to myth and, finally, superstition? *J Intensive Care Med.* 2005;20(4):199-211.

9. Pannu N, Wiebe N, Tonelli M; Alberta Kidney Disease Network. Prophylaxis strategies for contrast-induced nephropathy. *JAMA.* 2006;295(23):2765-2779.

10. Bagshaw SM, Cruz DN, Gibney RT, Ronco C. A proposed algorithm for initiation of renal replacement therapy in adult critically ill patients. *Crit Care.* 2009;13(6):317.

11. Bagshaw SM, Berthiaume LR, Delaney A, Bellomo R. Continuous versus intermittent renal replacement therapy for critically ill patients with acute kidney injury: a meta-analysis. *Crit Care Med.* 2008;36(2):610-617.

12. Schiffl H, Lang SM, Fischer R. Daily hemodialysis and the outcome of acute renal failure. *N Engl J Med.* 2002;346(5):305-310.

13. Ronco C, Bellomo R, Homel P, et al. Effects of different doses in continuous venovenous hemofiltration on outcomes of acute renal failure: a prospective randomised trial. *Lancet.* 2000;356(9223): 26-30.

14. Investigators RRTS, Bellomo R, Cass A, et al. Intensity of continuous renal-replacement therapy in critically ill patients. *N Engl J Med.* 2009;361(17):1627-1638.

15. Network VNARFT, Palevsky PM, Zhang JH, et al. Intensity of renal support in critically ill patients with acute kidney injury. *N Engl J Med.* 2008;359(1):7-20.

22

SEDATION AND ANALGESIA

Critical illness commonly causes distressing symptoms such as pain, anxiety, and delirium and can sometimes lead to dangerous agitation. The goal of this chapter is to highlight the key components of an effective approach to sedation and analgesia in critically ill patients.[1-3] Many times, adverse outcome in ICU is related to sedation and analgesia. It is not uncommon for a house officer to order sedatives, often on the basis of exhortation from a frustrated nurse with an unruly patient. By morning, the house officer may get an urgent call that his patient is now obtunded, not breathing, or in full cardiac arrest—as a consequence of injudicious, but well-meaning, overmedication. This chapter aims to provide the house officer with guidelines to avoid patient harm from well-intended efforts to control pain and agitation.

The House Officer's Guide to ICU Care: Fundamentals of Management of the Heart and Lungs, 3rd ed. © 2013 John A. Elefteriades, Curtis Tribble, Alexander S. Geha, Mark D. Siegel, and Lawrence S. Cohen, eds. Cardiotext Publishing, ISBN: 978-1-935395-68-3.

✚ AGITATION

First and foremost, the house officer must ascertain that there is no specific physical cause for the patient he is called to see to be agitated. **Life-threatening causes of agitation** must not be missed. Important examples **include respiratory failure, shock, sepsis, hypoglycemia, central nervous system catastrophes, and pain from myocardial infarction or intestinal ischemia.** A targeted physical exam, focused laboratory testing, and diagnostic imaging may reveal dangerous problems that might otherwise be hidden by sedatives. The other chapters in this book provide guidelines to assessment and management of these important physical conditions that may manifest as agitation. (See Figure 22.1.)

Other common causes of agitation may respond to non-pharmacologic interventions. Frustration over the inability to speak may be addressed with paper and pen. An uncomfortable bed position may respond to boosting or transfer to a chair. Some patients want their lips moistened or need to move their bowels. Directed questions, basic explanations, reassurance, and empiric interventions may be effective and prevent unnecessary medication use. In an era when nurses are overburdened by nearly overwhelming procedural and documentation responsibilities, such remediable patient-specific causes of agitation may be overlooked; it behooves the house officer to make an independent assessment before rushing to medicate.

Discomfort related to intubation and mechanical ventilation should be routinely considered. An optimally placed endotracheal tube should be positioned with its tip 5 cm above the carina. When placed too deeply, the tip may enter the right mainstem bronchus (Figure 22.2), potentially resulting in impaired gas exchange, over-inflation of the right lung and collapse of the left, sometimes leading to dyspnea and agitation. Alternatively, tubes placed too deeply may cause the tip to rub against the carina, inducing violent coughing and repeatedly setting off the ventilator's high-pressure alarm. A chest radiograph can identify the need for repositioning.

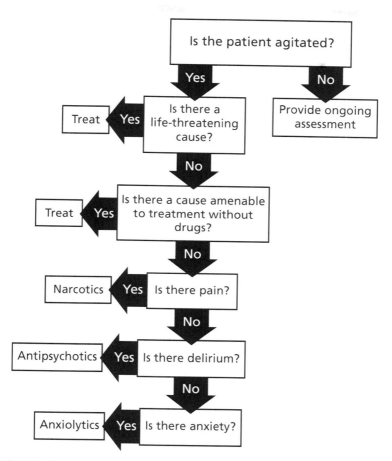

FIGURE 22.1

A systematic approach to evaluating and managing agitation in the ICU.

Patient-ventilator dysynchrony is also common.[4] Frequent causes include inadequate inspiratory flow rates and tidal volumes set too high or low. Frequent ventilator alarming, double triggering (ie, two consecutive breaths not separated by an exhalation), and ineffective triggering are all important signs that dysynchrony is occurring. Further evidence may be obtained by carefully studying graphic displays on the ventilator. Respiratory therapists are a valuable resource in most ICUs, helping to identify dysynchrony and

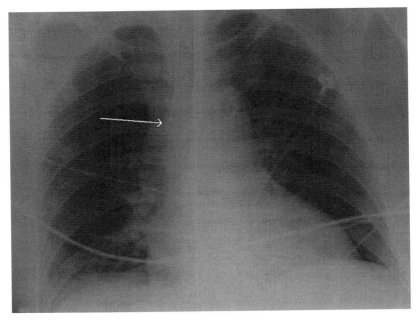

FIGURE 22.2

Chest radiograph of a patient with a malpositioned endotracheal tube. (The tube is too far in, having entered the right mainstem bronchus.)

adept at finding ventilator settings that foster patient comfort. Changing flow rates or ventilator modes may promote synchrony and help the patient relax. A sophisticated approach to setting the ventilator may even allow patients to tolerate intubation with minimal or no sedation.[5] Ideally, the house officer should see the intubated patient respiring comfortably, with the chest rising visibly and regularly with each machine breath; occasional spontaneous breaths may be interposed.

✚ PAIN, DELIRIUM, AND ANXIETY

Pain, delirium, and anxiety are exceedingly common in the ICU. Many of the house officer's calls will regard these phenomena. Pharmacologic treatment employs medications that are relatively

TABLE 22.1 Pharmacological Properties of Commonly Used Sedatives and Analgesics

Medication	Main Use	Peak (minutes)	Duration After Bolus (minutes)	Initial Dose
Fentanyl	Analgesia	2-5	30-45	25-100 mcg
Morphine	Analgesia	30	120-240	2-5 mg
Midazolam	Anxiolytic	2-5	30-120	0.5-2 mg
Lorazepam	Anxiolytic	15-30	360-480	0.5-2 mg
Haloperidol	Treatment of delirium	30	Variable	2-10 mg

Important note: It is vital to start treatment at the very low end of the dosage range until one sees the patient's response, especially in postoperative, elderly, debilitated, or hemodynamically unstable patients.

specific. (See Table 22.1.) As a rule, pain generally requires treatment with narcotics, delirium treatment with neuroleptic medications, and anxiety treatment with benzodiazepines. A relatively limited number of medications in each class can be employed to meet the needs of most patients. It behooves the house officer to become very familiar with the information in Table 22.1, so that he or she has a roster of drugs to use when called, and thereby can avoid toxicity in dosing.

Treatment of Pain

Pain is particularly common following trauma and surgery and after procedures such as chest tube placement. Certain illnesses such as cancer and arthritis frequently cause significant pain. Although many patients can report pain, some cannot, and it falls to the physician and nurse to identify the need for analgesia. Nurses commonly use pain assessment tools to identify discomfort when patients cannot communicate, looking for suggestive signs such as tearing, splinting, and knitting of the brow. Sometimes a beneficial response to empiric analgesia will support the diagnosis of pain in patients who cannot communicate. Also, of course, many procedures that we perform in the ICU (including chest tube placement and central venous and peripheral arterial cannulation) can be quite painful.

Some pain may respond to regional anesthesia (eg, nerve blocks and epidural catheters) or to moderately potent non-narcotic analgesics such as acetaminophen and nonsteroidal anti-inflammatory drugs (NSAIDs). More commonly, narcotics are required. Among the most common medications used are fentanyl and morphine, usually given intravenously (see Table 22.1). Meperidine (Demerol) is best avoided because metabolites may accumulate, particularly in renal failure, and lower the seizure threshold.

Dosed appropriately, narcotics can provide effective pain relief without inducing sedation, which generally occurs at higher doses. Narcotics lack anxiolytic effects but may exert a calming effect via effective analgesia. Class-specific side effects include respiratory depression, depressed gut motility, and hypotension. The latter is more common with morphine boluses, which promote histamine release. Decreased gut motility commonly causes ileus, and it is often wise to initiate a bowel regimen preemptively. Respiratory depression from narcotics may pose an obstacle to weaning some patients from the ventilator; in contrast, respiratory depression may be a useful property if suppression of the respiratory drive is needed for safe mechanical ventilation, for example in patients with severe acute respiratory distress syndrome (ARDS) or asthma.

The doses necessary for effective analgesia vary significantly. In general, lower doses are necessary in older patients, small individuals, those with liver disease, and patients who have not been treated previously. Please keep in mind also the tremendous impact of kidney disease; even for drugs considered to be hepatically metabolized, metabolites can be active and persist for long periods of time in case of depressed renal function.

Significant adverse synergy may occur when narcotics are combined with benzodiazepines, particularly respiratory depression and hypotension. Fentanyl acts rapidly and is particularly useful when quick onset is required, for example in anticipation of emergency procedures. A single dose of fentanyl wears off in less than an hour, so single doses are not ideal when pain is prolonged or recurrent. In such cases, continuous infusions of fentanyl or intermittent use of a longer-acting medication, such as morphine, is preferred.

Treatment of Delirium

Delirium is extremely common in the ICU, affecting the vast majority of patients requiring prolonged mechanical ventilation and those with underlying cognitive impairment.[6-8] The causes of delirium are multifactorial and include the direct and indirect effects of critical illness on the central nervous system as well as medications, particularly benzodiazepines. Clinical features of delirium include a waxing and waning mental status, inattention, and disorganized thinking. Several clinical tools have been developed to help diagnose delirium, among the best studied being the Confusion Assessment Method for ICU Patients or CAM-ICU,[9] which is simple and quickly performed at the bedside.

Most delirious patients have no outward manifestations and may evade diagnosis unless tests such as the CAM-ICU are performed routinely. A minority manifests hyperactive delirium, often with agitation that may require pharmacologic treatment to prevent untoward complications such as falls or self-extubation. It is best to avoid benzodiazepines in this population, since that class of drug may exacerbate or even cause delirium. Neuroleptic medications such as haloperidol (Haldol) are preferred. Although neuroleptics do not reverse delirium, they can suppress agitation. Unlike many other sedatives, antipsychotics do not induce respiratory depression. Typical doses of haloperidol are 2 to 10 mg given intravenously every 6 hours, with smaller doses employed initially in the elderly. An electrocardiogram should be performed to rule out a prolonged QTc interval when haloperidol is used to minimize the risk of torsade de pointes, particularly with higher doses. Haloperidol should be used cautiously in patients predisposed to seizures. Other medications such as olanzapine and quetiapine are potential alternatives if haloperidol is ineffective or not tolerated.

Treatment of Anxiety

Benzodiazepines are among the most commonly used medications in the ICU and, unfortunately, among the most often abused. At low doses, benzodiazepines provide anxiolysis and may induce a useful calming effect. At higher doses, benzodiazepines are the primary therapy used to treat delirium tremens (DTs) in patients with alcohol withdrawal.[10]

Although many varieties of benzodiazepine are available for clinical use, two of the most commonly used are midazolam and lorazepam. A bolus of midazolam (Versed) takes effect in less than 5 minutes, making it particularly useful for procedures such as intubation, cardioversion, and central line placement or when urgent treatment is needed. Midazolam wears off quickly, making it less useful for extended treatment. Although commonly used in a continuous infusion, midazolam has active metabolites that can lead to an undesired, prolonged clinical effect after the infusion is discontinued. Midazolam undergoes metabolism by the cytochrome P450 system, which can lead to prolonged sedation in patients with liver failure.

Lorazepam (Ativan) has a slower onset and is longer acting, making it less useful for immediate sedation but more appropriate for extended treatment. Lorazepam should generally be delivered intravenously with intermittent boluses. Occasional patients may need continuous infusions when repeated or high doses are required, for example for DTs. Unlike midazolam, lorazepam is metabolized in the liver by glucuronidation and is somewhat less affected by hepatic dysfunction.

Benzodiazepines are less likely to induce respiratory depression compared to narcotics, although respiratory depression can be induced when combined with narcotics or when benzodiazepines are used in patients with impaired respiratory drive. Benzodiazepines are generally well tolerated hemodynamically, although they may induce or exacerbate shock, particularly in patients with inadequate preload or those who are already hemodynamically tenuous. Benzodiazepines frequently induce amnesia and contribute significantly to cognitive impairment and an increased risk of delirium. In susceptible individuals, benzodiazepines can exacerbate rather than treat agitation. Benzodiazepines provide no analgesia, and a failure to respond to modest doses of benzodiazepines should raise suspicion that an alternative problem exists, such as delirium or pain, requiring different therapy.

✚ A WORD OF CAUTION REGARDING NARCOTICS, SEDATIVES, AND HYPNOTICS

It is not at all uncommon for narcotic, sedative, and hypnotic drugs to cause respiratory depression, hypotension, somnolence, loss of consciousness, cardiac arrest, or death. These drugs, among the most dangerous in the hospital, should be used with great care. The house officer should start with a very low dose, until he or she determines the response of the specific patient. The house officer should avoid standing orders and as needed (p.r.n.) orders, at least when he or she is first medicating a specific patient. The house officer should also avoid having a large roster of multiple drugs in these categories available for as-needed use in a specific patient; this takes control of these powerful medications out of your own hands.

✚ OTHER MEDICATIONS

Most ICU patients requiring sedation and analgesia can be effectively managed with narcotics, antipsychotics, and benzodiazepines. Occasional patients benefit from other medications such as propofol and dexmedetomidine. Propofol (Diprivan) is a rapidly acting sedative-hypnotic, generally given as a continuous infusion in mechanically ventilated patients.[2,3] Propofol works in less than a minute after it is initiated and wears off in within several minutes of discontinuing an infusion, even after hours of use. With very long duration (days) of administration, propofol can accumulate in fatty tissues and have a prolonged duration of action, even after discontinuation of the drip. Propofol is often useful when deeper sedation is required. Propofol has no analgesic properties, so a narcotic must be given if treatment of pain is required. Because of its rapid onset and potent sedative and respiratory depressant effects, propofol is generally reserved for use in intubated patients. Propofol is a strong vasodilator and largely contraindicated in patients with shock. Finally, because propofol is generally delivered in a lipid emulsion, careful aseptic technique must be used to avoid infection. At higher doses, the lipids may provide a significant number of calories, which must be considered when nutritional requirements are calculated.

Dexmedetomidine (Precedex) is an alpha-2 agonist with several unique properties, including easy arousal (even in the midst of infusions), a strong narcotic sparing effect, and absence of respiratory depression. A recent study suggested improved outcomes with dexmedetomidine compared to continuous infusions of midazolam, including less delirium and less time on the ventilator.[11] Future studies are needed to determine its role in the ICU, particularly given that effective care can be provided when less expensive, traditional drugs are used judiciously.

For patients requiring continuous infusions, **a daily sedation holiday** that allows patients to wake up to participate in activities (such as spontaneous breathing trials and physical and occupational therapy) appears to promote more rapid discontinuation of mechanical ventilation, decreased length of stay, better functional outcomes, and even improved long-term survival.

Occasional ICU patients require neuromuscular blockade. Standard practice, for compassion's sake, requires adequate sedation when neuromuscular blockade is used; this is important to avoid having a patient feel his paralysis while still awake. Paralyzing drugs are generally administered only to patients intubated and on mechanical ventilation. Specific ICUs have specific protocols for paralyzing medications. We use vecuronium at 5 to 10 mg total dose, which usually provides close to 1 hour of paralysis. Such treatment may be required in a critically ill patient who is fighting the respirator and thus impairing his ventilation or oxygenation, or in a patient actively bleeding.

✚ SUMMARY

A thoughtful approach to sedation and analgesia is critical to excellent ICU care. Most critically ill patients are at risk for pain, delirium, and/or anxiety, and agitation is a common problem. When assessing agitated ICU patients, it is essential to consider life-threatening problems requiring specific treatment, such as respiratory failure or shock. A nonpharmacologic approach can successfully address or mitigate many symptoms, particularly dysynchrony with the ventilator. When medication is required, a targeted approach should be used, using medications specifically geared to treat pain, delirium, or anxiety. Comfort can usually be achieved without excessive sedation, however. These medications are dangerous and must be used judiciously and with great respect.

REFERENCES

1. Jacobi J, Fraser GL, Coursin DB, et al. Clinical practice guidelines for the sustained use of sedatives and analgesics in the critically ill adult. *Crit Care Med.* 2002;30(1):119-141.
2. Honiden S, Siegel MD. Analytic reviews: managing the agitated patient in the ICU: sedation, analgesia, and neuromuscular blockade. *J Intensive Care Med.* 2010;25(4):187-204.
3. Siegel MD. Management of agitation in the intensive care unit. *Clin Chest Med.* 2003;24(4):713-725.
4. Epstein SK. Optimizing patient-ventilator synchrony. *Semin Respir Crit Care Med.* 2001;22(2):137-152.

5. Strøm T, Martinussen T, Toft P. A protocol of no sedation for critically ill patients receiving mechanical ventilation: a randomised trial. *The Lancet.* 2010;375(9713):475.

6. Ely EW, Siegel MD, Inouye SK. Delirium in the intensive care unit: an under-recognized syndrome of organ dysfunction. *Semin Respir Crit Care Med.* 2001;22(2):115-126.

7. McNicoll L, Pisani MA, Zhang Y, Ely EW, Siegel MD, Inouye SK. Delirium in the intensive care unit: occurrence and clinical course in older patients. *J Am Geriatr Soc.* 2003;51(5):591-598.

8. Misak CJ. The critical care experience: a patient's view. *Am J Respir Crit Care Med.* 2004;170(4):357-359.

9. Ely EW, Inouye SK, Bernard GR, et al. Delirium in mechanically ventilated patients: validity and reliability of the Confusion Assessment Method for the Intensive Care Unit (CAM-ICU). *JAMA.* 2001;286(21):2703-2710.

10. DeBellis R, Smith BS, Choi S, Malloy M. Management of delirium tremens. *J Intensive Care Med.* 2005;20(3):164-173.

11. Riker RR, Shehabi Y, Bokesch PM, et al. Dexmedetomidine vs midazolam for sedation of critically ill patients: a randomized trial. *JAMA.* 2009;301(5):489-499.

SUGGESTED FURTHER READING

De Cosmo G, Congedo E, Clemente A, Aceto P. Sedation in PACU: the role of propofol. *Curr Drug Targets.* 2005;6:741-744.
An excellent review of this important, useful, and potentially dangerous drug.

Honiden S, Siegel MD. Analytic reviews: managing the agitated patient in the ICU: sedation, analgesia, and neuromuscular blockade. *J Intensive Care Med.* 2010;25:187-204.
A thorough, up-to-date review of this topic.

Dunn WF, Adams SC, Adams RW. Iatrogenic delirium and coma: a "near miss." *Chest.* 2008;133(5):1217-1220.
A cautionary tale worth reading.

Additional instructions and background information on the diagnosis and treatment of delirium is available at http://www.icudelirium.org/

23

ADDITIONAL TOPICS

This chapter covers a number of subjects that do not merit separate chapters but are of enough significance to warrant the house officer's awareness. These topics are therefore discussed briefly and are grouped together in a single chapter.

✚ PROSTHETIC VALVES AND ANTICOAGULATION

Two general types of artificial heart valves are available: mechanical valves and bioprostheses. Mechanical valves are constructed from man-made materials. Bioprostheses are based mainly on biologic tissues from animals. Mechanical valves in the past included ball valves (like the Starr-Edwards) and tilting disc or "toilet seat" valves (like the Bjork-Shiley and Medtronic); currently, double-disk valves (St. Jude, Carbomedics) are most commonly used. Biologic valves are mainly of two types: one type is made from glutaraldehyde-fixed porcine aortic cardiac valves mounted on a sewing ring (Carpentier-Edwards and Hancock valves); the other type uses artificial leaflets constructed from glutaraldehyde-fixed bovine pericardium (Edwards pericardial valve).

It is important for the house officer to be aware that **a systolic flow murmur is normal following aortic valve replacement;** the prosthetic valve always creates some turbulence of flow that manifests as a murmur. (No artificial valve can re-create nature's normal laminar flow patterns.) No diastolic murmur should be audible, however; presence of a diastolic murmur would imply abnormal aortic regurgitation.

Likewise, no systolic murmur should be audible following mitral valve replacement; this would imply abnormal mitral regurgitation.

Mechanical valves should produce a crisp, mechanical closing sound. Loss of crispness, along with hemodynamic changes, would suggest a mechanical problem with leaflet closure. Biologic valves usually produce totally normal closure sounds.

The house officer often asks about anticoagulation practices with various prosthetic valves. Practices do vary regionally and from surgeon to surgeon. Several basic principles, however, can be enumerated. (The house officer can also consult the guidelines of the American Heart Association, at the websites[1,2] listed in the References.)

- **In general, no anticoagulation is required in the first 48 hours after surgery.** Clotting mechanisms are impaired for a period of time following cardiopulmonary bypass. Also, anticoagulation would not be safe until clot is well established at suture lines.
- **Anticoagulation is generally begun with warfarin (Coumadin) at about the time that chest tubes are removed.** This will produce a prolongation in clotting times within 2 to 3 days. We tend to give the first dose on the evening of postoperative day 1, and the chest tubes are removed on the morning of postoperative day 2.

- Many different schedules for coumadinization can be used effectively, as long as clotting times are followed. Some surgeons give 10 mg on the first day and 10 mg on the second and adjust according to clotting times thereafter.
- Most centers follow the INR (international normalized ratio) for coumadinization, aiming for an INR of 2.0 to 2.5 for aortic prostheses and 2.5 to 3.5 for mitral prostheses. The INR was developed to permit uniformity of results at various laboratories and throughout the world. The INR represents the ratio of the time it takes for the patient's blood to clot compared to that of a normal control. The house officer may wonder why the mitral valve requires a higher level of anticoagulation than the aortic. Remember that although the same total amount of flow passes through both the aortic and mitral valves (the cardiac output), the much larger mitral valve sees a much lower velocity of flow. The slower the velocity of blood flow, the higher the risk of thrombosis.
- **Bioprostheses, of themselves, do not require anticoagulation, regardless of mitral or aortic position.** That having been said, some surgeons use aspirin for aortic biologic prostheses, and many surgeons anticoagulate with Coumadin for at least 1 to 3 months after biologic mitral valve replacement.
- **Mechanical prostheses always require full anticoagulation with Coumadin, regardless of mitral or aortic position.**
- **Patients with a bioprosthetic mitral valve often require anticoagulation, not for the valve itself but for general cardiologic indications.** Most cardiologists would recommend anticoagulation, even without a prosthesis, for patients with mitral valve disease and atrial fibrillation, atrial thrombus, atrial dilatation, or history of arterial embolus. Most patients who come to mitral valve surgery meet one or more of these criteria.

- **Anticoagulation in a patient with a prosthetic mechanical valve should never be reversed acutely (by vitamin K or by fresh frozen plasma) without discussion with the responsible surgeon;** cases of sudden thrombosis of the mechanical prosthesis—a fatal phenomenon—have been reported with acute reversal of anticoagulation.
- Patterns for cessation and transitioning of anticoagulation in preparation for surgical procedures vary widely from center to center.[3] At our institution, for aortic valves, we simply stop the Coumadin 4 days preoperatively. The risk of stroke or valve thrombosis is very low. For mitral valves, where the risk of valve thrombosis or stroke is greater, we stop the Coumadin and admit the patient for IV heparin 2 days later; we then wait for the INR to normalize before proceeding to surgery. While these patterns are reasonable, it is best for the house officer to investigate the local policies at his or her institution.

✚ MAINTENANCE CARDIAC MEDICATIONS

Patients in the coronary care unit or those undergoing cardiac surgery often receive specific cardiac medications that fall into four general categories: digitalis glycosides, diuretics, antihypertensives and afterload-reducing medications, and antianginals. The house officer must be familiar with preoperative, perioperative, and postoperative management of these drugs around the time of cardiac surgery.

Digitalis

Digitalis is usually held the morning of surgery. The operating principle is to enter surgery with the patient somewhat underdigitalized, so that digitalis toxicity, especially with potassium fluxes, is not likely. As far as the putative inotropy of digitalis is concerned, the much more potent intravenous agents discussed in Chapter 7, Continuous Infusion Agents, are available, if required. In fact, one cannot even appreciate clinically the mild inotropic effect of digitalis postoperatively. For control of cardiac rate, digitalis can be administered postoperatively along the paradigm discussed in Chapter 2, Arrhythmias.

Usually digitalis will be resumed as preoperatively after surgery. If digitalis was given for arrhythmia control, it is likely to be useful as part of the postoperative regimen. If digitalis was given for preoperative congestive failure, it will usually be continued for at least 6 months postoperatively. Even after successful valve replacement for congestive heart failure, some ventricular dysfunction persists. A component of dysfunction may reverse over weeks to months; a certain component may be irreversible.

Diuretics

Diuretics are usually held the morning of surgery. The reasons are several. Diuretics deplete potassium; hypokalemia is very dangerous around the time of cardiac surgery. Volume status will be monitored invasively (by CVP or Swan-Ganz catheter) and adjusted accordingly. Fluid fluxes with cardiopulmonary bypass are so massive that omitting a preoperative diuretic is largely irrelevant.

As with digitalis, patients who were on diuretics chronically preoperatively will likely be placed on them postoperatively. Again, ischemic or valvular left ventricular dysfunction that required daily diuretics preoperatively is likely to persist to some degree postoperatively. The house officer will find that most surgeons use diuretics on an as-needed basis, depending on CXR appearance, weight gain, peripheral edema, and shortness of breath.

Antihypertensives

Antihypertensive medications are usually omitted on the morning of surgery. Potent intravenous agents (discussed in Chapter 7) are available to treat intraoperative or postoperative hypertension. For the powerful ACE and ARB agents, we often stop them 2 days in advance of surgery, to prevent unwanted postoperative hypotension from the "vasoplegia syndrome" (see Chapter 7, Continuous Infusion Agents).

Patients chronically hypertensive preoperatively will be so after recovery from surgery. At times, the specific antihypertensive drug protocol on discharge following surgery will need modification because of alteration in antianginal medications.

Nifedipine, a calcium antagonist with marked peripheral vasodilating properties, is very popular for acute or chronic blood pressure control. The usual dose is 10 to 30 mg orally 4 times daily.

The ACE inhibitors (angiotensin converting enzyme inhibitors) have become extremely popular as antihypertensive agents, especially because of demonstrated beneficial effects on symptomatic state and long-term survival in patients with compromised left ventricular function. These drugs bring about peripheral vasodilation by inhibiting formation of the vasoconstrictor angiotensin II. A major toxicity is azotemia, caused by disruption of normal autoregulation of glomerular blood flow, especially in patients with underlying renal artery disease. Another toxicity is hyperkalemia, resulting from inhibition of aldosterone. Specific agents and their dosage schedules are indicated in Table 23.1.

The ARBs are also very popular in the present era. The ARBs share the heart failure benefits of ACE inhibitors and are generally well tolerated. Table 23.2 shows commonly used ARBs and their dosages.

TABLE 23.1 ACE Inhibitors

Generic Name	Trade Name	Dose (mg)	Interval
Captopril	Capoten	6.25-50	b.i.d. to t.i.d.
Enalapril	Vasotec	2.5-10	b.i.d.
Lisinopril	Prinivil	10-40	q.d.
Fosinopril	Monopril	10-40	q.d.

TABLE 23.2   Angiotensin Receptor Blockers (ARBs)

Generic Name	Trade Name	Dose (mg)	Interval
Candesartan	Atacand	4-32	q.d.
Irbesartan	Avapro	75-300	q.d.
Telmisartan	Micardis	20-80	q.d.
Valsartan	Diovan	80-160	q.d. to b.i.d.
Losartan	Cozaar	25-50	b.i.d.

Antianginals

Three general classes of antianginal medications are in common use: nitrates, β-blockers, and calcium antagonists. The nitrates (nitroglycerine and nitroprusside are agents in this category), as discussed in Chapter 7, decrease preload, decrease afterload, and beneficially redistribute coronary flow by preventing coronary artery spasm and by dilating collateral vessels. Nitrates are available in several forms. The well-known nitroglycerin tablet is designed for emergency sublingual administration for an acute angina attack. Many longer-acting oral nitrate preparations are available (most incorporating isosorbide). Recently, nitroglycerin paste and time-release nitroglycerin patches (lasting up to 24 hours) have become popular.

The β-blockers improve the oxygen supply-demand relationship in the myocardium by limiting oxygen demand; this is done through a negative inotropic effect (a decrease in strength of cardiac contraction) and a negative chronotropic effect (a decrease in heart rate). Propranolol (Inderal) is the best known of these agents. A host of newer agents have become available that may offer an advantage in cardioselectivity (causing less bronchospasm from blocking of bronchial β-receptors) or in duration of action (allowing greater spacing of doses). Table 23.3 lists the available preparations, trade names, doses, and specific characteristics of these drugs for easy reference. Each internist or cardiologist has a particular preference and usage pattern for β-blockers. Table 23.3 will allow rapid

TABLE 23.3 β-Blockers

Generic Name	Trade Name	Dose (mg)	Interval	Specific Characteristics
Atenolol	Tenormin	50-100	q.d.	Cardioselective
Metoprolol	Lopressor	50-200	b.i.d.	Cardioselective
Nadolol	Corgard	40-240	q.d.	Nonselective
Pindolol	Visken	10-30	b.i.d.	Nonselective
Propranolol	Inderal	10-80	q.i.d.	Nonselective
Timolol	Blocadren	10-30	b.i.d.	Nonselective

assessment by the house officer, as patients may be referred for coronary care or cardiac surgery on any of the drugs in this class. (A number of newer preparations, not yet very widely used—including acebutolol, betaxolol, carteolol, and penbutolol—are, for purposes of simplification, omitted from Table 23.3.)

The calcium antagonists improve angina through mechanisms that are not totally clear. Decrease in myocardial oxygen demand and increase in myocardial oxygen supply via coronary artery dilatation or prevention of coronary artery spasm have been postulated.[4] Three calcium antagonists have been available for clinical use: diltiazem, nifedipine, and verapamil. These drugs, along with two newer ones, are summarized in Table 23.4. Again, individual cardiologists have individual preferences. Many of these drugs have become available in long-acting, sustained-release form, to allow the convenience of once-a-day dosage. (Felodipine and bepridil are omitted from Table 23.4, for simplification.)

In general, antianginals are continued up to the time of cardiac surgery, including morning doses. It has been found that abrupt withdrawal may precipitate an acute angina attack or infarction. Also, experience has shown that cardiac surgery can be performed safely with antianginals on board. (The feared suppression of contractile function after resumption of cardiac activity post-bypass did not occur.)

TABLE 23.4   Calcium Antagonists

Generic name	Trade Name(s)	Dose (mg)	Interval	Specific Characteristics
Diltiazem	Cardizem	30-90	t.i.d.	Relatively few side effects
Nifedipine	Procardia	10-30	t.i.d.	Potent vasodilator; dizziness; peripheral edema
Verapamil	Calan, Isoptin	40-120	t.i.d.	Constipating
Nicardipine	Cardene	20-40	t.i.d.	
Amlodipine	Norvasc	5-10	q.d.	

At our institution, on the morning of surgery, we continue nitrates. We continue the β-blocker and the calcium antagonist, generally at the same dosage. Local patterns of preoperative usage vary.

**In general, after revascularization, there is no need to con-
tinue antianginals.** Although a β-blocker or a calcium antagonist
may be chosen to treat or to prevent supraventricular tachycardia,
the indication in this setting is the arrhythmia, not angina. Also, the
β-blocker or calcium antagonist medications may be required for
blood pressure control, independently of their antianginal properties. A rare patient with known incomplete or inadequate revascularization may be continued on antianginals postoperatively for
treatment of ischemia. In matter of fact, most patients stay on a
β-blocker for blood pressure control alone, if not for general prophylaxis as well. Patients with congestive heart failure stay on
β-blockers as well as ACE inhibitors, as per recent American Heart
Association guidelines. (See References and Suggested Further
Reading at the end of this chapter.)

✚ ANTIPLATELET THERAPY

There exists some recent evidence[5-7] that antiplatelet treatment may
improve bypass graft patency, presumably by impairing clot formation at sites of intimal irregularity. Many cardiac surgeons routinely

administer antiplatelet agents postoperatively. Aspirin and/or dipyridamole (Persantine) are prescribed for this purpose. Dosage varies from surgeon to surgeon. In one study showing a beneficial effect on graft patency, dosage was aspirin 325 mg p.o. t.i.d. and Persantine 75 mg p.o. t.i.d. In that study, Persantine was begun preoperatively, and administration of both agents was implemented shortly postoperatively. Many centers have dropped the dipyridamole, using only a single aspirin tablet daily. The recently reported CASCADE trial[8] found no need to add the newer and more potent agent clopidogrel for protection of vein grafts after cardiac surgery; patency was excellent with aspirin alone.

Many surgeons also use antiplatelet therapy postoperatively in patients who have had a bioprosthetic valve implanted. Similar dosage is used.

✛ WOUNDS

The house officer should not instrument a median sternotomy wound without discussion with more senior team members. Not infrequently, a sternotomy wound has been needled or opened for insignificant reasons, only to lead to iatrogenic infection. A wound problem is never such an emergency that time cannot be taken to enlist an experienced opinion. However, any drainage or erythema should be reported to senior staff.

✛ FEVER

Thermoregulation is disordered for a period of time following cardiopulmonary bypass.[9] Almost uniformly, patients develop high fever during the first night after surgery. This does not signify sepsis. In fact, at our center, we do not become concerned about fevers until the third or fourth postoperative day.

🚻 NUTRITION

Most cardiothoracic patients, despite cardiac illness or undergoing major operative procedures, show little interference with gastrointestinal motility. By the morning after cardiac or thoracic surgery, most patients will be well enough to be extubated and can take nutrition orally several hours thereafter (when pharyngeal reflexes recover post-extubation). Diet can usually be advanced very rapidly. Nutrition thus does not represent a problem in most patients.

An occasional patient may require prolonged ventilatory assistance or be so severely ill that oral feeding is not possible. Nasogastric feeding is used in such patients, provided that gastrointestinal motility has resumed adequately. It is becoming popular to start early, so-called "trophic feedings" at a low level enterally and/or parenterally quite early (within 24 to 48 hours) in patients likely to be too ill to eat spontaneously; survival improvement has been demonstrated. It is important to use soft, small-caliber feeding tubes in intubated patients; **with an endotracheal tube in the trachea and a large or rigid feeding tube in the esophagus, erosion between the soft, posterior membranous trachea and the adjacent esophageal wall may result in tracheoesophageal fistula.**

It is important to start enteral feedings as early as possible, so that nutritional depletion will not be allowed to develop if the patient should require a prolonged cardiopulmonary recovery. In general, enteral feedings are preferred whenever the gut can be used; they are simple, are complete, and do not risk bloodstream infection. In unusual circumstances, a postoperative cardiac or thoracic patient may be so severely ill that gastrointestinal motility is impaired and enteral feedings are not possible. In such patients, parenteral hyperalimentation is appropriate. Many excellent reviews of this topic are available.[10] Meticulous technique is imperative to avoid bacteremia, especially in patients with prosthetic cardiac valves.

✚ RENAL FUNCTION

Renal function is so intimately related to hemodynamics that frequent reference to renal function has been made in preceding chapters. (See also Chapter 21, Acute Kidney Injury.) A number of key principles regarding renal functional assessment and management will be addressed specifically in this section.

Monitoring of renal function entails quantitation of urine output and measurement of blood urea nitrogen (BUN), creatinine, and electrolytes. The ICU patient will nearly always have an indwelling urinary catheter in the bladder. **An output of 30 mL/h of urine is sufficient (or 1/2 mL/kg of body weight/hour for children).** This output will allow adequate excretion of waste products. Urine output at this level is evidence of satisfactory renal blood flow, which in turn indicates adequate cardiac output. If urine output falls below 30 mL/h, the cause must be sought and corrected. With oliguria below this level, elevation in BUN and creatinine and abnormalities in serum electrolytes may follow with time.

It is well recognized that oliguria can have three major physiologic causes:

1. **In prerenal azotemia, renal blood flow is insufficient.** This insufficiency may result from decreased cardiac output, which may in turn be from hypovolemia or from pump failure.

2. **In postrenal azotemia, a mechanical obstruction blocks egress of urine from the kidney.** This may result from an anatomic obstruction in the ureters, bladder, or urethra; more commonly, in the ICU, obstruction occurs from mechanical occlusion of the urinary catheter by kinking, clotting, or displacement. It is wise to replace the urinary catheter as part of the evaluation of new oliguria in the ICU patient, so that mechanical factors are eliminated as concerns. Simply irrigating the catheter for assessment of patency can be misleading.

3. **In renal azotemia, dysfunction of the kidney itself causes oliguria.** Glomerulonephritis, interstitial nephritis, and "acute tubular necrosis" are common general causes.[11] Cardiopulmonary bypass, as is well appreciated, may injure the kidneys via many mechanisms.[12] Renal blood flow may be reduced during bypass, especially if atherosclerotic renal artery disease preexists. Nonpulsatile flow may not be as good for the kidneys as normal pulsatile flow. Microemboli to the kidneys may occur. Hemolysis may impose a hemoglobin load on the tubules, resulting in obstruction by casts. Low cardiac output and hypotension postoperatively may further injure the kidney. For all these reasons, true renal azotemia may occur following cardiac surgery. Postoperative renal dysfunction has been shown to be more common in patients with even mild preexisting renal insufficiency.[13]

Urine electrolytes and specific gravity can aid in differentiating prerenal from renal oliguria[11] (Table 23.5). In prerenal oliguria, specific gravity is greater than 1.015 and urine sodium is less than 10 mEq/L. Urine osmolality exceeds that of plasma by greater than two-fold, and urine-to-plasma ratios of BUN and creatinine exceed 20:1. Serum BUN level is more than ten times that of serum creatinine. All these relations are lost in acute renal parenchymal failure. In particular, specific gravity is low (approaching that of serum), sodium concentration is high (> 20 mEq/L), urine osmolality is less than 2 times that of serum, urine-to-plasma ratios of urea and creatinine are less than 10:1, and serum BUN usually does not exceed 10 times creatinine.

Once the cause of the oliguria is determined, appropriate treatment can be instituted. Prerenal oliguria requires optimization of cardiac output. Postrenal oliguria requires mechanical correction. True acute renal failure may require dialysis if severe. Dialysis may be performed peritoneally, if circumstances permit; alternatively, hemodialysis is possible even shortly after cardiac surgery. Continuous

TABLE 23.5 Urine Electrolytes in Oliguria

	Prerenal	Renal
Urine specific gravity	> 1.015	< 1.015
Urine sodium	< 10 mEq/L	> 20 mEq/L
Urine/plasma osmolality	> 2:1	< 2:1
Urine/plasma BUN Urine/plasma creatinine	> 20:1	< 20:1
Serum BUN/creatinine	> 10:1	≤ 10:1

ultrafiltration, which is cumbersome but hemodynamically "gentle," may be preferable early on for hemodynamically unstable patients. See Chapter 21, Acute Kidney Injury, for a full discussion of renal replacement therapies.

Because postoperative renal failure carries a high mortality, prevention is key. The surgeon will optimize renal protection during cardiopulmonary bypass. **The house officer can aid in prevention by optimizing cardiac output postoperatively** (thus ensuring adequate renal blood flow) **and by maintaining an adequate urine output at all times** (to clear debris from renal tubules).

Experience has shown that cardiac surgery can be performed reasonably safely even in patients with chronic renal failure requiring dialysis.[14]

One more point deserves emphasis. Nature's response to trauma or major surgery includes an outpouring of antidiuretic hormone (ADH) and aldosterone.[11] ADH promotes resorption of free water in the renal tubules, and aldosterone stimulates salt conservation. These hormones may lead to a physiologic oliguria with the electrolyte and chemistry profile of prerenal azotemia. This may occur despite adequate volume status and good myocardial function. In this setting, diuretics may be required to promote urinary flow and to prevent development of volume overload as fluids are administered.

✚ ACID-BASE BALANCE

Every house officer has probably discovered his or her own favorite references on the topic of acid-base balance. In the ICU patient, rapid evaluation of acid-base status is needed for prompt, appropriate treatment. In this section, we provide two tools to assist the house officer in rapid acid-base assessment: (1) the acid-base rule for assessing respiratory/metabolic components and (2) the acid-base nomogram.

The Acid-Base Rule

The acid-base rule for assessing respiratory/metabolic components can help the house officer quickly determine, without tables or charts, what the respiratory component of an acid-base disturbance is. If CO_2 is normal, that is, 40 mm Hg, no respiratory component exists; any disturbance must be metabolic. **In general, for every 10 mm Hg that CO_2 rises above 40 mm Hg, pH falls 0.05.** Thus if a patient's arterial blood gases (ABGs) show pH 7.30, pCO_2 of 60, and pO_2 of 75, pCO_2 is 20 mm Hg above normal; this will drop pH by 2 × 0.05, or 0.10. Normal pH is 7.40, so pH would be expected to be 7.30 just from the respiratory change. This patient thus has a pure respiratory acidosis. If another patient's ABGs showed pH 7.20, pCO_2 of 60, and pO_2 of 75, the acidosis would be disproportionate even after accounting for the CO_2 rise; this patient has a mixed respiratory and metabolic acidosis.

  In general, for every 10 mm Hg that CO_2 falls below 40 mm Hg, pH rises 0.10. Thus if a patient's ABGs show pH 7.60, pCO_2 of 20, pO_2 of 75, pCO_2 is 20 mm Hg below normal; this will raise pH by 2 × 0.10, or 0.20. Normal pH is 7.40, so pH would be expected to be 7.60 just from the respiratory change. This patient thus has a pure respiratory acidosis. If his pH were greater than 7.60, he would have a component of metabolic alkalosis as well.

This rule can be immensely valuable clinically. Respiratory abnormalities can be corrected by adjusting pCO_2 as outlined in Chapter 1, Ventilators and Respiratory Management. Metabolic abnormalities can be corrected accordingly. Metabolic acidosis can be corrected acutely by administering sodium bicarbonate. A general physiologic cause, often low cardiac output or diabetic ketoacidosis, must be sought and corrected appropriately. Metabolic alkalosis is not as common or as threatening as acidosis; usually, in the cardiac patient, alkalosis is of the hypokalemic, hypochloremic type (often brought on by excess diuresis) that requires salt and potassium replacement. The acid-base rule, although not perfect, is accurate enough for proper clinical decision making and intervention.

The Acid-Base Nomogram

The acid-base nomogram,[15] reproduced in Figure 23.1, **plots pH, serum bicarbonate (HCO_3), and pCO_2. On the nomogram, ranges for acute and chronic respiratory and metabolic alkalosis and acidosis are indicated.** This allows somewhat more precise assessment than the acid-base rule given earlier; in particular, the nomogram is useful for assessment of chronic states. The house officer needs merely to plot the pH, HCO_3, and pCO_2 obtained on ABG determination to ascertain to what category of acid-base abnormality a given patient's parameters usually correspond. Practice with the acid-base rule and the acid-base nomogram will give the house officer clinical facility in the often difficult problem of acid-base assessment.

✚ HEPARIN-INDUCED THROMBOSIS AND THROMBOCYTOPENIA

It is critically important that the house officer be familiar with the syndrome of heparin-induced thrombosis and thrombocytopenia (HITT), sometimes referred to as "heparin allergy."[16-19] Over the last two decades, it has become recognized that this is a common and very serious condition that can lead to devastating vascular

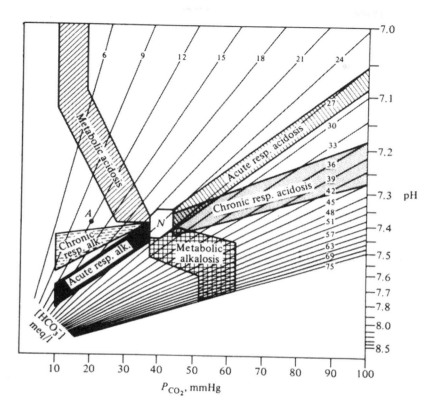

FIGURE 23.1

The acid-base nomogram.

Source: Reprinted with permission from Rose B. *Clinical Physiology of Acid-Base and Electrolyte Disorders.* New York, NY: McGraw-Hill; 1977.

complications. In fact, it is becoming clear that many of the patients who, prior to the recognition of this disorder, had unexplained limb ischemia or organ dysfunction actually suffered from heparin-related thrombosis.

In HITT, the patient is allergic to the administered heparin. Antibody adherence to the heparin molecule leads to platelet activation and widespread formation of intravascular thrombus, both venous and arterial. The widespread thrombosis leads to consumption of platelets and hence to the thrombocytopenia that characterizes the disorder.

The following points deserve emphasis:

- **The development of HITT requires at least two exposures to heparin,** the first producing sensitization and the second or subsequent doses leading to the syndrome in the presence of preformed antibody.
- **Up to 10% of patients who receive heparin have an immune response and are vulnerable to developing HITT with subsequent exposures.**
- **The severity of HITT varies widely.** The syndrome can vary from one of mild fall in platelet count without any clinical sequelae to one of widespread thrombosis, leading to venous thrombosis with pulmonary emboli and a variety of arterial thrombotic phenomena, including extremity thrombosis and limb loss, cerebral thrombosis with cerebral vascular accident, renal artery thrombosis with renal infarction and failure, hepatic artery thrombosis with hepatic necrosis and failure, and coronary artery or coronary graft thrombosis with myocardial infarction.
- **Many patients have an arterial intervention** (arterial stick, cardiac or peripheral vascular catheterization, cardiac or vascular surgery) **that triggers HITT-induced thrombosis in the involved artery.**
- **Cardiac surgical patients are especially prone to HITT,** as all have had an initial heparin exposure during catheterization and then receive massive doses of heparin for cardiopulmonary bypass. Many have had numerous prior exposures to heparin, "priming" the immune system for an exuberant, life-threatening response at the time of cardiac surgery.
- **Complete cessation of heparin is essential once the diagnosis is made or suspected.** No method of administration of heparin is safe, whether subcutaneous or intravenous. Switching from porcine to beef heparin is not necessarily effective. Low molecular heparin is not adequately safe as a substitute. Even the small amount of heparin in the

auto-flushes for arterial lines can trigger continuation of the HITT phenomenon and must be discontinued.

- In fact, in our ICU, as in many throughout the country, heparin is no longer used in these continuous flush lines; rather, straight saline is employed. Thus, additional heparin exposure is avoided. As HITT is an immunologic phenomenon, even trace amounts of heparin can trigger devastating consequences. Once heparin is stopped, some form of non-heparin-based anticoagulation is recommended, as with argatroban. Coumadin treatment is started after the platelet count has improved. Chances are that the advice of a hematologist will be sought for a specific, severe case in your ICU.

- **The full-blown HITT syndrome carries a very poor prognosis, with a mortality exceeding 50%.**

- **The key to limiting the damage from this devastating disorder is keeping a high index of suspicion and making an early diagnosis. The diagnosis should be entertained in any patient who manifests a fall in platelet count on heparin therapy.** The diagnosis should be suspected in any patient who develops evidence of limb ischemia unexpectedly postoperatively. The same is true for unexplained manifestations of cerebral, intestinal, hepatic, or renal ischemia.

- **A platelet aggregation test is available; this test, though definitive if positive, lacks sensitivity** (thought to be only about 50%). Nonetheless, the test should be ordered when the suspicion of HITT is raised. Recently, an enzyme-linked immunosorbent assay (ELISA) has become available that is highly sensitive in determining whether there are antibodies to heparin but is of uncertain value in determining if the patient has clinical HITT. Thus, the diagnosis of HITT, even in the present era, is largely clinical—and dependent on a high index of suspicion on the part of the house officer.

Illustrative Case

A 46-year-old male was admitted to an outlying hospital with an inferior-wall myocardial infarction in progress. He was given TPA (tissue plasminogen activator) with resolution of ischemic changes. He underwent cardiac catheterization, which revealed 95% stenoses of both the LAD (left anterior descending) and the RCA (right coronary artery). He was given continuous IV heparin. Over the next 48 hours he became desperately ill, with respiratory failure and limb ischemia. He was found to have suffered multiple pulmonary emboli. He developed ischemia of three limbs, including the leg through which the catheterization had been performed. He was found to have occlusion of both femoral arteries and one brachial artery.

He underwent operative thrombectomy of both femoral arteries and the one brachial artery. He required placement of an inferior vena caval filter for repeated pulmonary emboli. He developed anuric renal failure. Thrombocytopenia had developed.

A test for heparin antibodies was positive. HITT was recognized and heparin discontinued. Coumadin was substituted. Pulmonary failure resolved, as did renal failure. Cardiac status remained stable.

The patient was transferred after recovery to our institution, where he successfully underwent coronary artery bypass, with two internal mammary artery bypass grafts, one to the LAD and one to the RCA. Anticoagulation for the procedure was achieved through the use of ancrod (snake venom) to avoid heparin administration.

This case is a vivid demonstration of the protean consequences of HITT. Many patients, especially if HITT is not recognized, do not survive the multiple serious insults consequent to HITT. This case is described to heighten the house officer's index of suspicion regarding HITT.

A very high proportion of ICU patients currently receive heparin, which is popular for treatment of myocardial ischemia; many patients have invasive arterial catheterizations or cardiac surgical procedures; and nearly all patients have indwelling lines that require continuous automatic flushing—hopefully non-heparin containing. The house officer with a high index of suspicion will likely make a life-saving diagnosis of HITT during a year in an ICU environment.

REFERENCES

1. http://www.acc.org/qualityandscience/clinical/guidelines/valvular/valvularpocketguide.pdf
2. http://www.americanheart.org/presenter.jhtml?identifier=3040028
3. Whitlock PR, Crowther MA, Warkentin TE, Blackall MH, Farrokhyar F, Teoh KH. Warfarin cessation before cardiopulmonary bypass: lessons learned from a randomized controlled trial of oral vitamin K. *Ann Thorac Surg.* 2007;84:108-109.
4. Feldman RL. Using calcium antagonists in rest and effort angina. *Drug Ther.* 1983;(January):43-60.
5. Chesebro J, Clements I, Foster V, et al. A platelet-inhibitor-drug trial in coronary-artery bypass operations. *N Engl J Med.* 1982;307:73-78.
6. Goldman S, Copeland J, Moritz T, et al. Starting aspirin therapy after operation: effects on early graft patency. *Circulation.* 1991;84:520-526.
7. Gavaghan TP, Gebski V, Baron DW. Immediate postoperative aspirin improves vein graft patency early and late after coronary artery bypass graft surgery: a placebo-controlled, randomized study. *Circulation.* 1991;83:1526-1533.
8. Kulik A, Le May MR, Voisine P, et al. Aspirin plus clopidogrel versus aspirin alone after coronary artery bypass grafting: the clopidogrel after surgery for coronary artery disease (CASCADE) trial. *Circulation.* 2010;122:2680-2687. Epub 2010 Dec 6.
9. Wilson AP, Treasure T, Gruneberg RN, et al. Should the temperature chart influence management in cardiac operations? Result of a prospective study in 314 patients. *J Thorac Cardiovasc Surg.* 1988;96:518-523.

10. Dudrick S, Rhoads J. Metabolism in surgical patients: protein, carbohydrate, and fat utilization by oral and parenteral routes. In: Sabiston D, ed. *Davis-Christopher textbook of surgery*. Philadelphia: WB Saunders; 1977:150-177.

11. Geha, AS. Acute renal failure in cardiovascular and other surgical patients. *Surg Clin North Am*. 1980;60:1151-1166.

12. Edmunds L, Stephenson L. Cardiopulmonary bypass for open heart surgery. In: Glenn W, Baue A, Geha A, et al, eds. *Thoracic and Cardiovascular Surgery*. 4th ed. Norwalk, CT: Appleton-Century-Crofts; 1983:1091-1105.

13. Abel R, Buckley M, Austen W. Acute postoperative renal failure in cardiac surgical patients. *J Surg Res*. 1976;20:341-348.

14. Love J. *Cardiac Surgery in Patients with Chronic Renal Disease*. Mt Kisco, NY: Futura; 1982.

15. Rose B. *Clinical Physiology of Acid-Base and Electrolyte Disorders*. New York: McGraw-Hill; 2011.

16. Makhoul RG, Greenberg CS, McCann RL. Heparin-associated thrombocytopenia and thrombosis: a serious clinical problem and potential solution. *J Vasc Surg*. 1986;4:522-528.

17. Walls JT, Curtis JJ, Silver D, Boley TM. Heparin-induced thrombocytopenia in patients who undergo open heart surgery. *Surgery*. 1990;4:686-693.

18. Shabtsila E, Lip GY, Chong BH. Heparin-induced thrombocytopenia. A contemporary clinical approach to diagnosis and management. *Chest*. 2009;135:1651-1654.

19. Mayo Clinic Medical Laboratories. http://www.mayomedical laboratories.com/test-catalog/Clinical+and+Interpretive/81904

SUGGESTED FURTHER READING

Patel VP, Bong M, Di Cesare PE. Heparin-induced thrombocytopenia and thrombosis. *Am J Orthop*. 2007;36:255-260.
  Plain talk, but clear and helpful.

Walls JT, Curtis JJ, Silver D, Boley TM. Heparin-induced thrombocytopenia in patients who undergo open heart surgery. *Surgery*. 1990;4:686-693.
  An excellent review of the topic of heparin-induced thrombosis and thrombocytopenia; recommended for all readers, regardless of specialty.

SELF-ASSESSMENT QUIZZES

TEST 1

1) Which measurement is the most reasonable proxy for volume status?

A. pulmonary capillary wedge pressure
B. pulmonary arterial diastolic pressure
C. left ventricular end-diastolic pressure
D. central venous pressure
E. right ventricular end-diastolic pressure

2) Which is NOT a common indication for intra-aortic balloon counter-pulsation (IABP)?

A. status post open heart surgery with reduced CO off cardiopulmonary bypass
B. angina refractory to medical treatment
C. cardiogenic shock status post myocardial infarction
D. ventricular septal rupture
E. acute mitral regurgitation (as with papillary muscle rupture)
F. acute aortic dissection resulting in cardiac tamponade

3) What is the mechanism of action of aprotinin?

A. plasmin/kallikrein inhibitor
B. factor VIIa inhibitor
C. potentiates AT3's effects
D. binds to and promotes degradation of vWF
E. inhibits matrix metalloproteinase activity

The House Officer's Guide to ICU Care: Fundamentals of Management of the Heart and Lungs, 3rd ed. © 2013 John A. Elefteriades, Curtis Tribble, Alexander S. Geha, Mark D. Siegel, and Lawrence S. Cohen, eds. Cardiotext Publishing, ISBN: 978-1-935395-68-3.

4) What is the correct initial therapy for cardiac tamponade?

  A. pericardiocentesis
  B. subxiphoid pericardiotomy
  C. inotropic support
  D. volume administration to maximize CVP
  E. cardiac catheterization

5) What is the appropriate initial FiO_2 setting after major surgery, such as open heart surgery?

  A. .50
  B. .75
  C. 1.0
  D. 1.5

6) What is the first-line drug for ventricular ectopic beats?

  A. lidocaine
  B. adenosine
  C. digitalis
  D. verapamil

7) A 62-year-old patient, postoperative day 1 status post coronary artery bypass graft ×3, is found to be in new atrial fibrillation. The patient has a pulse of 130/min and BP 136/78, with no angina and no disturbance of consciousness. What is the level of urgency of atrial fibrillation in this patient?

  A. Level III, requires direct current (DC) cardioversion
  B. Level II, requires digitalis plus verapamil
  C. Level I, requires digitalis, with or without β-blockers or calcium antagonists

8) A 74-year-old patient, postoperative day 2 status post coronary artery bypass graft ×4, is found to be in atrial fibrillation. The patient has a pulse rate of 158 and BP 63 (discernible by palpation only), accompanied by angina and an impaired level of consciousness. What is the level of urgency of atrial fibrillation in this patient?

   A. Level III, requires direct current (DC) cardioversion
   B. Level II, requires digitalis plus verapamil
   C. Level I, requires digitalis

9) What is the risk of inducing ventricular fibrillation with asynchronous cardioversion?

   A. 2 to 5%
   B. 25%
   C. 60%
   D. 80%

10) A 70-year-old patient was admitted to the ICU after mitral valve repair surgery a few hours ago. You notice that his RA pressure, RVEDP, PADP, and PCWP are between 19 to 22 mm Hg. Also, his BP is 90 systolic, his cardiac index is only 2.1, and his urine output is low. Also, you note that his chest tube drainage has been between 125 and 350 cc/h. You suspect the Swan readings may be spurious, so you check with your senior resident about repositioning the Swan-Ganz catheter. He tells you he will be there immediately to assess the patient with you. What is the senior resident most concerned about?

   A. pulmonary embolus
   B. ventricular septal rupture
   C. cardiac tamponade
   D. mitral regurgitation

ANSWERS

1) **A.** pulmonary capillary wedge pressure

   Pulmonary capillary wedge pressure (PCWP) most accurately reflects volume state. With the catheter "wedged" in the pulmonary radicles (balloon inflated) only the pulmonary capillaries separate the catheter tip from the left atrium, the chamber for which we really wish to measure pressure.

2) **F.** acute aortic dissection resulting in cardiac tamponade

   The conditions listed in answer choices A through E are very appropriate scenarios for institution of intra-aortic balloon counterpulsation (IABP). In acute aortic dissection, not only is IABP not directly beneficial or relevant, but passing the IABP catheter in face of an acute aortic dissection would be dangerous.

3) **A.** plasmin/kallikrein inhibitor

   Aprotinin has complex modes of action, but its immune inhibition is well appreciated and underlies many of the beneficial effects other than improved coagulation (such as less pulmonary toxicity from cardiopulmonary bypass). Aprotinin does not affect the other processes listed.

4) **D.** volume administration to maximize CVP

   Paradoxically, although the CVP is high in tamponade, one must give more volume. In tamponade, "the heart can't pump, because the heart can't fill." So we have to provide a higher driving force for filling—via volume administration. The other listed modalities are all useful in appropriate circumstances. Pericardiocentesis can be very useful, especially in non-hemorrhagic effusion and tamponade (hemorrhagic fluid in the pericardial space may be hard to draw via needle). Subxiphoid pericardiotomy (an incision into the pericardium just below the xiphoid process) can be literally life-saving in trauma—instantly relieving the pressure on the heart and restoring hemodynamics. Inotropic support may be beneficial, even though decreased inotropy is not the core issue, because with the low flow of cardiac tamponade, it may be necessary to artificially support blood pressure so that the heart can maintain its own perfusion.

5) **C.** 1.0

An FiO_2 of 1.0, that is, pure oxygen, is appropriate for most patients returning to ICU after major cardiac surgery. This initial setting will ensure an adequate pO_2 initially. There may be atelectasis, secretions, edema of the lungs, pneumothorax, or a whole host of other abnormalities that depress pO_2 in this setting. The high initial FiO_2 provides a safety margin. Once the first ABG is checked, the FiO_2 can be decreased. O_2 toxicity is not relevant for short intervals of high FiO_2.

6) **A.** lidocaine

Lidocaine is an excellent, time-tested drug for suppressing ventricular ectopic beats. It is a safe drug. Myocardial depression is rarely seen. Seizures can occur with very large doses, but these are self-limited and relatively benign in an intubated and ventilated patient. The drugs in answer choices B through D have no role for ventricular ectopic beats. Amiodarone would be another good response; however, amiodarone is more toxic than lidocaine (vasodilation, negative inotropy, bradycardia with loading dose) and may be best left until the house officer has more experience or has direction from more senior team members.

7) **C.** Level I, requires digitalis, with or without β-blockers or calcium antagonists

Level I is the lowest of the three urgency categories. This patient's atrial fibrillation is relatively slow, well tolerated hemodynamically, and asymptomatic clinically. Treatment can proceed without IV β-blockers or calcium channel antagonists or DC cardioversion. The digitalis may be given IV, of course.

8) **A.** Level III, requires direct current (DC) cardioversion

This patient is in trouble. His atrial fibrillation is very rapid—too rapid to generate good ventricular ejection—so his blood pressure is vanishingly low. His angina signifies that his heart is struggling for blood to meet the very high contraction rate. Drifting in and out of consciousness is an indication that global perfusion is very low. This patient will have a cardiac arrest if his atrial fibrillation is not corrected immediately. DC cardioversion is indicated. Do not hesitate under such circumstances!

The cardioversion should be done in synchronous mode (so that it coordinates with the patient's native heart rate to avoid an iatrogenic R-on-T phenomenon) and with 200 J (urgent situation).

9) **A.** 2 to 5%

While the risk of inducing ventricular fibrillation with an asynchronous cardioversion for atrial fibrillation is low, there is no reason to take this risk (unless the patient is in an arrest or near-arrest), so synchronize your cardioversion in most circumstances.

10) **C.** cardiac tamponade

Equalized pressures are a classic finding in cardiac tamponade (all the chambers take on the pressure in the pericardial space). The relative hypotension, low cardiac output, and oliguria all go along with marginal cardiac function, quite possibly due to tamponade. The relatively high chest tube outputs raise concern that blood may be accumulating in the pericardial space. Chances are that the senior resident will perform a stat echo exam to visualize any pericardial collections of fluid or clot; alternatively, he may appropriately and justifiably call his attending and suggest that they explore the patient surgically to rule out and relieve any tamponade.

TEST 2

1) A 68-year-old female is admitted to the ICU with severe angina and dyspnea leading to cardiogenic shock. She receives an intra-aortic balloon pump to augment her cardiac function. Her care is transferred to you from the previous team, and on examination, you hear a loud systolic murmur. What murmur is this likely to be?

A. aortic regurgitation
B. mitral regurgitation
C. mitral stenosis
D. tricuspid regurgitation

2) The ABG values come back on one of your ventilated patients, and the pCO_2 is 50 mm Hg. The ventilation is not adequate for this patient. Which of the following should you do?

A. decrease PEEP
B. increase FiO_2
C. decrease minute volume
D. increase respiratory rate

3) A patient is admitted to the ICU for acute dyspnea, and there is a question of a concomitant MI. On examination, you hear a harsh systolic murmur radiating to the carotids. An echocardiogram reveals a critically stenotic aortic valve < 0.7 cm² in diameter for which an operation is essential. The patient develops chest pain. Which medication is contraindicated?

A. digoxin
B. lidocaine
C. dobutamine
D. nitroglycerin
E. metoprolol

4) The efficiency of oxygenation is monitored daily in a seriously ill patient in the ICU. Calculate the alveolar-arterial oxygen difference given the following parameters: $pH_2O = 47$, $pCO_2 = 40$, Patm = 760, and $paO_2 = 400$.

   A. 273
   B. 447
   C. 367
   D. 190

5) You are walking through the step-down unit, you hear an alarm, and you see ventricular fibrillation on the monitor. You should check the patient for consciousness and check for a pulse If consciousness or pulse is absent, which of the following should you perform?

   A. synchronized cardioversion
   B. asynchronous defibrillation at 100 J
   C. asynchronous defibrillation at 100 ma
   D. asynchronous defibrillation at 200 J

6) Which of the following is a complete list of the factors that directly affect cardiac output?

   A. heart rate
   B. heart rate, preload, and afterload
   C. heart rate, preload, afterload, ventricular distensibility, and contractility
   D. heart rate, preload, afterload, pulmonary capillary wedge pressure

7) Which of the following describes the most common site(s) for the initial tear in an aortic dissection?

   A. between the innominate and left carotid arteries
   B. 1 cm before the innominate artery
   C. 4 cm above the aortic valve or immediately after the subclavian artery
   D. at the level of the diaphragm and immediately distal to the renal arteries

8) You are a physician working at a military hospital in a war zone. A patient with a gunshot wound to the chest is brought to the emergency department. You hear a sucking noise coming from the wound. What is the first intervention you should implement?

A. intubate and apply positive pressure ventilation
B. place an occlusive dressing
C. administer blood transfusion
D. place a chest tube

9) You are called by the nursing staff because one of the patients in the cardiothoracic ICU has a systolic pressure of 58 mm Hg. What is the best intervention to implement first?

A. dobutamine
B. calcium chloride
C. vasopressin
D. epinephrine

10) Using the acid-base rule, calculate the pH of a patient with a pCO_2 of 20 mm Hg.

A. 7.70
B. 7.60
C. 7.50
D. 7.20

ANSWERS

1) **B.** mitral regurgitation.

Cardiogenic shock in the face of an acute MI can indeed be due to acute mitral regurgitation due to papillary muscle rupture (or severe dysfunction). This is the correct answer. The other options are not really pertinent (and aortic regurgitation and mitral stenosis do not produce systolic murmurs). Other possible explanations for this woman's precarious hemodynamic state include simply a very extensive MI, affecting much of her left ventricular muscle (40% or more), or an acute ventricular septal defect (VSD). Cardiac echo or cardiac catheterization will usually be diagnostic.

2) **D.** increase respiratory rate

The CO_2 directly reflects the adequacy of ventilation. In this case, ventilation is inadequate. You need to increase respiratory rate or tidal volume. The other answers are inappropriate.

3) **D.** nitroglycerin

Nitroglycerin is contraindicated because a patient with critical aortic stenosis is markedly preload dependent. Nitroglycerin will decrease preload. Then there may not be enough blood going forward through the aortic valve to maintain blood pressure and consciousness. Syncope or cardiac arrest may ensue. The medications in answers A, B, C, and E are not contraindicated.

4) **A.** 273

Remember our formula. The formula essentially first calculates the partial pressure of oxygen in the alveolus by subtracting the contributions from water vapor and carbon dioxide. Next, the arterial PO_2 is subtracted from that number, yielding the alveolar-arterial PO_2 difference. (See below.) This parameter enables the house officer to follow the efficiency of oxygenation on a quantitative basis from day to day. These calculations require brief administration of 100% oxygen through the endotracheal tube during the conduct of the test.

$$p(A - a)O_2 = pAO_2 - paO_2$$
$$= (Patm - pH_2O - pCO_2) - paO_2$$
$$= (760 - 47 - 40) - 400$$
$$= 673 - 400$$
$$= 273$$

5) **D.** asynchronous defibrillation at 200 J

It is crucial to check for consciousness; it is not uncommon for disconnected leads, or even a patient brushing her teeth, to cause electrical tracings that look for all the world like rapid ventricular tachycardia or ventricular fibrillation. An unconscious patient rules out an artifactual trace. It is crucial also to feel for a pulse, as another check that the heart has really stopped. Once you have done these two simple checks, you must spring immediately into action. An asynchronous defibrillation at maximum energy is essential. You do not need to waste precious time synchronizing. You do not want to waste precious time ramping up on the energy level. You must give it everything you've got immediately. The chance of success diminishes with each passing second. Current bi-phasic defibrillators have a maximum energy setting of 200 J; ma is a designation for a pacing current and has nothing to do with defibrillation.

6) **C.** heart rate, preload, afterload, ventricular distensibility, and contractility

The other lists are incomplete. Ventricular distensibility and contractility are important as well, in addition to the "big 3" of heart rate, preload, and afterload.

7) **C.** 4 cm above the aortic valve or immediately after the subclavian artery

In Type A, or ascending aortic dissection, the initiating tear is usually located in the proximal ascending aorta, about 4 cm above the aortic valve. In Type B, or descending aortic dissection, the initiating tear is usually located in the proximal descending aorta, just beyond the subclavian artery.

8) **B.** place an occlusive dressing

Placing an occlusive dressing will "defuse" the sucking chest wound. The soldier will no longer lose tidal volume moving air in and out of the nonrespiratory exchange pleural space. You may well need to transfuse, to place a chest tube, and to intubate, but that remains to be seen.

9) **B.** calcium chloride

This patient is in trouble. You will, of course, evaluate the rhythm, assess the fluid status, make certain that the patient is oxygenating and ventilating well, and check for bleeding. But first you must do something to correct the BP immediately while your assessment progresses. Calcium chloride is a good first choice. Calcium will raise the BP, by both vasoconstriction and positive inotropy. Calcium does not cause arrhythmias or undue tachycardia. Calcium does not usually cause overcorrection or severe hypertension. You can give one amp of calcium chloride (1 g) by IV push with relative impunity. Once you have the BP restored to a life-sustaining range, you can carry out further assessments. In extremely serious situations like the vignette in this question, it is not a bad idea to have one staff member call for senior help while you are giving calcium and making an assessment; if not, and if your measures are not immediately effective, you will have a cardiac arrest on your hands very shortly. Remember to call early for help, while your immediate therapies are being implemented. The other vasoconstrictors and inotropes listed as possible remedies among the answers to this question may be appropriate later, but calcium is the best immediate choice.

10) **B.** 7.60

Remember that the body blunts the pH change of hypercarbia better than it does with hypocarbia. Here we have severe hypocarbia. The acid-base rule tells us that the pH rises 0.10 for each 10 mm Hg drop in pCO_2. Therefore, the answer is 7.60.

$$2 \times 0.10 = 0.20$$
$$7.40 + 0.20 = 7.60$$

TEST 3

1) A 70-kg male patient in the cardiothoracic ICU produces 80 mL of urine over 4 hours. What is the minimum acceptable urine output for this patient, and is the current rate sufficient?

- A. 40 mL/h, current rate sufficient
- B. 35 mL/h, current rate insufficient
- C. 20 mL/h, current rate sufficient
- D. 10 mL/h, current rate sufficient

2) Which of the following is first priority in a patient with a massive hemothorax?

- A. place a chest tube
- B. emergent trip to the OR
- C. administer IV fluids
- D. administer blood

3) Which of the following is NOT an indication for intra-aortic balloon pump (IABP) placement?

- A. pulmonary edema from aortic regurgitation
- B. recent cardiopulmonary bypass surgery
- C. refractory angina
- D. refractory life-threatening ventricular arrhythmias
- E. cardiogenic shock

4) What is the primary goal in the management of acute atrial fibrillation?

- A. rate control
- B. restoration of sinus rhythm
- C. anticoagulation
- D. increase inotropy

5) Which of the following acute valvular insufficiencies would benefit most from insertion of an intra-aortic balloon pump?

   A. aortic regurgitation
   B. pulmonary regurgitation
   C. mitral regurgitation
   D. tricuspid regurgitation

6) The adequacy of ventilation can be quantified using the alveolar-arterial O_2 difference, or the A-a gradient. When breathing 100% O_2, alveoli will only contain water vapor with a partial pressure of 47 mm Hg and CO_2 with a partial pressure of 40 mm Hg. Given that the sum of all partial pressures in the alveolus must equal atmospheric pressure (Patm), and the normal A-a gradient is usually 60 to 80 mm Hg, what is the normal arterial PO_2 in a patient breathing 100% O_2?

   A. 100 to 120 mm Hg
   B. 200 to 220 mm Hg
   C. 300 to 320 mm Hg
   D. 600 to 620 mm Hg
   E. 700 to 720 mm Hg

7) When the arterial PO_2 is less than 60 mm Hg, the hemoglobin saturation is less than 90% and severe hypoxia exists. In postoperative patients presenting with hypoxia shortly after arrival in ICU, what is the best initial treatment?

   A. increasing positive end-expiratory pressure (PEEP; or Rafferty maneuver)
   B. increasing FiO_2
   C. increasing tidal volume
   D. increasing respiratory rate

8) What is the characteristic murmur of mitral regurgitation?

A. blowing, holosystolic murmur maximal at the cardiac apex

B. blowing, diastolic murmur at the left sternal border

C. holosystolic murmur at the lower left sternal border that increases with inspiration

D. harsh, crescendo-decrescendo murmur, best heard at the right upper sternal border, radiating to the carotids

9) What are the 4 most dangerous complications of aortic dissection?

A. rupture, tamponade, pleural effusion, and aortic stenosis

B. pleural effusion, tamponade, rupture, and mitral regurgitation

C. rupture, tamponade, branch occlusion, and aortic regurgitation

D. aortic regurgitation, aortic stenosis, mitral regurgitation, and mitral stenosis

10) Which of the following major physiologic types of injury due to chest trauma is NOT lethal within the first few minutes?

A. airway obstruction

B. esophageal perforation

C. tension pneumothorax

D. flail chest

E. sucking chest wound

F. massive hemothorax

G. cardiac tamponade

ANSWERS

1) **B.** 35 mL/h, current rate insufficient

   Remember that we like to see at least ½ to 1 cc of urine per kilogram per hour. Lower amounts of urine usually imply hypoperfusion or renal dysfunction. So the minimal acceptable output is 35 mL/h [0.5 mL × 70 kg × 1 h = 35 mL/h]. The current rate of output is only 20 mL/h [80 mL / 4 h = 20 mL/h] and is therefore insufficient.

2) **D.** administer blood

   By definition, a patient with massive hemothorax has lost blood—a lot of blood. Remember that one pleural space can hold the entire blood volume. So administer blood. A chest tube, IV fluids, and a trip to the OR may be in the offing, but the immediate response is blood administration.

3) **A.** pulmonary edema from aortic regurgitation

   These are all fine indications for the IABP, with the exception of aortic insufficiency. Not only does the IABP not improve aortic insufficiency, but it actually hurts: the augmented pressure in diastole forces more blood back into the heart through the regurgitant aortic valve. Significant aortic insufficiency is a relatively strong contraindication to use of the IABP. (In cardiac parlance, the terms *insufficiency* and *regurgitation* are used interchangeably in describing valve function.)

4) **A.** rate control

   An excessively high rate (say, above 125 bpm) will tax the heart (via increased O_2 demands) and decrease BP (via decreased ventricular filling time). The very sensitive heart in the early hours or days after major cardiac surgery may be intolerant of these stresses. You want to control the rate. In most cases, you are not aiming for conversion to normal sinus rhythm, as this may not "hold"—many patients early after cardiac surgery go into and out of atrial fibrillation repeatedly. Anticoagulation is not an early concern. Inotropy is usually not a problem.

5) **C.** mitral regurgitation

The IABP has a dramatically beneficial effect on acute mitral insufficiency. When the IABP collapses in systole, it creates a low-pressure space in the aorta into which the left ventricle can easily eject blood, so the stroke volume passes more preferentially forward into the aorta (where we want it to go) rather than backward into the left atrium (where we do not want it to go). The IABP is relatively contraindicated in aortic insufficiency. The IABP is not of direct benefit in pulmonary or tricuspid regurgitation.

6) **D.** 600 to 620 mm Hg

$$\text{Arterial } PO_2 = \text{Atmospheric pressure} - PH_2O - PCO_2 - \text{A-a gradient}$$
$$= 760 \text{ mm Hg} - 47 \text{ mm Hg} - 40 \text{ mm Hg} - 60 \text{ mm Hg}$$
$$= 613 \text{ mm Hg}$$

7) **A.** increasing positive end-expiratory pressure (PEEP; or Rafferty maneuver)

Hypoxia early after open heart surgery is usually due to atelectasis. Remember that the lungs have been "down" for hours during cardiopulmonary bypass. The best treatment, usually instantaneously raising PO_2, is to expand the atelectatic lung segments. This can usually be accomplished by PEEP or by the Rafferty maneuver (very strong Valsalva maneuver, to the point that BP falls briefly).

8) **A.** blowing, holosystolic murmur maximal at the cardiac apex

A blowing, holosystolic murmur maximal at the cardiac apex, often radiating into the axilla, is characteristic of mitral regurgitation. Answer B describes the characteristic murmur of aortic insufficiency; C describes that of tricuspid insufficiency; and D describes the murmur of aortic stenosis.

9) **C.** rupture, tamponade, branch occlusion, and aortic regurgitation

These are the 4 life-threatening complications of aortic dissection.

10) **B.** esophageal perforation

All of the others are the key injuries capable of early lethality. Esophageal perforation can certainly occur from trauma, but it is not immediately lethal, as it does not have immediate dire physiologic consequences. If esophageal injury is not diagnosed, sepsis will supervene ultimately, but not immediately.

House Officer's Guide to ICU Care— Emergency Response Sheet

Management of Urgent Bradyarrhythmia

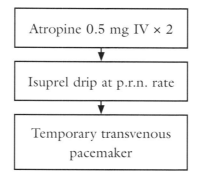

Intropic Agents

Generic Name (Trade Name)	Activity	Dilution	Dose Range
Norepinephrine (Levophed)	α > β	2 mg/250 mL (8 µ/mL)	0.02-0.2 µg/kg/min
Epinephrine (Adrenalin)	α and β	1 mg/250 mL (4 µ/mL)	0.01-0.1 µg/kg/min
Dopamine (Inotropin)	α and β	200 mg/250 mL (800 µg/mL)	1-30 µg/kg/min
Dobutamine (Dobutrex)	α and β	250 mg/250 mL (1,000 µug/mL)	1-30 µg/kg/min
Isoproterenol (Isuprel)	β	1 mg/250 mL (1000 µg/mL)	0.01-0.1 µg/kg/min
Milrinone (Primacor)	NA	1 mg/mL	0.375-0.75 µg/kg/min
Vasopressin (Pitressin)	NA	5g/250 mL	0.01-0.1 u/min (or 0.6-6 u/h)
Phenylephrine (Neosynephrine)	α	5mg/250 mL	0.5-9 µg/kg/min

Bolus Agents for the House Officer's "Bag of Tricks" for Initial Response to Hypotensive Bouts

Calcium Chloride	1 amp	1 g
Epinephrine	1 cc	0.1 mg (of 1:10,000 sol'n)
Pitressin	1-2 u	
Phenylephrine	2-5 mg	

The House Officer's Guide to ICU Care: Fundamentals of Management of the Heart and Lungs, 3rd ed. © 2013 John A. Elefteriades, Curtis Tribble, Alexander S. Geha, Mark D. Siegel, and Lawrence S. Cohen, eds. Cardiotext Publishing, ISBN: 978-1-935395-68-3.

Afterload-reducing Agents Used by Continuous Infusion

Generic Name (Trade Name)	Arterial or Venous Predominance	Dilution	Dose Range
Sodium nitropruside (Nipride)	Arterial	100 mg/250 mL	1-10µg/kg/min
Nitroglycerine (TNG)	Venous	200 µg/mL	1-5 µg/kg/min

Essential Drugs in Cardiac Arrest

Drug	Available Forms	Dose	Use(s)	Disadvantage(s)
Sodium bicarbonate (NaHCO$_3$)	50 mL ampule (44 mEq/ ampule)	1 mL/kg	Corrects acidosis	Considerable salt load
Atropine	0.4-0.5 mg/ mL (vial) or 1 mg/10 mL (ampule)	0.4-0.5 mg; repeat × 1 prn	Corrects bradycardia	
Lidocaine	100 mg/10 mL (ampule)	1 mg/kg	Corrects ventricular ectopy	Seizures, myocardial depression
Amiodarone		150 mg load 1 mg/min to follow	Corrects ventricular ectopy	Potent vasodilator, negative inotrope
Calcium chloride (CaCl)	1 g/10 mL (ampule)	2.5-10 mL	Augments contractility	Ventricular irritability
Epinephrine	1:10,000 solution (ampule)	1-10 mL	Augments contractility; restores electrical activity in asystole; enhances defibrillation	Ventricular irritability
Norepinephrine	4 mg/4 mL (ampule)	Give by continuous infusion at 0.02-0.2 µug/kg/min	Augments contractility; restores arteriolar tone and increases BP to improve coronary perfusion following restoration of cardiac rhythm	Generalized vasoconstriction, increased afterload
Vasopressin		1-2 units bolus	Increases blood pressure	Can overshoot and cause hypertension

INDEX

Page numbers followed by *f* or *t* refer to figures or tables

A

AAI mode, 70, 70*t*, 74
abciximab (ReoPro), 245, 284
ABG. *See* arterial blood gas
Abiomed AB5000 Ventricle, 181, 182*f*
absorption atelectasis, 21
ACE. *See* angiotensin converting enzyme
acebutolol, 438
acid-base nomogram, 446, 447*f*
acid-base rule, 445–446
acidosis, contractility and, 129
acidosis, respiratory, 4, 15
  arrhythmias and, 31
activated clotting time (ACT), 284–285, 287–288
acute aortic dissection. *See* aortic dissection
acute aortic transection. *See* aortic transection
acute coronary ischemia
  angina, unstable, 231*t*, 232–237, 234*t*
  non-ST-segment elevation myocardial infarction (NSTEMI), 231*t*, 232–237, 234*t*
  ST-segment elevation myocardial infarction (STEMI), 231*t*, 237–248, 238*f*, 239*t*, 241*t*, 242*f*, 244*f*, 246*t*
acute kidney injury (AKI)
  acronyms associated with, 410*t*
  AKIN criteria, 410, 410*t*, 411*t*

categories/classification of, 411, 412*t*
diagnosis of, 410–413
prevention and treatment for, 413–417
renal replacement therapy, 414–417, 415*t*
Acute Kidney Injury Network (AKIN)
  criteria, 410, 410*t*, 411*t*
acute renal failure (ARF), acronyms associated with, 410*t*
acute respiratory distress syndrome (ARDS)
  post-pneumonectomy, 378
  protocol, 15–16
acute tubular necrosis (ATN), 411, 412
adenosine, atrial flutter and, 48–49
ADH. *See* antidiuretic hormone
Adrenalin. *See* epinephrine
afterload, cardiac output and, 123, 129–130, 152
afterload-reducing agents
  clevidipine (Cleviprex), 158
  nicardipine (Cardene), 158
  nitroglycerine (TNG), 152, 153*t*, 155–158, 156*f*
  nitroprusside (Nipride), 152, 153–155, 153*t*
  purpose of, 152
Aggrastat. *See* trofiban
agitation, 420–422, 421*f*
air embolism
  systemic, 322–325, 323*f*
  venous, 325
air leaks
  chest tubes and assessment of, 346–348

The House Officer's Guide to ICU Care: Fundamentals of Management of the Heart and Lungs, 3rd ed. © 2013 John A. Elefteriades, Curtis Tribble, Alexander S. Geha, Mark D. Siegel, and Lawrence S. Cohen, eds. Cardiotext Publishing, ISBN: 978-1-935395-68-3.